Interventional Pain Medicine for Women's Health

Comprehensive Treatment Strategies

Edited by
Anita Gupta, DO, MPP, PharmD, FASA
Anesthesiology and Pain, Adjunct Assistant Professor
Johns Hopkins School of Medicine
Baltimore, MD

Medicine, Professor
University of California School of Medicine
Riverside, CA

Anesthesiology and Pain, Professor
Loma Linda School of Medicine
Loma Linda, CA

OXFORD
UNIVERSITY PRESS

OXFORD
UNIVERSITY PRESS

Oxford University Press is a department of the University of Oxford.
It furthers the University's objective of excellence in research, scholarship,
and education by publishing worldwide. Oxford is a registered trade mark of
Oxford University Press in the UK and in certain other countries.

Published in the United States of America by Oxford University Press
546 Fifth Avenue, New York, NY 10036, United States of America.

CIP data is on file at the Library of Congress
ISBN 978-0-19-782047-6

DOI: 10.1093/med/9780197820476.001.0001

Printed by Integrated Books International, United States of America

The manufacturer's authorized representative in the EU for product safety is
Oxford University Press España S.A. of Parque Empresarial San Fernando de Henares,
Avenida de Castilla, 2 – 28830 Madrid (www.oup.es/en or product.safety@oup.com).
OUP España S.A. also acts as importer into Spain of products made by the manufacturer.

MIX
Paper
FSC FSC® C183721

For Mom, who has loved me unconditionally.
This book is for you, for always believing in me,
For showing me the meaning of resilience, courage, and gentleness.
Thank you for being my greatest inspiration.

Contents

Foreword by Marsha B. Henderson

One of the most brilliant women I know, Dr. Anita Gupta, has stepped up to the challenge of offering not only timely information, but a bold, clear-eyed vision of what women's pain care can and should be.

For far too long, women's pain has lived in the shadows—reduced to reproductive health alone or filtered through the lens of short-term or inadequate care. Despite countless women reporting chronic physical pain throughout their lives the medical system has repeatedly failed to take their voices seriously. This failure has left too many women feeling invisible in exam rooms, misunderstood by practitioners, and underserved by research.

Dr. Anita Gupta's groundbreaking new book, *Interventional Pain Management for Women's Health* changes that.

With evidence-based strategies, actionable insights, and a voice that empowers, Dr. Gupta and her colleagues help to chart a new path forward. This work equips patients to advocate for themselves and challenges the medical community to listen more closely, respond more effectively, and deliver care that honors the full complexity of women's pain health.

What makes this work especially powerful is the expertise and leadership behind it. Under the editorial guidance of Dr. Anita Gupta, a globally recognized expert in pain medicine and a trailblazer in women's health, this book elevates the conversation with authority and compassion. Dr. Anita Gupta has dedicated her career to closing the gap in pain care, and her vision has brought together a multidisciplinary body of knowledge that is both scientifically rigorous and urgently relevant.

This book is not just a contribution—it is a breakthrough. It will be a lifeline for many and a call to action for all. Whether you are a clinician, policymaker, educator, advocate, or someone seeking to better understand your own health—this book is a vital tool. It empowers readers with knowledge, grounded in science and empathy, and it reminds us that health is not a privilege for a few, but a right for all.

May this work spark meaningful conversation, deepen understanding, and, most importantly, inspire collective action to advance equitable, effective pain management for women—now and in the years to come.

Let this be the moment we stop asking women to "push through the pain" and start asking how we can better understand, support, and heal it.

—Marsha B. Henderson (Retired)
Associate Commissioner for Women's Health,
U.S. Food and Drug Administration

Foreword by Arunma Oteh

Around the world, millions of women live with chronic, unrelenting pain—often in silence and without access to effective treatment. This reality is not only a health crisis but also a development challenge. Women's health has long been a cornerstone of global development policy, and yet, within this critical domain, pain management remains a profoundly unmet need. Too many women face systemic barriers to care, from inadequate diagnostic tools and treatment pathways to deeply rooted biases in medical research and healthcare delivery.

Chronic pain disrupts education, employment, caregiving, and community participation—directly impacting economic growth and social stability. As a global institution committed to reducing poverty and advancing equity, we recognize that sustainable development is impossible without addressing the health burdens that disproportionately affect women. Pain is one of the most disabling conditions worldwide, yet interventional pain management—evidence-based, cost-effective, and potentially life-changing—remains inaccessible to most women, especially in low- and middle-income countries.

This book fills an urgent and long-overlooked gap. It brings together expert voices, clinical insight, and policy perspectives to shine a light on the role of interventional pain management in women's health. It calls for a paradigm shift: one where pain is not normalized, dismissed, or endured but treated with urgency, innovation, and dignity. This timely and essential work is led by Dr. Anita Gupta, a world-renowned expert in pain medicine and a visionary leader in women's health. With decades of groundbreaking clinical, academic, and global health experience, Dr. Anita Gupta brings unmatched expertise and credibility to this field. The editor's dedication to closing the gap in pain care has been transformative—not only for patients, but for practitioners and policymakers worldwide.

As leaders, clinicians, researchers, and advocates, we have a responsibility to prioritize women's pain not only as a medical issue but also as a matter of global development. I commend the editor and contributing authors for this important contribution and encourage policymakers, practitioners, and partners to take its message forward. We must do better—and together, we can.

—Arunma Oteh,
Academic, University of Oxford
Former World Bank Vice President & Treasurer

Preface

Pain is a universal human experience, yet it remains deeply personal and uniquely complex, especially for women. Despite advances in medicine, the understanding and treatment of pain in women are often inadequate, overlooked, or misunderstood. This discrepancy reflects a significant unmet need in healthcare that demands urgent attention specific to pain treatment.

Women experience pain differently from men, influenced by biological, hormonal, psychological, and social factors. Conditions such as chronic pelvic pain, fibromyalgia, migraine, and autoimmune diseases disproportionately affect women and often lead to persistent suffering. Unfortunately, women's pain is frequently underdiagnosed, undertreated, or dismissed, resulting in diminished quality of life and substantial societal costs across the world.

As an anesthesiologist, advanced interventional pain management procedures offer an opportunity to address this unmet need. These procedures offer targeted, minimally invasive procedures that can significantly alleviate both acute and chronic pain when conventional treatments fall short. However, despite its promise, this approach remains underutilized and under researched in women's health. The gap in awareness, clinical guidelines, and tailored interventions highlights a critical void in contemporary pain management strategies.

This volume to address this area aims to begin to bridge that gap by presenting comprehensive insights into the unique characteristics of women's pain and the vital role that interventional pain management can play in addressing it. Through multidisciplinary perspectives, evidence-based practices, and real-world clinical experiences, we explore how to better recognize, diagnose, and treat pain in women using advanced interventional pain techniques. There is much more work to be done. This volume is simply a starting point for work ahead and a hope to inspire more experts in this area to help women suffering around the world.

As the editor, I am deeply committed to advancing women's health and empowering clinicians and patients with the knowledge needed to improve human health. It is my hope that this work will stimulate greater dialogue, research, and clinical health innovation, ultimately ensuring that women around the world receive the compassionate, safe, and effective pain care they deserve today and much ahead in the future. I want to thank the many contributors, experts, medical students, and volunteers around the world who have helped shape this volume: without their commitment and efforts *Interventional Pain Medicine for Women's Health* would not have come to fruition. I hope this volume is a starting point for the much-needed work ahead.

—Anita Gupta, DO, MPP, PharmD, FASA

Acknowledgments

This volume is the culmination of sustained scholarly effort made possible through the support and contributions of numerous individuals and institutions.

We are deeply indebted to our mentors, colleagues, and collaborators for their intellectual guidance, constructive feedback, and ongoing engagement, all of which helped shape this manuscript. We also gratefully acknowledge the many contributors who generously shared their expertise, time, and insights, enhancing the rigor and clarity of this work.

We extend our sincere appreciation to the editorial and publishing teams at Oxford University Press, led by Caroline Smith and Paulina dos Santos Major, for their professionalism, patience, and commitment to excellence throughout the development of this volume. Their coordination and stewardship of multidisciplinary contributions were instrumental to its completion.

We express our gratitude to the Gates Foundation, Milken Institute, and the World Economic Forum for their dedicated initiatives global. Their commitment to advancing research on health innovation and women's health was instrumental shaping the development of this work.

We are especially grateful to the volunteers, medical students, illustrators, and research scholars whose dedication and insight strengthened both the scholarly rigor and accessibility of this volume.

We also express our sincere gratitude to our communities, families, and friends for their enduring support, encouragement, and patience throughout this journey.

We acknowledge the use of digital tools to support the editorial and technical processes including language refinement, reference standardization, and the preparation of supplementary text, in accordance with Oxford University Press policies. The authors have carefully reviewed and verified all content, and retain full responsibility in collaboration with OUP for the accuracy, integrity, and validity of this work.

Contributors

Katherine Adams, MD, University of Kansas Medical Center, Kansas City, KS

Ahmed Alassal, MD, CNIM, MHA, Professor, Clinical Anatomy, University of California, Riverside, CA

Farah Alvi, MD, Clinical Associate, Obstetrics and Gynecology, University of Chicago Medicine, Chicago, IL

Suwarna Anand, MD, Anesthesiology, University of Mississippi Medical Center, Jackson, MS

Magdalena Anitescu, MD, PhD, FASA, Professor, Director, Chief, Anesthesiology and Pain Medicine, University of Chicago Medicine, Chicago, IL

Farrukh A. Ansari, MD, Anesthesiology and Pain, OrthoNY Orthopedic Injury Clinic, Albany, NY

Punthitra Arpornsuksant, MD, Anesthesiology, Johns Hopkins School of Medicine, Baltimore, MD

Nyla K. Azam, MD, Associate Professor, Albany Medical Health System, Albany, NY

Dhiresh Bandaru, BS, University of California School of Medicine, Riverside, CA

Anuj Bapodra, MD, Anesthesiology and Pain, Beth Israel Deaconess Medical Center, Boston, MA

Chadwick Barker, DO, Anesthesiology, Maimonides Medical Center, New York, NY

Antje Barreveld, MD, Associate Professor, Anesthesiology, Tufts University School of Medicine, Newton, MA

Mohammad Husain Bawany, MD, Assistant Professor, Pain Medicine, Columbia University, New York Presbyterian Hospital, New York, NY

Niranjana Bienkowska, BA, University of California School of Medicine, Los Angeles, CA

Alejandra Cardenas Rojas, MD, Physical Medicine and Rehabilitation, Johns Hopkins School of Medicine, Baltimore, MD

Melissa Chao, MD, Assistant Professor, Anesthesiology and Pain, Columbia University, New York Presbyterian Hospital, New York, NY

Nathaniel Co, BS, University of California School of Medicine, Riverside, CA

Rosalynn R. Z. Conic, MD, PhD, MPH, Physical Medicine and Rehabilitation, University of Florida, Gainesville, FL

Stephanie Crimmel, MD, Anesthesiology, Johns Hopkins School of Medicine, Baltimore, MD

Carla Demerdjian, MS, California University of Science and Medicine, Colton, CA

Laura Douglass, MD, Assistant Professor, Director, Obstetrics and Gynecology, University of Chicago Medicine, Chicago, IL

Benjamin Allen Fujita-Howie, MD, Anesthesiology, Columbia University Irving Medical Center – New York Presbyterian Hospital, New York, NY

Patrick George, BS, University of Kansas Medical Center, Kansas City, KS

Katherine Gohres, MD, MBA, Anesthesiology, University of Chicago Medicine, Chicago, IL

Vahid Grami, MD, Anesthesiology and Critical Care Medicine, Assistant Professor, Johns Hopkins Medicine, Baltimore, MD

Anita Gupta, DO, MPP, PharmD, FASA, Adjunct Assistant Professor, Anesthesiology and Pain, Johns Hopkins School of Medicine, Baltimore, MD; Professor, University of California School of Medicine, Riverside, CA; Professor, Anesthesiology and Pain, Loma Linda School of Medicine, Loma Linda, CA

Kelsey Gustafson, MD, University of Kansas Medical Center, Kansas City, KS

Amna Haider, DO, Physical Medicine and Rehabilitation, Johns Hopkins School of Medicine, Baltimore, MD

Don Hoang, MD, Penn State Hershey Medical Center, Hershey, PA

Ankur Jain, DO, Physical Medicine and Rehabilitation, Johns Hopkins School of Medicine, Baltimore, MD

Aparna Jindal, MD, Assistant Professor, Interventional Pain Division, University of Arkansas for Medical Sciences, College of Medicine, Little Rock, AR

Sarafina Kankam, MD, Anesthesiology and Pain Medicine, University of Kansas Medical Center, Kansas City, KS

Meera Kirpekar, MD, Clinical Associate Professor, Director of Pelvic Pain, Anesthesiology and Pain Medicine, New York University Grossman School of Medicine, New York, NY

Lynn Kohan, MD, Chief, Pain Division, Professor, Anesthesiology, Pain Management, University of Virginia, Charlottesville, VA

Karishma Kondapalli, MD, Anesthesiology, University of Chicago Medicine, Chicago, IL

Kenzo Lacuarta, BA, Hackensack Meridian School of Medicine, Nutley, NJ

Danielle Levin, MD, Anesthesiology, Pain Medicine, Penn Medicine Princeton Medical Center, Plainsboro, NJ

Gerard Limerick, MD, PhD, Assistant Professor, Physical Medicine and Rehabilitation, Johns Hopkins University School of Medicine, Baltimore, MD

Jessie J. Liu, BA, Harvard Medical School, Boston, MA

Catherine Lowe, BS, University of California School of Medicine, Riverside, CA

O. Sandra Madueke-Laveaux, MD, Associate Professor, Obstetrics and Gynecology, University of Chicago Medicine, Chicago, IL

Yehuda Masturov, MD, Maimonides Medical Center, New York, NY

Ankita Mathur, MD, New York University—Langone Health, New York, NY

Leena Mathew, MD, Professor of Anesthesiology, Chief—Pain Division, Pain Fellowship Program Director, Columbia University, New York Presbyterian Hospital, New York, NY

Sharon Marie Mathew, BS, UQ-Ochsner Clinical School, New Orleans, LA

Joseph A. McGuire, MD, Anesthesiology and Pain Medicine, West Virginia University School of Medicine, Morgantown, WV

Jason Mizrahi, MD, Johns Hopkins University School of Medicine, Baltimore, MD

Shawana S. Moore, PhD, DNP, APRN, WHNP-BC, FNAP, FAAN, FNPWH, Associate Professor, Program Director, Nell Hodgson School of Nursing, Emory University, Atlanta, GA

Jessica Opoku-Anane, MD, MS, Associate Professor, Section Chief, Obstetrics and Gynecology, Robert Wood Johnson Medical School, New Brunswick, NJ

Ioana Pasca, MD, FASA, Associate Professor, Associate Program Director, Anesthesiology, Riverside University Health System, Moreno Valley, CA

Alopi M. Patel, MD, FASA, Associate Professor, Anesthesiology and Pain Medicine, Robert Wood Johnson Medical School, New Brunswick, NJ

Raj Patel, MD, Anesthesiology, University of Chicago Medicine, Chicago, IL

Grace Park, MD, Stony Brook University, Stony Brook, NY

Insiyyah Patanwala, MD, Assistant Professor, Obstetrics and Gynecology, University of Chicago Medicine, Chicago, IL

Sudheer Potru, DO, FASAM, Director, Complex Pain Clinic, Atlanta VA Healthcare System, Atlanta, GA

Anand Prem, MD, Professor, Medical Director, Anesthesiology, University of Mississippi Medical Center, Jackson, MS

Kavya Rajan, Research Scholar, Alpharetta, GA

Chitra Ramasubbu, MD, Medical Director, Anesthesiology and Pain, Nova Spine and Pain Care, Alpharetta, GA

Anesh Rugnath, MD, Associate Professor, Program Director, Cardiothoracic Anesthesia Fellowship, University of Mississippi Medical Center, Jackson, MS

Eliot Sadik, MD, Johns Hopkins University School of Medicine, Baltimore, MD

Gary Schwartz, MD, Vice Chair, Anesthesiology and Pain, Maimonides Medical Center, New York, NY

Jarna R. Shah, MD, Associate Professor, Anesthesiology and Pain, Saint Louis University, St. Louis, MO

Loren Shamalov, BS, City University of New York School of Medicine, New York, NY

Sumedha Shastry, Research Scholar, Cornell University, Ithaca, NY

Borys Shturman, MD, Anesthesiology, Maimonides Medical Center, New York, NY

Tanvee Singh, MD, Assistant Professor, Anesthesiology and Pain Medicine, Columbia University Irving Medical Center – New York Presbyterian Hospital, New York, NY

Priyanka Singla, MD, Assistant Professor, Department of Anesthesiology and Pain Medicine, University of Virginia, Charlottesville, VA

Peter Sloane, MD, Anesthesiology, University of Chicago Medicine, Chicago, IL

Sophie E. Smith, BA, Robert Wood Johnson Medical School, New Brunswick, NJ

Jay Srinivas, Research Scholar, San Diego, CA

Shaan Srinivas, Research Scholar, San Diego, CA

Hirsch K. Srivastava, MD, Anesthesiology and Pain Medicine, Columbia University Irving Medical Center, New York Presbyterian Hospital, New York, NY

James Sturvidant, MD, Anesthesiology, University of Mississippi Medical Center, Jackson, MS

Michael Suarez, DO, Physical Medicine and Rehabilitation, Johns Hopkins School of Medicine, Baltimore, MD

Joanna Sung, BS, University of California School of Medicine, Riverside, CA

Rachel Sunico, MD, Olive View Medical Center/ UC Los Angeles, Los Angeles, CA; UC Irvine, Orange, CA

Sejal Tamakuwala, MD, Assistant Professor, Gynecology and Obstetrics, Emory University School of Medicine, Atlanta, GA

Kimberly Templeton, BA, Professor; Vice Chair, University of Kansas Medical Center, Kansas City, KS

Birpartap S. Thind, MD, MHA, Anesthesiology, Riverside Community Hospital, Riverside, CA

Thanh Thanh Tran, BS, University of California School of Medicine, Riverside, CA

Huy Truong, DO, Western University of Health Sciences College, Glendale, AZ

Trevor Van De Water, MD, Johns Hopkins School of Medicine, Baltimore, MD

Richard Vaglienti, MD, MBA, FASA, Associate Professor, Director, Pain Medicine, West Virginia University, Morgantown, WV

Archana Venkatesan, BS, Medical College of Georgia, Augusta, GA

Rishika Voruganti, BS, Rutgers Robert Wood Johnson Medical School, New Brunswick, NJ

Patricia Wang, MD, Assistant Professor, Anesthesiology, Columbia Anesthesiology—New York Presbyterian Hospital, New York, NY

PART I

INTRODUCTION TO PAIN IN WOMEN

1

Advancing Pain Care for Women

A Comprehensive Overview

Birpartap S. Thind and Anita Gupta

Sex Differences in Pain Prevalence

Migraine, musculoskeletal pain, temporomandibular disorders, fibromyalgia, neuropathic pain, irritable bowel syndrome, rheumatoid arthritis, and osteoarthritis are common pain conditions that occur markedly more frequently in women than in men. Moreover, several chronic pain conditions—including endometriosis, interstitial cystitis, vulvodynia, and pelvic girdle pain—are exclusive to women.

These epidemiologic data support the expectation that, on average, women report greater pain than men and therefore may require increased clinical attention and treatment.

Underrecognition and Undertreatment of Women's Pain

Despite this higher burden of pain, longitudinal studies consistently demonstrate that women's pain is underrecognized and undertreated compared with men's pain. The reasons for this persistent discrepancy are multifactorial and rooted in long-held, antiquated beliefs that unfortunately remain prevalent in modern medical practice.[1]

Sex differences in pain experience are influenced by a wide range of factors, including anatomical, physiological, neural, hormonal, psychological, social, and cultural variables.[2] Women demonstrate increased pain sensitivity and a higher risk of developing chronic pain conditions, findings that have been well documented in the literature.[3] However, rather than being used to guide more individualized care, these differences have too often resulted in biased and suboptimal treatment. Proper recognition of sex-based differences should instead be leveraged to improve pain management strategies for women.

Molecular, Physiological, and Pharmacologic Differences

Differences at the molecular and physiological levels play an important role in shaping sex-specific pain experiences. Variations in drug absorption, distribution, metabolism, and excretion can lead to a wide range of clinical responses to medications, including opioid analgesics—ranging from no effect to optimal analgesia to intolerable adverse effects.

In women, the endogenous opioid system and other hormonal systems significantly influence pain sensitivity and responsiveness to analgesics.[4] For example, women have been shown to respond differently to kappa opioid receptor agonists, such as pentazocine, likely due to genetic and hormonal factors.[5] Pain sensitivity in women also fluctuates across the menstrual cycle, with increased sensitivity observed during the luteal phase.[6]

In many cases, women may require different dosing strategies to achieve effective analgesia. However, until recently, many pain medications were studied predominantly in male populations, thus limiting knowledge about appropriate dosing and efficacy in women.[7]

Neurobiological and Hormonal Influences on Pain Processing

Emerging research indicates that pain is perceived and processed differently in the nervous systems of women and men. One key explanation for these differences lies in the influence of sex hormones and their relative concentrations. Sex hormones modulate nociceptive transmission in both the central and peripheral nervous systems.

Testosterone appears to exert a primarily antinociceptive and protective effect, which may partially explain sex-based differences in pain perception and transmission.[8] These biological differences have important implications for the development of sex-specific pharmacologic and nonpharmacologic pain management strategies.[9]

Systemic Bias and Delays in Acute Pain Care

The urgency to better understand pain physiology in women is underscored by the reality that pain is experienced within a healthcare system affected by systemic bias. Women presenting with acute conditions frequently receive delayed or inadequate care. For example, female patients presenting to the emergency department with acute myocardial infarction experience longer wait times, receive less aggressive treatment, and are less likely to be admitted than male patients.[10]

Similarly, women presenting with acute chest pain or abdominal pain in emergency settings are less likely to receive timely analgesia or opioid prescriptions.[11] These delays not only exacerbate acute suffering but also contribute to poorer long-term outcomes.

Diagnostic Delays and Psychologization in Chronic Pain

Biases against women persist in the management of chronic pain. Conditions such as endometriosis and fibromyalgia are often diagnosed years after symptom onset due to limited awareness and a tendency to psychologize women's symptoms.[10] As a result, women's pain complaints are frequently dismissed, minimized, or labeled as "psychological" or "all in their head."[12,13]

This failure to diagnose and treat pain perpetuates a vicious cycle. Studies demonstrate that women are more likely than men to receive referrals for mental health care or antidepressants for pain management, whereas men are more frequently prescribed opioids.[10] These patterns reinforce distorted perceptions of women's pain among healthcare providers.

Credibility, Stereotypes, and the Perception of Pain

Women are often perceived as less credible reporters of their own pain, a perception linked to stereotypes portraying women as overly emotional or unreliable narrators of suffering.[10]Even when women and men report identical pain levels, women's pain is significantly underestimated.[10]

These biases highlight the urgent need for systemic reform in pain assessment and management. Recognizing this, the International Association for the Study of Pain (IASP) adopted an updated definition of pain: "An unpleasant sensory and emotional experience associated with, or resembling that associated with, actual or potential tissue damage."[14]

Systemic Changes Needed to Address Disparities

While redefining pain is an important step, meaningful progress requires concrete action to dismantle entrenched biases. Without systemic change, women's pain will continue to be dismissed, minimized, or misdiagnosed, perpetuating centuries-old stereotypes.[15]

Key areas for reform include:

- *Advancing inclusion of women in research.* Historically, women have been underrepresented in clinical trials, thus limiting evidence-based care. The National Institutes of Health's 2016 mandate to include sex as a biological variable marked progress, but further efforts are needed.[16]
- *Women's health education and training.* Medical curricula must include comprehensive education on sex and gender differences in pain perception and management, as well as training to recognize and mitigate bias.[17]
- *Patient-centered approaches.* Individualized pain assessments and shared decision-making improve outcomes and ensure that women's experiences are validated.[3]
- *Addressing implicit bias.* Healthcare systems should implement standardized protocols and decision-support tools to reduce subjectivity in pain assessment and treatment.[10]
- *Innovative therapies and interventions.* Emerging evidence suggests sex-based differences in pain mechanisms, such as microglial and T-cell involvement, may lead to novel, sex-specific therapies.[4]

Conclusion

Disparities in pain management for women arise from complex biological, systemic, and cultural factors. Addressing these inequities requires a multifaceted approach that acknowledges sex differences, confronts systemic bias, and promotes individualized care. Women's pain must be recognized and treated with the same urgency and legitimacy afforded to men. Only through sustained systemic change can long-standing barriers to equitable pain care be dismantled.

References

1. Mogil JS. Sex differences in pain and pain inhibition: Multiple explanations of a controversial phenomenon. Nat Rev Neurosci. 2012;13(12):859–866. doi:10.1038/nrn3360
2. Casale R, Atzeni F, Bazzichi L, et al. Pain in women: A perspective review on a relevant clinical issue that deserves prioritization. Pain Ther. 2021;10(1):287–314. doi:10.1007/s40122-021-00244-1
3. Bartley EJ, Fillingim RB. Sex differences in pain: A brief review of clinical and experimental findings. Br J Anaesth. 2013;111(1):52–58. doi:10.1093/bja/aet127
4. Fillingim RB, King CD, Ribeiro-Dasilva MC, Rahim-Williams B, Riley JL 3rd. Sex, gender, and pain: A review of recent clinical and experimental findings. J Pain. 2009;10(5):447–485. doi:10.1016/j.jpain.2008.12.001
5. Mogil JS, Sternberg WF, Kest B, Marek P, Liebeskind JC. Sex differences in the antagonism of swim stress-induced analgesia: Effects of gonadectomy and estrogen replacement. Pain. 1993;53(1):17–25. doi:10.1016/0304-3959(93)90050-7
6. Riley JL 3rd, Robinson ME, Wise EA, Myers CD, Fillingim RB. Sex differences in the perception of noxious experimental stimuli: A meta-analysis. Pain. 1998;74(2–3):181–187. doi:10.1016/s0304-3959(97)00199-1
7. Soldin OP, Mattison DR. Sex differences in pharmacokinetics and pharmacodynamics. Clin Pharmacokinet. 2009;48(3):143–157. doi:10.2165/00003088-200948030-00001
8. Fischer L, Clemente DR, Tambeli CH. The protective role of testosterone in the development of temporomandibular joint pain. J Pain. 2007;8(4):316–324. doi:10.1016/j.jpain.2006.10.003
9. Greenspan JD, Craft RM, LeResche L, et al. Studying sex and gender differences in pain and analgesia: A consensus report. Pain. 2007;132(suppl 1):S26–S45. doi:10.1016/j.pain.2007.10.014
10. Samulowitz A, Gremyr I, Eriksson E, Hensing G. "Brave men" and "emotional women": A theory-guided literature review on gender bias in health care and gendered norms towards patients with chronic pain. Pain Res Manag. 2018;2018:6358624. doi:10.1155/2018/6358624
11. Chen EH, Shofer FS, Dean AJ, et al. Gender disparity in analgesic treatment of emergency department patients with acute abdominal pain. Acad Emerg Med. 2008;15(5):414–418. doi:10.1111/j.1553-2712.2008.00100.x
12. Goldberg DS. Dismissing women's pain: The implicit biases of clinical judgment. Bioethics. 2024;38(4):345–353. doi:10.1111/bioe.13271
13. Pearson, C. (2022, February 16). How doctors dismiss women's pain. The Washington Post. https://www.washingtonpost.com/health/2022/02/16/how-doctors-dismiss-womens-pain/
14. Raja, S. N., Carr, D. B., Cohen, M., Finnerup, N. B., Flor, H., Gibson, S., Keefe, F. J., Mogil, J. S., Ringkamp, M., Sluka, K. A., Song, X. J., Stevens, B., Sullivan, M. D., Tutelman, P. R., Ushida, T., & Vader, K. (2020). The revised International Association for the Study of Pain definition of pain: concepts, challenges, and compromises. *PAIN, 161*(9), 1976–1982. https://doi.org/10.1097/j.pain.0000000000001939
15. Hoffmann DE, Tarzian AJ. The girl who cried pain: A bias against women in the treatment of pain. J Law Med Ethics. 2001;29(1):13–27. doi:10.1111/j.1748-720x.2001.tb00037.x
16. National Institutes of Health. (2015). Notice: NOT-OD-15-102: Consideration of sex as a biological variable in NIH-funded research. U.S. Department of Health and Human Services. https://grants.nih.gov/grants/guide/notice-files/NOT-OD-15-102.html
17. Moretti C, De Luca E, D'Apice C, et al. Gender and sex bias in prevention and clinical treatment of women's chronic pain: Hypotheses of a curriculum development. Front Med (Lausanne). 2023;10:1189126. doi:10.3389/fmed.2023.1189126

2

Defining Pain and Its Unique Impact on Women's Health

Gerard Limerick, Eliot Sadik, Alejandra Cardenas Rojas, and Amna Haider

Definitions and Types of Pain

Approximately 25% of emergency department visits for pain are estimated to progress into chronic pain.[1] This has led to growing interest in understanding the mechanisms underlying this transition, including the distinct signaling pathways involved at each stage. Acute pain (pain lasting less than 6 months) typically results from a rapid inflammatory response to injury, whereas chronic pain (pain lasting longer than 6 months) is characterized by a persistent inflammatory state. Various factors—such as gender, genetic predisposition, and comorbid conditions—play a role in influencing both the onset and persistence of pain.[2]

While pain can be classified as *acute* or *chronic*, it may also be classified by underlying pathophysiology (Table 2.1). Nociceptive pain is defined by the International Association for the Study of Pain (IASP) as "pain that arises from actual or threatened damage to non-neural tissue that is due to activation of nociceptors."[3]. *Nociceptive pain* occurs when noxious stimuli trigger the generation of an action potential in the peripheral nervous system. This action potential is propagated through afferent fibers, up the spinal cord to the thalamus and, finally, the cerebral cortex.[4] This contrasts with the classification of *nociplastic pain*, which the IASP defines as "pain arising from altered nociception despite no clear evidence of actual or threatened tissue damage or evidence of disease to the somatosensory system." In this type of pain, pain pathways are activated without a clear inciting stimulus. It should be noted that nociplastic pain can occur in combination with nociceptive pain. A third classification of pain is *neuropathic pain*, which the IASP defines as "pain caused by a lesion or disease of the somatosensory nervous system."[3] Neuropathic pain can be further subdivided into central and peripheral pain. Central neuropathic pain occurs with a lesion or disease in the central nervous system. Examples include thalamic pain syndrome, poststroke pain, and pain after spinal cord injury. Peripheral neuropathic pain involves a lesion or disease in the peripheral somatosensory nervous system. This includes pain states such as postherpetic neuralgia, painful diabetic neuropathy, and complex regional pain syndrome (CRPS).

Last, pain may also be classified by the fiber type involved in propagating the pain signals. Somatic pain is defined as "pain carried along the sensory fibers" and is usually "discrete and intense" in nature.[4] This contrasts with visceral pain, which is "carried by sympathetic fibers" and is "diffuse and poorly localized" in nature.[4] However, when sympathetic nonadrenergic neurons in the periphery interact with primary afferent neurons, this can create a maintenance loop of pain. This is referred to as *sympathetically maintained pain*.[4]

Table 2.1 Types of pain and characteristics

Classification basis	Pain type	Definition/Pathophysiology (IASP-based)	Characteristics/Examples
Duration	Acute	Pain resulting from a rapid inflammatory response to injury, typically lasting <6 months.	Clear inciting event; protective function.
	Chronic	Pain characterized by a persistent inflammatory state, typically lasting >6 months.	Transition influenced by genetics, gender, and comorbidities.
Pathophysiology	Nociceptive	Pain arising from actual or threatened damage to non-neural tissue due to activation of nociceptors.	Triggered by noxious stimuli; action potential propagates through peripheral to central nervous system.
	Nociplastic	Pain arising from altered nociception despite no clear evidence of actual/threatened tissue damage or disease of the somatosensory system.	Activated pathways without clear stimulus; dysfunction in pain processing.
	Neuropathic	Pain caused by a lesion or disease of the somatosensory nervous system.	Central (e.g., poststroke) or Peripheral (e.g., postherpetic neuralgia).
Fiber type	Somatic	Pain carried along sensory fibers.	Usually discrete and intense in nature.
	Visceral	Pain carried by sympathetic fibers.	Usually diffuse and poorly localized in nature.
	Sympathetically maintained	A maintenance loop created by the interaction of sympathetic non-adrenergic neurons and primary afferent neurons in the periphery.	Persistence of pain beyond normal healing time.

How Pain Affects Women Differently Compared to Men

Women generally exhibit a lower pain threshold and tolerance to acute stimuli, including thermal (heat, cold), pressure, and electrical pain, when compared to men.[5–7] Lund and colleagues found that only women—but not men—showed increased electrical pain thresholds following high-frequency transcutaneous electrical nerve stimulation (TENS) and that pain modulation responses were more variable among women.[8] These differences appear to be influenced by mood-related factors. Goffaux et al. showed that the sex differences could be attributed to cortical, but not spinal nociceptive processing and that controlling for trait anxiety eliminated these sex differences, indicating a key role for emotional factors.[9] Additionally, there is evidence for sex-specific modulation of cold pain by transient receptor potential melastatin 8 (TRPM8), an ion channel that regulates both innocuous and noxious cold sensations at the level of the trigeminal or dorsal root ganglia.[10] Therefore, these findings underscore a sex difference in acute pain perception driven by both neurobiological mechanisms and emotional modulation.

Chronic pain conditions such as fibromyalgia, knee osteoarthritis, migraine, and other musculoskeletal conditions have been shown to have an increased central sensitization pattern. Women with chronic pain have greater temporal summation of pain (increase pain amplification with repeated noxious stimuli) than do men, indicating enhanced central sensitization.[11] Guekos et al. confirmed that healthy women had more experimentally induced central sensitization (heat temporal summation protocol) compared to men.[12]

Women have also been shown to have a pro-nociceptive conditioned pain modulation (CPM) profile, meaning that, while an initial painful stimulus often inhibits the discomfort of a second painful stimulus, in some women, the initial stimulus *facilitates* rather than inhibits pain. Firouzian et al. showed that pain unpleasantness and salience of the conditioning stimuli were correlated with reduced CPM efficiency, particularly in women.[13] These findings reinforce the existence of sex-based differences in central pain processing and descending inhibitory pathways.

Biological Factors

Body fat composition appears to affect central and peripheral mechanisms of pain sensitivity.[14] Women typically have more subcutaneous fat than men, especially in the femoral region. Increased levels of subcutaneous fat are associated with elevated inflammatory markers such as C-reactive protein (CRP), interleukin (IL)-6, and leptin, all of which can influence pain perception.[15] Sex hormones such as estrogen and progesterone play a crucial role in the development and maintenance of chronic pain in women.[16] Hormonal fluctuations, especially during the menstrual cycle, may exacerbate numerous chronic pain conditions such as cluster headaches, migraines, fibromyalgia, irritable bowel syndrome, temporomandibular joint (TMJ) disorders, and rheumatoid arthritis.[16] Low estrogen levels have also been associated with a reduction of endogenous opioid activity, thereby increasing pain perception. Conversely, estrogen increases serotonin synthesis and reduces its reuptake and metabolism, which may improve pain tolerance. Progesterone, another sex hormone, inhibits pro-inflammatory cytokines and promotes anti-inflammatory cytokines, which may reduce pain perception. It is also associated with reduced pain severity in patients with fibromyalgia. Additionally, elevated levels of prolactin, another neuroimmune hormone, are associated with migraines and chronic pain in females.[17]

Social Factors

Psychosocial factors influence chronic pain in the female population.[18] Female patients report experiencing more pain when tested by male practitioners, whereas male patients report less pain when tested by female practitioners. Additionally, peer influence may also play a role in pain perception. Male patients demonstrate higher levels of pain tolerance when friends are present, while no such effect is observed in females.[18] Furthermore, the impact of stress on pain processing differs by sex. Elevated stress levels in females have a greater impact on pain perception when compared to males. In females, exposure to childhood and adolescent stress leads to increased visceral sensitivity and elevated expression of stress-induced genes in the amygdala, a phenomenon not observed in males.[16]

References

1. Friedman BW, Ochoa Abril L, Naeem F et al. Predicting the transition to chronic pain 6 months after an emergency department visit for acute pain: A prospective cohort study. J Emerg Med. 2020;59(6):805–811.
2. Gregus AM, Levine IS, Eddinger KA, Yaksh TL, Buczynski MW. Sex differences in neuroimmune and glial mechanisms of pain. Pain. 2021;162(8):2186–2200.
3. IASP Taxonomy Working Group. Pain terms: A current list with definitions and notes on usage. IASP. 2011;209–214. https://www.iasp-pain.org/resources/terminology/
4. Benzon HT, Raja SN, Fishman SM, Liu SS, Cohen SP, Hurley RW, eds. *Essentials of Pain Medicine*, 4th ed. Elsevier, 2018.
5. Fillingim RB, King CD, Ribeiro-Dasilva MC, Rahim-Williams B, Riley JL. Sex, gender, and pain: A review of recent clinical and experimental findings. J Pain. 2009;10(5):447–485.
6. Racine M, Tousignant-Laflamme Y, Kloda LA, Dion D, Dupuis G, Choinière M. A systematic literature review of 10 years of research on sex/gender and experimental pain perception - Part 1: Are there really differences between women and men? Pain. 2012;153(3):602–618.
7. Doehring A, Bangert M, Sibilia V et al. Effect sizes in experimental pain produced by gender, genetic variants and sensitization procedures. PloS One. 2011;6(3):e17724.
8. Lund I, Lundeberg T, Kjellgren A, Bove G. Gender differences in electrical pain threshold responses to transcutaneous electrical nerve stimulation (TENS). Neurosci Lett. 2005;375(2):75–80.
9. Goffaux P, Redmond WJ, Rainville P, Marchand S. Sex differences in perceived pain are affected by an anxious brain. Pain. 2011;152(9):2065–2073.
10. Wei C, Kim B, McKemy DD. Transient receptor potential melastatin 8 is required for nitroglycerin- and calcitonin gene-related peptide-induced migraine-like pain behaviors in mice. Pain. 2022;163(12):2380–2389.
11. Nijs J, Clark J, Malfliet A et al. Central sensitisation in chronic pain conditions: Latest discoveries and their potential for precision medicine. Lancet Rheumatol. 2021;3(5):e383–e392.
12. Guekos A, Saxer J, Salinas Gallegos D, Schweinhardt P. Healthy women show more experimentally induced central sensitization compared with men. Pain. 2024;165(6):1413–1424.
13. Firouzian S, Osborne NR, Cheng JC et al. Individual variability and sex differences in conditioned pain modulation and the impact of resilience, conditioning stimulus pain unpleasantness and salience. Pain. 2020;161(8):1847–1860.
14. Tashani OA, Astita R, Sharp D, Johnson MI. Body mass index and distribution of body fat can influence sensory detection and pain sensitivity. Eur J Pain. 2017;21(7):1186–1196.
15. Berwal D, Branisteanu DD, Glickman M, Sagar A, Pilitsis JG. The sex-dependent impact of adipose tissue and inflammation on chronic pain: A cross-sectional study from the all of us research program. Cytokine. 2024;179:156614.
16. Mogil JS. Qualitative sex differences in pain processing: Emerging evidence of a biased literature. Nat Rev Neurosci. 2020;21(7):353–365.
17. Sorge RE, Totsch SK. Sex differences in pain. J Neurosci Res. 2017;95(6):1271–1281.
18. Meints SM, Edwards RR. Evaluating psychosocial contributions to chronic pain outcomes. Prog Neuropsychopharmacol Biol Psychiatry. 2018;87(Pt B):168–182.

3

Foundations of Interventional Pain Treatment in Women

Multimodal and Comprehensive Approaches

Priyanka Singla, Jessie J. Liu, and Antje Barreveld

Introduction

The etiology of chronic pelvic pain (CPP) is often multifactorial and challenging to manage. Treating pelvic pain requires careful workup and a comprehensive multimodal approach for treatment.[1] This chapter discusses interventional pain management techniques to provide diagnostic as well as complementary strategies for a multidisciplinary approach to the management of pelvic pain.

Overview of Interventional Pain Management Procedures

Interventional pain management techniques can be used for diagnostic evaluation as well as treatment of CPP.[1] The interventional techniques include injections and neuromodulation techniques based on the pathophysiology of the symptoms and disease.

The etiologies of CPP are often multifactorial and can be related to various urological, gastrointestinal, musculoskeletal, gynecological, neurological, and psychosocial conditions.[2] These systems-based causes can be further grouped into visceral, somatic, neuropathic, and psychosocial categories.[3,4]

Central sensitization plays an important role, adding another layer of complexity for diagnosis and treatment. The risk of central sensitization is associated with prolonged pain, making delays in seeking care critical to address.[5] Viscero-viscero and viscero-somatic cross-sensitization can also be present, where a repeated nociceptive stimulus from one organ leads to a secondary pain sensation in another organ innervated by the same dorsal root ganglion, or referred to abdominopelvic myofascial trigger points, respectively.[6,7]

A diagnostic injection is an injection of a local anesthetic agent to localize the cause of pain.[8] It targets specific pain generators such as muscles, nerves, or joints.[8] For example, positive response to a pudendal nerve block is one of the five essential criteria for diagnosis of pudendal neuralgia due to pudendal nerve entrapment.[9] A positive response to diagnostic injection points toward the cause of pain but is not an indicator for efficacy of therapeutic injections or longer-term relief.[8] A therapeutic injection, on the other hand, may provide long-lasting relief.

Medications used for therapeutic injections include steroids, botulinum toxin, platelet-rich plasma, dextrose, alcohol, and or local anesthetics.[8] Neuromodulation techniques such as spinal cord stimulation (SCS) and dorsal root ganglion (DRG) stimulation involve stimulation of the nervous system by electrical current and have been used successfully to treat visceral, somatic, and neuropathic CPP.[10,11] Table 3.1 provides an overview of interventional techniques used for management of CPP.

Integrating Comprehensive, Multidisciplinary Approaches

The treatment of a multifactorial condition such as CPP should ideally involve multidisciplinary, long-term care from providers in primary care, gynecology, pain management, gastroenterology, urology, physiotherapy, and mental health.[17]

Before a treatment regimen is initiated, patients should receive education on nongynecologic contributors to CPP, including neurological and psychological aspects, because enhancing patients' awareness of their perception of pain in conjunction with adjuvant therapies such as cognitive behavioral therapy (CBT) can empower patient self-care and significantly improve outcomes.[3,5,16] Combination mind–body therapies are recommended over single-agent pharmacotherapy or surgery.[16]

Clinical Vignette

73-year-old woman presents with a chief complaint of intractable, chronic bladder and pelvic pain with extreme urinary frequency. The patient presents with a long-standing, debilitating history of pelvic pain primarily localized to the bladder area, with radiation to the vagina and rectum. She reports severe urinary frequency, exceeding 50 voids per day. She describes the pain quality as a combination of intense burning and sharp spasms.

Functional Status

Functional impairment is severe because the patient is unable to sit due to mechanical pressure exacerbating the pain. She utilizes a bed pan while driving to alleviate pressure on the vagina and rectum.

Psychosocial Status

The chronicity and intensity of the pain have led to significant psychological distress. The patient has expressed suicidal ideation ("thoughts of not living anymore") and has proactively requested a radical cystectomy from her urologist to mitigate symptoms.

Diagnostic Impression

The patient's presentation is likely a multifactorial, centralized pain syndrome. The differential diagnosis and contributing components include:

Table 3.1 Interventional treatment options for chronic pelvic pain (CPP)[3-5,8,11–15]

	Intervention	Indications	Complications/Adverse effects
Myofascial	Trigger point injections (local anesthetic, saline, steroids, dry needling)	Myofascial pain, pelvic floor myofascial pain, e.g., transvaginal approach	Risks of vascular or nerve injury, steroid reactions, procedural pain Botox: temporary incontinence
	Botulinum toxin injections	Myofascial pelvic floor dysfunction refractory to Physical therapy	
Joint injections	Sacroiliac (SI) joint injection	Low back, pelvic pain	Procedural pain, medication reaction
	Hip injection	Groin, gluteal and low back pain	
Nerve blocks	Superior hypogastric plexus block (SHPB)	Chronic nonmalignant and cancer-related pelvic pain (descending colon, rectum, internal sex organs, uterus, bladder, urethra, perineum, prostate), e.g., interstitial cystitis, urethral pain, endometriosis	Risk of infection, retroperitoneal hematoma, bowel/bladder/sexual dysfunction, epidural/intrathecal injections
	Ganglion impar block (GIB)	Pain associated with distal pelvic viscera and perineal structures (genitals, rectum, anus, perineum), e.g., coccydynia, refractory pudendal neuralgia	Rectal perforation, epidural injection, sciatic nerve impingement, cauda equina syndrome, risk of infection and bleeding; fluoroscopy-guided trans-sacrococcygeal technique preferred
	Pudendal nerve block	Pain from perineum, external genitalia, internal vagina, or rectum, e.g., pudendal neuralgia	Temporary sciatic nerve numbness, bleeding, infection, nerve injury
	Ilioinguinal/genitofemoral nerve block	Pain in groin radiating to vagina	Bleeding, infection, nerve injury
	Obturator nerve block	Pain in genitals radiating to inner thigh	
	Anterior abdominal cutaneous nerve block	Pain over abdominal skin	
Neuromodulation	Spinal cord stimulation (SCS)	Severe refractory visceral pelvic pain	Superficial skin infection, lead migration, headache from CSF leak; seen in 10% of patients
	Dorsal root ganglion stimulation (DRG)	Chronic visceral pelvic pain (majority of pelvis and perineum) refractory to more conservative therapies	
	Sacral neuromodulation (SNM)	Pelvic pain below S2, e.g., generalized CPP, interstitial cystitis, vulvodynia, pudendal neuralgia, SI joint pain	
	Peripheral neuromodulation (Peripheral nerve stimulation)	Neuropathic pain of peripheral nerve. e.g., Pudendal neuralgia, Ilioinguinal neuralgia	Infection, nerve damage, lead fracture, lead migration, allergic reaction to adhesive patch

- **Central sensitization:** Likely complex, centralized pain processing resulting from long-standing pelvic dysfunction.
- **Neuropathic component:** Suggestive of pudendal neuralgia or related neuropathy given burning radiation to the vagina and rectum.
- **Myofascial component:** Significant pelvic floor muscle dysfunction, likely involving spasm of the levator ani and obturator internus muscles.
- **Visceral component:** Possible underlying interstitial cystitis/bladder pain syndrome (IC/BPS), currently manifested as extreme frequency and spasm.

Goals of Treatment and Multimodal Therapeutic Approach

Due to the complexity of centralized pain, a multimodal, multidisciplinary treatment plan is required to address the functional, physical, and psychological aspects of the patient's suffering. Treatment for this patient requires a high-intensity, patient-centered approach. While interventional techniques (obturator internus injections) have shown promise, the postprocedural flare highlights the fragility of her sensitized nervous system. Concurrent focus on medication optimization, pelvic floor physical therapy, and intensive psychological support is imperative for functional improvement and risk mitigation regarding suicidal ideation. Treatment plan is summarized in Table 3.2.

Table 3.2 Clinical vignette: Goals of treatment and multimodal therapeutic approach in chronic bladder pain

Modality	Intervention strategy	Rationale
Pharmacotherapy	Oral agents: Optimization of gabapentinoids, tricyclic antidepressants (TCAs), or serotonin and norepinephrine reuptake inhibitors (SNRIs). Suppositories: Valium/baclofen pelvic suppositories.	Address central sensitization and neuropathic pain. Target localized pelvic floor myofascial spasm with reduced systemic side effects.
Interventional radiology/Pain	Targeted injections: Levator ani/obturator internus muscle injections (local anesthetic +/ - botulinum toxin). Pudendal nerve blocks.	Alleviate acute pelvic floor spasm. *Note: Patient reported significant relief previously but experienced a paradoxically intense flare for 3 days postprocedure, a known potential response.*
Physical therapy	Pelvic floor physical therapy (PT): Internal and external myofascial release, biofeedback.	Address myofascial component, improve tissue mobility, and retrain muscles to reduce bracing.
Psychological care	Therapeutic support: Cognitive behavioral therapy (CBT), referral to pain psychology, and support group participation.	Address suicidal ideation, bracing behavior, and improve coping mechanisms for chronic pain.
Behavioral/Lifestyle	Relaxation and functional rehabilitation: Introduction of sewing (as mentioned by patient) and other pacing techniques.	Promote parasympathetic activation and gradual re-engagement with functional activities (e.g., sitting retraining).

References

1. Nagpal AS, Moody EL. Interventional management for pelvic pain. Phys Med Rehabil Clin N Am. 2017;28(3):621–646.
2. Ayorinde AA, Macfarlane GJ, Saraswat L, Bhattacharya S. Chronic pelvic pain in women: An epidemiological perspective. Womens Health (Lond Engl). 2015;11(6):851–864.
3. American College of Obstetricians and Gynecologists. Chronic pelvic pain. Obstet Gynecol. 2020;135(3):e98–e109.
4. Smith SE, Eckert JM. Interventional pain management and female pelvic pain: Considerations for diagnosis and treatment. Semin Reprod Med. 2018;36(2):159–163.
5. Dydyk AM, Singh C, Gupta N. Chronic pelvic pain. StatPearls. 2025. Accessed January 2026. https://www.ncbi.nlm.nih.gov/books/NBK554585/
6. Carey ET, McClurg AB. Evaluation and medical management of chronic pelvic pain. Semin Intervent Radiol. 2023;40(4):372–378.
7. Yosef A, Ahmed AG, Al-Hussein T, Abdellah MS, Cua G, Bedaiwy MA. Chronic pelvic pain: Pathogenesis and validated assessment. Middle East Fertility Society Journal. 2016;21(4):205–221.
8. Facing Pelvic Pain. A guide to facing pelvic pain (for men, women & children). https://www.facingpelvicpain.org/about-the-book. Accessed July 27, 2025
9. Labat JJ, Riant T, Robert R, Amarenco G, Lefaucheur JP, Rigaud J. Diagnostic criteria for pudendal neuralgia by pudendal nerve entrapment (Nantes criteria). Neurourol Urodyn. 2008;27(4):306–310.
10. Xiang H, Zhang T, Al-Danakh A, Yang D, Wang L. Neuromodulation in chronic pelvic pain: A narrative review. Pain Ther. 2022;11(3):789–816.
11. Yang CC. Neuromodulation in male chronic pelvic pain syndrome: Rationale and practice. World J Urol. 2013;31(4):767–772.
12. Vorenkamp K, Yi P, Kemp A. Sympathetic blocks for visceral pain. Phys Med Rehabil Clin N Am. 2022;33(2):475–487.
13. Huntzinger J, Selassie M. Interventional pain management in the treatment of chronic pelvic pain. Curr Urol Rep. 2023;24(4):165–171.
14. Torres JE, Nagpal AS, Iya A, McGeary D, Srinivasan M. Interventional treatment options for women with pelvic pain. Curr Phys Med Rehabil Rep. 2020;8(3):229–239.
15. Wie C, Ghanavatian S, Pew S, Kim A, Strand N, Freeman J, et al. Interventional treatment modalities for chronic abdominal and pelvic visceral pain. Curr Pain Headache Rep. 2022;26(9):683–691.
16. Lamvu G, Carrillo J, Ouyang C, Rapkin A. Chronic pelvic pain in women: A review. JAMA. 2021;325(23):2381–2391.

4
Epidemiology and Prevalence of Pain in Women

Catherine Lowe and Ioana Pasca

Prevalence

The past several decades have seen an increase in attention toward the epidemiology of pain syndromes in women. Globally, there is a higher prevalence of pain in women when compared to men.[1,2] According to the Centers for Disease Control (CDC) National Health Interview Survey (NHIS), women in the United States experience chronic pain or pain that often affects the ability to perform daily work and life activities at a significantly higher rate than that experienced by men. An estimated one out of four women in the United States experienced chronic pain in 2023, an increase from the same survey in 2019.[3]

Large-scale population estimates that amalgamate broad sources of data provide insight into the implications of pain syndromes. The Global Burden of Disease Study found that females disproportionately experienced higher disability-adjusted life-year (DALY) rates of low back pain and headache disorders, including migraine, than males.[4] Several chronic pain conditions are experienced at a higher rate by women than men including chronic low back pain,[5] fibromyalgia,[6] chronic tension-type headache,[7] irritable bowel syndrome,[8] temporomandibular disorders,[9] and interstitial cystitis.[10] Additionally, women assigned female at birth may experience pain syndromes unique to their biological sex, including endometriosis, vulvodynia, childbirth, and menstrual pain. Endometriosis, for instance, is estimated to affect 10% of the global female population and is associated with a significantly increased comorbidity including chronic pelvic pain and infertility.[11]

Demographics

Certain demographic factors are associated with pain in both men and women. In the United States, increased age, comorbid depression, lower educational attainment, and housing in less urbanized areas have been shown to be risk factors for pain.[12] According to the aforementioned NHIS survey, the highest percentage of adults reporting chronic pain were American Indian and Alaska native individuals, followed by non-Hispanic White, non-Hispanic other and multiple races, non-Hispanic Black, Hispanic, and Asian respondents. Biopsychosocial factors, such as lower socioeconomic status (SES) and psychological distress, are also significant risk factors for chronic pain.[13] When controlling for SES and other comorbidities in older adults, Black and Hispanic Americans report higher pain intensity than White Americans, with Black individuals also reporting significantly higher levels of pain-related disruption with family–home responsibilities, work, sexual behavior, and daily self-care.[14] Given the likely compounding effects of gender, race, ethnicity, and SES on pain, recognition by healthcare providers of the intersection and co-factors that may encompass a woman's identity and health is essential.

Morbidity

Diagnostic and treatment decisions by a patient's medical team have been implicated in the experience of pain syndromes among women, including delayed treatment and/or under-treatment of pain. Conditions associated with pain, such as fibromyalgia, may present with nonspecific and less traditionally recognized signs and symptoms. Nontraditional symptoms and societal perceptions of women's pain may lead to lack of timely and appropriate diagnosis and care.[15] A recent survey of individuals in the United Kingdom with endometriosis found that the average time from first contact with the healthcare system for their symptoms to formal diagnosis of endometriosis was almost 9 years. In the same survey, almost 80% of respondents reported being told by their clinician that they were exaggerating their symptoms.[16]

Population-based studies shed light on adverse health outcomes associated with specific pain conditions. A Finnish study of women with endometriosis aged 50 and younger found this population was at higher risk of hospital-based diagnoses such as infectious diseases, pain-causing diseases, and respiratory diseases than their counterparts without endometriosis.[11] Additionally, endometriosis and fibromyalgia are associated with psychological distress, including depression and anxiety.[17–19]

Analgesic prescribing practices also differ between men and women. When analyzing electronic medical records of emergency departments, Guzikevits and colleagues found that females presenting with a pain-related complaint received less analgesic treatment when compared to males, a finding consistent across all age groups and pain scores.[20] Another study found that women presenting to the emergency department with chest pain were evaluated later than men and were triaged less acutely than men with the same complaint. Women were additionally less likely to undergo electrocardiography and to be admitted to the hospital for their symptoms.[21]

Negative health consequences associated with pain are not limited to adult women. Dorn et al.[22] found that samples of adolescent females experiencing intense menstrual symptoms reported more depression, anxiety, and smoking than those with less symptoms. Furthermore, early-onset menarche was associated with chronic pain in the neck, abdomen, arms, and widespread pain syndrome later in life.[23] Awareness of this data is essential for healthcare providers because normalization and dismissal of gynecological pain may pose a unique risk factor for females in the development of further adverse health outcomes.

Mortality

Population-based studies linked severe chronic pain with increased risk of 10-year all-cause mortality, independent of sociodemographic factors. A Danish population study found all-cause mortality was increased among women who reported widespread musculoskeletal pain.[24] Another prospective population study of women in Norway found increased mortality risk with widespread pain and accompanying feelings of anxiety and/or fear.[25] Diagnosis of fibromyalgia has been associated with heightened risk of all-cause mortality and significantly higher risk of suicide than in those without fibromyalgia.[26] These findings necessitate the need for further population and subpopulation studies specific to mortality in women to meet the needs of advancing healthcare equity.

Various etiologies contribute to the increased prevalence of pain syndromes and differences in pain perception in women versus men, including a complex interplay among inflammation, genetics, neurologic, and hormonal influences.[27, 28, 29] Given these molecular complexities and demographic differences, the intersection of these various processes remain poorly understood, requiring the development of specific therapeutic strategies that are inclusive for women of all backgrounds.

References

1. Tsang A, Von Korff M, Lee S, et al. Common chronic pain conditions across world regions: Gender and age differences and comorbidity with depression-anxiety disorders. J Pain. 2008;9(10):883–891.
2. Zimmer Z, Fraser K, Grol-Prokopczyk H, Zajacova A. A global study of pain prevalence across 52 countries: Examining the role of country-level contextual factors. Pain. 2022;163(9):1740–1750. doi:10.1097/j.pain.0000000000002557
3. Lucas JW, Sohi I. Chronic pain and high-impact chronic pain in U.S. adults, 2023. Centers for Disease Control and Prevention. November 21, 2024. Accessed July 19, 2025. https://www.cdc.gov/nchs/products/databriefs/db518.htm
4. Patwardhan V, Gil GF, Arrieta A, et al. Differences across the lifespan between females and males in the top 20 causes of disease burden globally: A systematic analysis of the Global Burden of Disease Study 2021. Lancet Public Health. 2024;9(5):e282–e294. doi:10.1016/S2468-2667(24)00053-7
5. Meucci RD, Fassa AG, Faria NM. Prevalence of chronic low back pain: Systematic review. Rev Saude Publica. 2015;49:1. doi:10.1590/S0034-8910.2015049005874
6. Ruschak I, Montesó-Curto P, Rosselló L, et al. Fibromyalgia syndrome pain in men and women: A scoping review. Healthcare (Basel). 2023;11(2):223. doi:10.3390/healthcare11020223
7. Stovner LJ, Hagen K, Linde M, et al. The global prevalence of headache: An update, with analysis of the influences of methodological factors on prevalence estimates. J Headache Pain. 2022;23:34. doi:10.1186/s10194-022-01402-2
8. Lovell RM, Ford AC. Effect of gender on prevalence of irritable bowel syndrome in the community: Systematic review and meta-analysis. Am J Gastroenterol. 2012;107(7):991–1000. doi:10.1038/ajg.2012.131
9. Zieliński G, Pająk-Zielińska B, Ginszt M. A meta-analysis of the global prevalence of temporomandibular disorders. J Clin Med. 2024;13(5):1365. doi:10.3390/jcm13051365
10. Hanno P, Cervigni M, Choo MS, et al. Summary of the 2023 report of the International Consultation on Incontinence Interstitial Cystitis/Bladder Pain Syndrome (IC/BPS) Committee. Continence. 2023;8:101056. doi:10.1016/j.cont.2023.101056

11. Rossi HR, Uimari O, Terho A, et al. Increased overall morbidity in women with endometriosis: A population-based follow-up study until age 50. Fertil Steril. 2023;119(1):89–98. doi:10.1016/j.fertnstert.2022.09.361
12. Lautenbacher S. Experimental approaches in the study of pain in the elderly. Pain Med. 2012;13 Suppl 2:S44–S50. doi:10.1111/j.1526-4637.2012.01326.x
13. Zajacova A, Grol-Prokopczyk H, Zimmer Z. Pain trends among American adults, 2002–2018: Patterns, disparities, and correlates. Demography. 2021;58(2):711–738. doi:10.1215/00703370-8977691
14. Yang Y, Reid MC, Grol-Prokopczyk H, Pillemer K. Racial-ethnic disparities in pain intensity and interference among middle-aged and older U.S. adults. J Gerontol A Biol Sci Med Sci. 2022;77(2):e74–e81. doi:10.1093/gerona/glab207
15. Zhang L, Berkel T, Combs D, et al. Gender biases in estimation of others' pain. J Pain. 2022;22(9):1048–1059. doi:10.1016/j.jpain.2021.11.002
16. Endometriosis UK. "Dismissed, ignored and belittled": The long road to endometriosis diagnosis in the UK. March 2024. Accessed July 19, 2025. https://www.endometriosis-uk.org/sites/default/files/2024-03/Endometriosis%20UK%20diagnosis%20survey%202023%20report%20March.pdf
17. Pope CJ, Sharma V, Sharma S, Mazmanian D. A systematic review of the association between psychiatric disturbances and endometriosis. J Obstet Gynaecol Can. 2015;37(11):1006–1015. doi:10.1016/S1701-2163(16)30050-0
18. Smorgick N, Marsh CA, As-Sanie S, Smith YR, Quint EH. Prevalence of pain syndromes, mood conditions, and asthma in adolescents and young women with endometriosis. J Pediatr Adolesc Gynecol. 2013;26(3):171–175. doi:10.1016/j.jpag.2012.12.004
19. Cetingok S, Seker O, Cetingok H. The relationship between fibromyalgia and depression, anxiety, anxiety sensitivity, fear avoidance beliefs, and quality of life in female patients. Medicine (Baltimore). 2022;101(39):e30868. doi:10.1097/MD.0000000000030868
20. Guzikevits M, Gordon-Hecker T, Rekhtman D, et al. Sex bias in pain management decisions. Proc Natl Acad Sci U S A. 2024;121(33):e2401331121. doi:10.1073/pnas.2401331121
21. Banco D, Chang J, Talmor N, et al. Sex and race differences in the evaluation and treatment of young adults presenting to the emergency department with chest pain. J Am Heart Assoc. 2022;11(10). doi:10.1161/JAHA.121.024199
22. Dorn LD, Negriff S, Huang B, et al. Menstrual symptoms in adolescent girls: Association with smoking, depressive symptoms, and anxiety. J Adolesc Health. 2009;44(3):237–243. doi:10.1016/j.jadohealth.2008.07.018
23. Lund CI, Engdahl B, Rosseland LA, et al. The association between age at menarche and chronic pain outcomes in women: The Tromsø Study, 2007 to 2016. Pain. 2022;163(9):1790–1799. doi:10.1097/j.pain.0000000000002579
24. Holmberg T, Davidsen M, Thygesen LC, et al. Mortality among persons experiencing musculoskeletal pain: A prospective study among Danish men and women. BMC Musculoskelet Disord. 2020;21:666. doi:10.1186/s12891-020-03620-8
25. Nitter AK, Forseth KØ. Mortality rate and causes of death in women with self-reported musculoskeletal pain: Results from a 17-year follow-up study. Scand J Pain. 2013;4(2):86–92. doi:10.1016/j.sjpain.2012.12.002

26. Treister-Goltzman Y, Peleg R. Fibromyalgia and mortality: A systematic review and meta-analysis. RMD Open. 2023;9(3):e003005. doi:10.1136/rmdopen-2023-003005
27. Bartley EJ, Fillingim RB. Sex differences in pain: A brief review of clinical and experimental findings. Br J Anaesth. 2013;111(1):52–58. doi:10.1093/bja/aet127
28. Campbell CM, Edwards RR. Ethnic differences in pain and pain management. Pain Manag. 2012;2(3):219–230. doi:10.2217/pmt.12.7
29. Oakley Browne MA, Posada-Villa J, Seedat S, Watanabe M. Common chronic pain conditions in developed and developing countries: Gender and age differences and comorbidity with depression-anxiety disorders. J Pain. 2008;9(10):883–891.

5
Biological Sex Differences in Pain Experience

Perception, Diagnosis, and Treatment

Rachel Sunico and Don Hoang

Introduction

Chronic pain affects more women than men. Yet women are underrepresented in chronic pain research, and there are limited studies regarding the relationship between chronic pain and sex differences. Decades of research describing sex differences in experimental and clinical pain have not found direct mechanisms to explain this variability. Rather, these differences arise from complex interactions among biological, psychological, cultural, and social factors, and further studies are required to understand how these differences contribute to sex disparities in pain management.[1]

Sex Differences in Pain Perception

Experimental Pain Studies

Women show greater pain perception in several experimental settings.[1] Overall, studies regarding sex differences in pain sensitivity vary in their methodology and thus have varied findings.[2] Response to pressure pain shows the largest sex difference, with lower female pain threshold and tolerance. Similarly, the electric pain threshold is also lower in females. Meanwhile, no significant differences are seen with ischemic pain tolerance, threshold, or perceived intensity. Inconsistent results regarding heat and cold pain were also seen across studies, showing either lower pain thresholds or no difference in females. Mice studies have shown increased mechanical allodynia and cold sensitivity in HIV-induced neuropathic pain and allodynia in chemotherapy-induced peripheral neuropathy.[1]

Pain modulation also has key sex differences: temporal summation of pain, a key factor in the wind-up phenomenon in chronic pain pathophysiology, is more pronounced in females.[1,3] On the other hand, there are no sex differences in spatial summation of pain.[1] Mouse models also show sex differences in analgesic medication responses: male and female mice respond differently to sumatriptan in mechanical hyperalgesia, selective serotonin reuptake inhibitors (SSRIs) only produce analgesia in females, and calcium channel inhibitors only produce anti-nociceptive effects in females.[4] Animal studies have also shown stronger opioid analgesic effects in males.[4] However, overall studies regarding sex differences in opioid and nonopioid analgesic responses have been inconsistent, requiring further investigation.[1]

Clinical Pain Conditions

Clinical sex differences exist in several contexts, most discussed is disease prevalence. Approximately 50% of chronic pain conditions are more prevalent in women, while only 20% are more prevalent in men.[5] Females generally experience a higher prevalence of neuropathic pain, headache, osteoarthritis-related knee and hip pain, abdominal pain of unknown etiology, temporomandibular joint (TMJ) pain, and oral pain.[1,4,6] Similarly, there is a higher prevalence of back pain in females, although this difference diminishes with age. Clinically, female patients exhibit higher pain perception and lower pain thresholds.[4,6] They have increased sensitivity to noxious stimuli and lower pain tolerance.[4] This is also seen with higher levels of acute postoperative and postprocedural pain in females. There are no sex differences seen with cancer pain intensity or pain-related disability.[1] While chronic pain is generally more prevalent and intense in females, the prevalence of various pain disorders can also differ depending on age. Sex differences typically appear between 12 and 14 years of age. For example, migraines are more common in males prior to puberty but rapidly increase in prevalence in females during adolescence.[1]

Factors Influencing Pain Perception

Biological Mechanisms

Gonadal hormones likely explain these biological differences in pain perception; however, this relationship is rather complex. Studies regarding the role of estradiol on pain perception in females have shown varied results. Testosterone, on the other hand, plays a consistent role in anti-nociception in males.[6] It is more likely that it is the *fluctuation* of estrogen levels that leads to increased pain in females, as noted by studies on female pain during conditions in which there are changes in hormone levels such as the menstrual cycle, menopause, or hormone therapy.

Menstrual cycle phases have been suggested to be associated with differences in pain threshold (see Figure 5.1).[6] Fibromyalgia is associated with the luteal phase.[2] Heat pain and pressure pain thresholds are decreased in the ovulatory phase. Hyperalgesia and lower pain thresholds occur in the middle of the menstrual cycle, when estradiol levels drop.[6] Decreased estrogen levels during menopause also come with decreased prevalence of certain painful conditions such as headaches.[2] Hormone supplements have also been shown to have varying effects on presence of pain, and one study showed lower pain ratings in women on oral contraceptive therapy compared to men.[1,6] Nongonadal hormone neurotransmitters, such as dopamine, serotonin, and N-methyl-D-aspartate (NMDA), that play key roles in pain modulation, pain processing, and pain perception have been shown to have varying activities depending on sex.[1] The exact mechanism between hormones and pain is likely complex and consists of both direct effects on tissue targets as well as indirect downstream effects that are difficult to measure.[1,4]

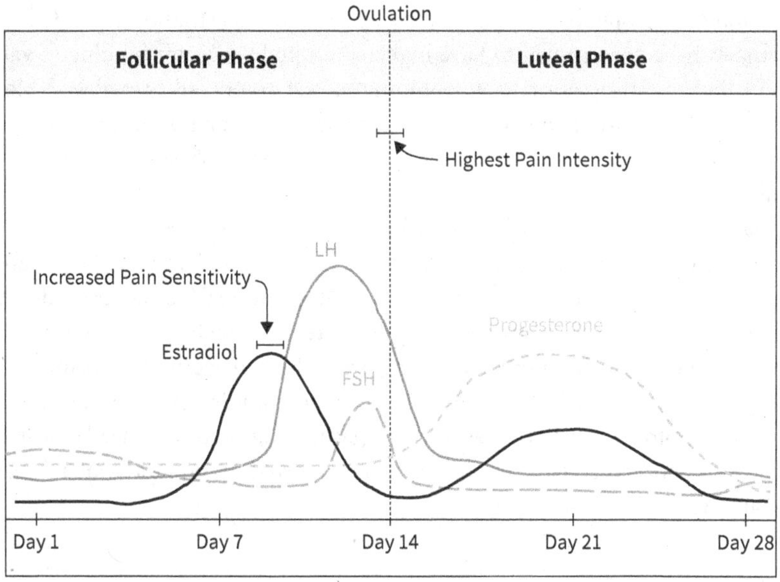

Figure 5.1 Female sex hormone level trends during the menstrual cycle.
Reproduced from Athnaiel O, Cantillo S, Paredes S, Knezevic NN. The role of sex hormones in pain-related conditions. Int J Mol Sci. 2023;24(3):1866.

Psychosocial and Cultural Factors

Gender roles may contribute to these differences, specifically the masculine gender norm of increased pain tolerance as opposed to feminine norm of accepting pain as a normal part of life.[1] Endorsed masculinity is associated with a higher pain threshold and tolerance and lower pain ratings. A study found that women were more sensitive to pain, less enduring of pain, and more willing to report pain compared to men, but these sex differences in pain threshold were no longer significant when controlling for willingness to report pain.[3] There are also sex differences in cognitive performance in the presence of pain. Males experiencing pain showed longer response times, enhanced interoceptive accuracy, reduced attention to external social events, and slower information processing speed.[7]

Mood and affective disorders are also contributing factors. While anxiety and depression prevalence are higher in females, the relationship between the pain and anxiety is stronger in males.[1,3,4] Pain coping processes also differ between sexes. Women use more pain coping strategies, such as behavioral activities, positive self-statements, social and emotional support, and problem-focused coping.[3] However, women tend to have higher levels of catastrophizing, which may mediate sex differences in pain-related outcomes, clinical pain, and experimental pain.[3] Women also responded more to focusing on the affective components of pain, while men focused on the sensory components of pain.[2]

Treatment Considerations

There are known sex differences in opioid receptor activity in various regions of the central nervous system. In the spinal cord, there are differences in kappa-opioid receptor density, and mu- and kappa-opioid receptor activity modulation is estradiol-dependent.[1,4] In the brain, females have been shown to have higher mu-opioid receptor binding in various regions, and higher mu-opioid receptor binding at rest compared to males.[3,4] Males have higher endogenous mu-opioid release in the amygdala, a region responsible for modulating the sensory and affective component of pain, whereas women showed suppression of tonic endogenous opioid release.[2,4]

A key factor to take into consideration when inspecting sex differences in pain diagnosis and treatment is the presence of gender and sex bias. Women are less likely than men to receive invasive and noninvasive diagnostic and interventional cardiac procedures. While women consume less opioids postoperatively, they are more likely to be prescribed sedatives as opposed to men, who are more likely to be prescribed analgesics for postoperative pain after cardiac surgery.[1,2] Women tend to experience more minimization or dismissal of their chronic pain symptoms, also known as "medical gaslighting," which can lead to worse mental health outcomes and potentially negative effects on morbidity and mortality if disease management and treatment are delayed.[8]

Conclusion

Research has found sex differences in pain perception in both the experimental and clinical setting. Sexually dimorphic responses to pain can be explained by a complex interplay among biological, psychological, and societal factors. More studies are necessary to clarify how these differences affect pain management outcomes between males and females.

References

1. Fillingim RB, King CD, Ribeiro-Dasilva MC, Rahim-Williams B, Riley JL 3rd. Sex, gender, and pain: A review of recent clinical and experimental findings. J Pain. 2009;10(5):447–485. doi:10.1016/j.jpain.2008.12.001
2. Pieretti S, Di Giannuario A, Di Giovannandrea R, et al. Gender differences in pain and its relief. Ann Ist Super Sanita. 2016;52(2):184–189. doi:10.4415/ANN_16_02_09
3. Meints SM, Edwards, RR. Evaluating psychosocial contributions to chronic pain outcomes. Prog Neuropsychopharmacol Biol Psychiatry. 2018;87(Pt B):168–182. doi:10.1016/j.pnpbp.2018.01.017
4. Presto P, Mazzitelli M, Junell R, Griffin Z, Neugebauer V. Sex differences in pain along the neuraxis. Neuropharmacology. 2022;210:109030. doi:10.1016/j.neuropharm.2022.109030
5. Palacios-Cena D, Albaladejo-Vicente R, Hernandez-Barrera V, et al. Female gender is associated with a higher prevalence of chronic neck pain, chronic low back pain, and migraine: Results of the Spanish national health survey, 2017. Pain Med. 2021;22(2):382–395. doi:10.1093/pm/pnaa368

6. Athnaiel O, Cantillo S, Paredes S, Knezevic NN. The role of sex hormones in pain-related conditions. Int J Mol Sci. 2023;24(3):1866. doi:10.3390/ijms24031866
7. González-Roldán AM, Bustan S, Kamping S, Flor H, Anton F. Pain and related suffering reduce attention toward others. Pain Pract. 2023;23(8):873–885. doi:10.1111/papr.13260
8. The Lancet Rheumatology. Time to listen to women about their pain. Lancet Rheumatol. 2024;6(6):e329. doi:10.1016/S2665–9913(24)00126–7

6

Diagnoses, Pathophysiology, and Interventional Pain Treatment in Women

Loren Shamalov, Yehuda Masturov, and Gary Schwartz

Introduction

Chronic pain is defined as debilitating pain lasting longer than 3 months that has a profound impact on daily functioning.[1] A 2021 survey reported that 20.9% of US adults experienced chronic pain,[1] although studies report prevalence from 11% to 40% depending on population and definition criteria.[2,3] Taking into account the higher rates of acute and chronic pain conditions in women,[2,4] it is imperative that pain management physicians are cognizant of women's pain. In this chapter, an overview of the available interventional strategies in women's pain management is provided.

Background

The etiologies of female acute and chronic pain are widespread and multifactorial. Chronic pelvic pain afflicts roughly 26% of women,[5–7] similar to the prevalence of migraines and back pain.[6] Labor pains remain a consistent, common cause of intense pain experienced by women.[8] Postmastectomy pain syndrome, defined as a chronic, neuropathic pain condition that develops soon after mastectomy/lumpectomy, affects an estimated 28.2% of women who undergo surgical management for breast cancer.[9] Other etiologies of female pain are less defined, as in fibromyalgia, which results in potentially debilitating symptoms with complex etiologies.[10]

Epidemiology and Risk Factors

The strongest clinical risk factor associated with chronic pain is presence of acute or chronic pain in different sites on the body.[2] Female sex is an independent risk factor across most pain conditions, with women showing higher prevalence rates for fibromyalgia, migraine, and chronic pelvic pain. Additional established risk factors include increased age, comorbid physical and mental conditions, low socioeconomic status, and smoking.[3]

Pathophysiology

Pain mechanisms vary depending on the etiology. Nociceptive pain involves direct tissue damage and inflammation, while neuropathic pain results from nerve injury or dysfunction.

Labor pain is characterized by visceral pain transmitted through the posterior nerve root ganglia at T10 through L1 and somatic pain transmitted through the pudendal nerve (S2–S4).[11] Pelvic pain is primarily neuropathic with invasion of the obturator, pudendal, ilioinguinal, iliohypogastric, genitofemoral, or lateral femoral cutaneous nerves.[12] However, due to viscero-viscero cross-sensitization, in which activity in one organ hypersensitizes another organ,[13] it may be difficult to distinguish between visceral and somatic sources of pain.[5]

The etiology of chest wall pain in the setting of postmastectomy pain syndrome is multifactorial. One possible cause is muscle spasticity due to mastectomy, radiation, or reconstruction.[14,15] In the setting of chest wall neuropathic pain, a multitude of causes may be considered. The intercostobrachial nerve provides sensation to the axilla, lateral chest wall, and medial upper arm.[16] The anterolateral chest wall is supplied by the lateral cutaneous branches of the thoracic intercostal nerves of T2–T9, the long thoracic nerve, and the thoracodorsal nerve and is a target of therapy.[17] Back pain is commonly mediated by nociceptors and is due to a variety of structural causes ranging from herniated intervertebral discs to ligamentous strains.[18]

Diagnosis and Assessment

Initial evaluation warrants obtaining a comprehensive history. Patient work-up should include, but is not limited to, onset, progression, location, frequency, and severity of the pain.[5,7] Review of past medical history should include medical conditions, past surgeries, and any other associated symptoms.[5] Incorporation of the biopsychosocial model into patient history is paramount to obtaining the full scope of the patient's experience[7]: pain management physicians should be mindful to inquire about psychological history, social history, current or past substance use, and mental health.[7,18]

The next step in evaluation is a focused physical exam to identify the primary sources of pain. The physician should first obtain a general assessment of the patient, including their mood, affect, current pain levels, mobility, and gait.[5] Patients presenting with pelvic pain should subsequently receive an abdominal examination. Initial visualization of the abdomen should be performed, followed by testing for any pain trigger points with a cotton swab.[5,7] External visual and neurosensory examination should be performed on the vulva and perineum, with follow-up single-digit vaginal exam to evaluate for localized causes of pelvic tenderness.[5] The physical exam for back pain typically involves a visual inspection followed by a variety of provocative maneuvers, such as the straight leg raising test for lumbar disk herniation, to narrow the back pain differential.[19]

Diagnostic imaging studies have limited utility in the evaluation of pelvic pain and are largely specific to the presenting symptoms.[5,7] A pregnancy test should be obtained in all reproductive-aged females, with subsequent imaging obtained as needed. Back pain can be further worked up with x-rays or MRI, with limited utility of laboratory testing.[19]

Treatment Options

Chronic Pelvic Pain Interventions

Interventional procedures for chronic pelvic pain have not been widely accepted due to a paucity of studies substantiating their use. Botulinum toxin injections may be useful for decreasing myofascial pain secondary to muscle hyperspasticity by blocking presynaptic acetylcholine release.[15,20–22] A superior hypogastric nerve block is an established approach for intractable pelvic pain,[23,24] classically performed under a fluoroscopy-guided, two-needle technique with injection of typical neurolytic agents.[23] Ultrasound and CT scan-guided approaches have also been described in the literature.[25,26] Ganglion impar blocks are scarcely utilized to treat vulvar, rectal, and anal pain due to high failure rates.[24] Transcutaneous nerve stimulation is an emerging treatment for chronic pelvic pain,[27] with sacral neuromodulation being described as an effective treatment for chronic pelvic pain.[6] Myofascial trigger point injections are also effective in treating chronic pelvic pain secondary to endometriosis.[12]

Abdominal Pain Interventions

Celiac plexus block (CPB) is a well-described technique that is effective in the management of abdominal pain secondary to malignancy.[24,28] Typically conducted under fluoroscopic guidance,[29] it may also be performed under CT or ultrasound guidance with injection of preferred neurolytic or anesthetic agent.[24,28] Splanchnic nerve block is considered in abdominal pain refractory to CPB or with distorted celiac plexus anatomy.[30]

Fibromyalgia Interventions

Fibromyalgia is a functional somatic disorder that is typically managed with conservative, noninvasive pharmacologic and nonpharmacologic interventions. However, patients with limited response to pharmacotherapy and psychotherapy have shown significant improvements with electrical neuromodulation.[31]

Back Pain Interventions

Interventional therapies are considered step-up treatment from conservative therapy for chronic lower back pain. Epidural steroid injections remain a mainstay of therapy[32,33] due to improved pain outcomes. However, intraarticular steroid injections are not effective in alleviating back pain symptoms.[34] Thoracic medial branch blocks are useful for the diagnosis and management of thoracic pain.[35] Biological therapies, basivertebral nerve ablation, and multifidus muscle stimulation are also effective interventions for chronic back pain.[34]

Labor Pain Interventions

Neuraxial regional anesthesia is utilized by a majority of women during labor.[8,36] It provides adequate pain control and may be delivered via an epidural, spinal, combined spinal-epidural, and dural-puncture epidural technique with or without ultrasound assistance.[8,36] Of the available neuraxial anesthetic techniques, lumbar epidural insertion is considered the gold standard and should be pursued first in the management of labor pain. Patients may control their anesthetic dose via patient-controlled analgesia, thus allowing for adequate management of breakthrough pain.[8]

Chest Wall Pain Interventions

For postmastectomy pain syndrome and generalized chest wall pain, botulinum toxin injections have shown to improve patient symptoms by decreasing muscle spasticity.[15] Intercostobrachial nerve blocks are used to relieve medial upper arm, axilla, and lateral chest wall pain.[16] Serratus plane blocks are an effective treatment for anterolateral chest wall pain.[17] Additional interventions include myofascial trigger point injections[37] and nerve blocks targeting the pectoralis major, pectoralis minor, and erector spinae muscles.[14,38,39]

Patient-Centered Approaches

Patients experiencing chronic pain are neglected by clinicians[40] and preemptively dismissed. Hence, physicians should encourage patients to recount their stories and discuss their functional limitations. This establishes a therapeutic alliance that defines goals of care and sets realistic goals for pain improvement, resulting in improved patient outcomes.

Clinical Pearls

- History-taking is imperative to evaluation of female pain.
- Evaluating the etiology of a patient's pain is key to appropriate intervention selection.
- Interventional pain management techniques are generally considered when the patient is unresponsive to conservative therapy.

Conclusion

Managing pain in women requires understanding of sex-specific presentations and a comprehensive assessment to guide appropriate, evidence-based intervention selection. Intervention success requires knowledge of available techniques, establishment of therapeutic alliance, and patient-centered goals of care. Given the complexity of women's pain conditions, physicians must couple thorough patient evaluations with available interventional therapies to optimize patient outcomes.

References

1. Rikard SM, Strahan AE, Schmit KM, Guy GP, Jr. Chronic pain among adults – United States, 2019–2021. MMWR Morb Mortal Wkly Rep. 2023;72(15):379–385. doi:10.15585/mmwr.mm7215a1

2. Mills SEE, Nicolson KP, Smith BH. Chronic pain: A review of its epidemiology and associated factors in population-based studies. Br J Anaesth. 2019;123(2):e273–e283. doi:10.1016/j.bja.2019.03.023
3. Fayaz A, Croft P, Langford RM, Donaldson LJ, Jones GT. Prevalence of chronic pain in the UK: A systematic review and meta-analysis of population studies. BMJ Open. 2016;6(6):e010364. doi:10.1136/bmjopen-2015-010364
4. Osborne NR, Davis KD. Sex and gender differences in pain. Int Rev Neurobiol. 2022;164:277–307. doi:10.1016/bs.irn.2022.06.013
5. Lamvu G, Carrillo J, Ouyang C, Rapkin A. Chronic pelvic pain in women: A review. JAMA. 2021;325(23):2381–2391. doi:10.1001/jama.2021.2631
6. Greig J, Mak Q, Furrer MA, Sahai A, Raison N. Sacral neuromodulation in the management of chronic pelvic pain: A systematic review and meta-analysis. Neurourol Urodyn. 2023;42(4):822–836. doi:10.1002/nau.25167
7. Meisenheimer ES, Carnevale AM. Chronic pelvic pain in women: Evaluation and treatment. Am Fam Physician. 2025;111(3):218–229.
8. Nanji JA, Carvalho B. Pain management during labor and vaginal birth. Best Pract Res Clin Obstet Gynaecol. 2020;67:100–112. doi:10.1016/j.bpobgyn.2020.03.002
9. Capuco A, Urits I, Orhurhu V, et al. A comprehensive review of the diagnosis, treatment, and management of postmastectomy pain syndrome. Curr Pain Headache Rep. 2020;24(8):41. doi:10.1007/s11916-020-00876-6
10. Sarzi-Puttini P, Giorgi V, Marotto D, Atzeni F. Fibromyalgia: An update on clinical characteristics, aetiopathogenesis and treatment. Nat Rev Rheumatol. 2020;16(11):645–660. doi:10.1038/s41584-020-00506-w
11. Njogu A, Qin S, Chen Y, Hu L, Luo Y. The effects of transcutaneous electrical nerve stimulation during the first stage of labor: A randomized controlled trial. BMC Pregnancy Childbirth. 2021;21(1):164. doi:10.1186/s12884-021-03625-8
12. Plavnik K, Tenaglia A, Hill C, Ahmed T, Shrikhande A. A Novel, Non-opioid treatment for chronic pelvic pain in women with previously treated endometriosis utilizing pelvic-floor musculature trigger-point injections and peripheral nerve hydrodissection. PMR. 2020;12(7):655–662. doi:10.1002/pmrj.12258
13. Schwartz ES, Gebhart GF. Visceral pain. Curr Top Behav Neurosci. 2014;20:171–197. doi:10.1007/7854_2014_315
14. Murugappan A, Khanna A. Interventional treatment options for post-mastectomy pain. Curr Oncol Rep. 2023;25(10):1175–1179. doi:10.1007/s11912-023-01435-z
15. Zehm A, Kamdar M. Palliative uses of botulinum neurotoxin #324. J Palliat Med. 2017;20(3):300–302. doi:10.1089/jpm.2016.0498
16. Wijayasinghe N, Duriaud HM, Kehlet H, Andersen KG. Ultrasound guided intercostobrachial nerve blockade in patients with persistent pain after breast cancer surgery: A pilot study. Pain Physician. 2016;19(2):E309–18.
17. Zocca JA, Chen GH, Puttanniah VG, Hung JC, Gulati A. Ultrasound-guided serratus plane block for treatment of postmastectomy pain syndromes in breast cancer patients: A case series. Pain Pract. 2017;17(1):141–146. doi:10.1111/papr.12482
18. Allegri M, Montella S, Salici F, et al. Mechanisms of low back pain: A guide for diagnosis and therapy. F1000Res. 2016. doi:10.12688/f1000research.8105.2
19. Casiano, V. E., Sarwan, G., Margetis, K., & Singh, C. (2026). Back pain. *StatPearls*. https://www.ncbi.nlm.nih.gov/books/NBK538173/

20. Knapman BL, Li FG, Deans R, Nesbitt-Hawes E, Maheux-Lacroix S, Abbott J. Botulinum toxin for the management of pelvic floor tension myalgia and persistent pelvic pain: A systematic review and meta-analysis. Obstet Gynecol. 2024;143(1):e7–e17. doi:10.1097/aog.0000000000005388
21. Meister MR, Brubaker A, Sutcliffe S, Lowder JL. Effectiveness of botulinum toxin for treatment of symptomatic pelvic floor myofascial pain in women: A systematic review and Meta-analysis. Female Pelvic Med Reconstr Surg. 2021;27(1):e152–e160. doi:10.1097/spv.0000000000000870
22. Spruijt MA, Klerkx WM, Kelder JC, Kluivers KB, Kerkhof MH. The efficacy of botulinum toxin a injections in pelvic floor muscles in chronic pelvic pain patients: A systematic review and meta-analysis. Int Urogynecol J. 2022;33(11):2951–2961. doi:10.1007/s00192-022-05115-7
23. Urits I, Schwartz R, Herman J, et al. A comprehensive update of the superior hypogastric block for the management of chronic pelvic pain. Curr Pain Headache Rep. 2021;3:13. doi:10.1007/s11916-020-00933-0
24. Wie C, Ghanavatian S, Pew S, et al. Interventional treatment modalities for chronic abdominal and pelvic visceral pain. Curr Pain Headache Rep. 2022;26(9):683–691. doi:10.1007/s11916-022-01072-4
25. Gofeld M, Shankar H, Benzon H. Fluoroscopy and ultrasound-guided sympathetic blocks. In: Benzon H, Raja SN, Fishman SM, Liu SS, Cohen SP, eds. *Essentials of Pain Medicine*. Elsevier: 2018;789–804. doi:10.1016/B978-0-323-40196-8.00084-X
26. Yang X, You J, Tao S, Zheng X, Xie K, Huang B. Computed tomography-guided superior hypogastric plexus block for secondary dysmenorrhea in perimenopausal women. Med Sci Monit. 2018;24:5132–5138. doi:10.12659/msm.906970
27. Cottrell AM, Schneider MP, Goonewardene S, et al. Benefits and harms of electrical neuromodulation for chronic pelvic pain: A systematic review. Eur Urol Focus. 2020;6(3):559–571. doi:10.1016/j.euf.2019.09.011
28. Urits I, Jones MR, Orhurhu V, et al. A comprehensive review of the celiac plexus block for the management of chronic abdominal pain. Curr Pain Headache Rep. 2020;24(8):42. doi:10.1007/s11916-020-00878-4
29. An JW, Choi EK, Park CH, Choi JB, Ko DK, Lee YW. Alternative method of retrocrural approach during celiac plexus block using a bent tip needle. Korean J Pain. 2015;28(2):109–115. doi:10.3344/kjp.2015.28.2.109
30. Ahmed A, Arora D. Fluoroscopy-guided neurolytic splanchnic nerve block for intractable pain from upper abdominal malignancies in patients with distorted celiac axis anatomy: An effective alternative to celiac plexus neurolysis – A retrospective study. Indian J Palliat Care. 2017;23(3):274–281. doi:10.4103/ijpc.Ijpc_28_17
31. Cheng Y-C, Hsiao C-Y, Su M-I, Chiu C-C, Huang Y-C, Huang W-L. Treating fibromyalgia with electrical neuromodulation: A systematic review and meta-analysis. Clin Neurophysiol. 2023;148:17–28. doi:10.1016/j.clinph.2023.01.011
32. Kennedy DJ, Zheng PZ, Smuck M, McCormick ZL, Huynh L, Schneider BJ. A minimum of 5-year follow-up after lumbar transforaminal epidural steroid injections in patients with lumbar radicular pain due to intervertebral disc herniation. Spine J. 2018;18(1):29–35. doi:10.1016/j.spinee.2017.08.264
33. Manchikanti L, Knezevic NN, Boswell MV, Kaye AD, Hirsch JA. Epidural injections for lumbar radiculopathy and spinal stenosis: A comparative systematic review and meta-analysis. Pain Physician. 2016;19(3):E365–410.

34. Mekhail N, Eldabe S, Templeton E, Costandi S, Rosenquist R. Pain management interventions for the treatment of chronic low back pain: A systematic review and meta-analysis. Clin J Pain. 2023;39(7):349–364. doi:10.1097/ajp.0000000000001116
35. Manchikanti L, Knezevic E, Knezevic NN, et al. The effectiveness of medial branch blocks and radiofrequency neurotomy in managing chronic thoracic pain: A systematic review and meta-analysis. Pain Physician. 2023;26(5):413–435.
36. Smith A, Laflamme E, Komanecky C. Pain management in labor. Am Fam Physician. 2021;103(6):355–364.
37. Khoury AL, Keane H, Varghese F, et al. Trigger point injection for post-mastectomy pain: A simple intervention with high rate of long-term relief. NPJ Breast Cancer. 2021;7(1):123. doi:10.1038/s41523-021-00321-w
38. Tulgar S, Ahiskalioglu A, De Cassai A, Gurkan Y. Efficacy of bilateral erector spinae plane block in the management of pain: Current insights. J Pain Res. 2019;12:2597–2613. doi:10.2147/jpr.S182128
39. Ueshima H, Otake H, Hara E, Blanco R. How to use pectoral nerve blocks effectively: An evidence-based update. Asian J Anesthesiol. 2019;57(2):28–36. doi:10.6859/aja.201906_57(2).0002
40. Till SR, Nakamura R, Schrepf A, As-Sanie S. Approach to diagnosis and management of chronic pelvic pain in women: Incorporating chronic overlapping pain conditions in assessment and management. Obstet Gynecol Clin North Am. 2022;49(2):219–239. doi:10.1016/j.ogc.2022.02.006

PART II

HEADACHE AND CRANIOFACIAL PAIN

7

Anatomical Considerations of the Female Head and Neck in Pain Syndromes

Niranjana Bienkowska and Anita Gupta

Introduction

A solid understanding of head and neck anatomy is a prerequisite for healthcare professionals who conduct patient examinations, establish diagnoses, and treat a variety of pain conditions involving the head and neck region. Sex-related anatomical, physiological, and biomechanical differences have been shown to influence the presentation, severity, and response to treatment of head and neck disorders. Acknowledging these differences is essential for precise diagnosis and effective management of pain syndromes and conditions that disproportionately affect women.[1]

Skull

The skull consists of 22 bones and provides a rigid, protective shell for the brain and associated structures, including the cerebrum, cerebellum, brainstem, and orbits.[2] Structurally and functionally, the skull is divided into two primary components: the calvaria and the skull base.[2]

Calvaria

The upper portion of the skull, known as the calvaria, protects the cerebral cortex and cerebellum. It is composed of the occipital bone along with other cranial bones that together form a protective dome over the brain.[2]

Skull Base and Neurovascular Foramina

The skull base forms the floor of the cranial cavity and provides critical structural support for the brain. It contains multiple neurovascular foramina—openings and canals that allow cranial nerves and blood vessels to pass between the cranial cavity and the rest of the body. The carotid and vertebral arteries are the most significant contributors to cerebral blood flow and volume and supply the brain's circulatory system.[3] Due to its proximity to these major vessels and neural structures, the skull base is of clinical relevance in vascular and pain-related disorders.[3]

Cranial Nerves and Musculature

The facial and scalp muscles are striated muscles that are largely under voluntary control. These muscles receive motor innervation from several cranial nerves, including the oculomotor (CN III), trigeminal (CN V), facial (CN VII), glossopharyngeal (CN IX), vagus (CN X), spinal accessory (CN XI), and hypoglossal (CN XII) nerves.[4] Dysfunction or abnormal stimulation of these nerves may result in facial pain, headache syndromes, and other neuromuscular disorders.

The fontanelles and cranial sutures are membranous structures composed of softer connective tissue that join the bones of the skull. These structures allow for growth and structural flexibility during development.[2]

Anatomy of the Neck

The neck is an anatomically and functionally complex region that serves as a critical conduit for neurovascular structures as well as the respiratory and digestive tracts. Its organization and topography are essential for understanding both normal physiological function and pathological processes.[5]

Cervical Triangles

For anatomical and clinical purposes, the neck is divided into anterior and posterior cervical triangles. The anterior neck is further subdivided into four clinically significant triangles: the submental, submandibular, carotid, and muscular triangles. The posterior neck contains two important subtriangles: the occipital triangle and the subclavian triangle.[5] These subdivisions help identify anatomical landmarks and assist clinicians in the evaluation of neck pathology.

Fascial Layers

The neck is enveloped by layers of fascia, classified as superficial and deep cervical.[6] These fascial planes compartmentalize anatomical structures, provide structural support, and influence the direction and spread of infection, inflammation, and pain.[6]

Sex Differences in Head and Neck Anatomy

Sex differences are evident throughout head and neck anatomy. In general, women have smaller head, facial, and neck dimensions compared with men.[7] Women also exhibit a

Table 7.1 Sex-based differences in head and neck pain: Anatomical and neurobiological factors in women

Category	Characteristic (Female) Smaller cervical vertebrae	Characteristic (Male) Larger cervical vertebrae
Skull/Cervical spine	Less muscle mass	Larger skull size
Musculature	Lower neck strength Smaller cross-sectional neck area	Greater neck strength Larger neck strength
Larynx	Less prominent thyroid cartilage ("Adam's Apple")	More prominent thyroid cartilage ("Adam's Apple")
Brain volume/Neurons	8–15% smaller total brain volume Fewer neurons	Larger total brain volume; more neurons
Cortical thickness	Thinner global cortical thickness	Thicker global cortical thickness

smaller cross-sectional neck area, smaller cervical vertebrae, reduced neck muscle area, and decreased neck muscle mass and strength.[8] These biomechanical differences may contribute to specific injury patterns and pain syndromes involving the cervical region (Table 7.1).

Additionally, the female larynx is typically less prominent, resulting in a less visible or absent "Adam's apple." This anatomical difference may influence airway assessment and surgical considerations.[9]

Neuroanatomical Sex Differences

Sex differences in neuroanatomy have been described, with males demonstrating approximately 8–15% greater total brain volume, larger intracranial volume, a greater number of neurons, and increased global cortical thickness compared with females.[10] These differences may contribute to sex-specific patterns of neurological disease and variations in pain processing.

Hormonal Influences on Anatomy and Pain

Sex differences in head and neck anatomy and physiology are further modified by female reproductive hormones, particularly estrogen and progesterone. These hormones play important roles in neurological development, synaptic plasticity, and pain modulation.[11] Their effects on the central nervous system are thought to contribute to the increased prevalence of depression, anxiety, and chronic pain conditions observed in females.[12] Chronic conditions such as depression and anxiety frequently coexist with head and neck pain, further complicating clinical presentation and management.[13]

Clinical Implications

An understanding of female-specific anatomical and physiological differences of the head and neck, including neuroanatomical and hormonal influences, is essential for clinicians (Table 7.2). This knowledge underpins accurate physical examination, diagnosis, and management of women with head and neck pain. By incorporating sex-specific considerations into clinical practice, greater precision and effectiveness in the treatment of pain conditions affecting women can be achieved.[1]

Table 7.2 Common head and neck pain conditions

Condition	Pain characteristics	Common causes/ Triggers	Relevant anatomical structures
Tension-type headache	Dull, pressure-like, bilateral pain	Stress, muscle tension, poor posture	Scalp muscles, cervical muscles, occipital region
Migraine	Throbbing, pulsating, unilateral ± aura	Hormonal changes, light/noise sensitivity, triggers	Trigeminovascular system, cerebral cortex
Cluster headache	Severe, unilateral, around the eye, episodic	Circadian rhythm dysfunction, alcohol	Hypothalamus, trigeminal nerve, autonomic system
Temporomandibular joint disorder (TMJ/ TMD)	Jaw or facial pain, clicking, limited jaw movement	Bruxism, jaw misalignment, arthritis	TMJ, masseter muscle, trigeminal nerve
Cervicogenic headache	Pain radiating from neck to head, often unilateral	Neck injury, cervical spine arthritis	C2–C3 nerves, upper cervical spine, neck muscles
Occipital neuralgia	Sharp, shooting pain at back of head/neck	Nerve compression, trauma	Greater/lesser occipital nerves
Trigeminal neuralgia	Sudden, electric-shock-like facial pain	Vascular compression, multiple sclerosis	Trigeminal nerve (CN V)
Glossopharyngeal neuralgia	Sharp pain in throat, ear, or back of tongue	Swallowing, talking, tumors	Glossopharyngeal nerve (CN IX)
Sinus headache	Pressure pain in cheeks, forehead, or nose area	Sinus infection, allergies	Frontal, maxillary sinuses, trigeminal nerve
Whiplash-associated disorder	Neck pain/stiffness, headache, dizziness	Motor vehicle accidents, rapid neck movement	Cervical muscles, ligaments, intervertebral joints
Myofascial pain syndrome	Localized muscle pain with trigger points	Muscle overuse, stress, posture	Sternocleidomastoid, trapezius, neck muscles
Postconcussive headache	Diffuse head pain, worsened by activity	Traumatic brain injury (TBI), concussion	Cerebral cortex, meninges, cervical spine

References

1. Institute of Medicine (US) Committee on Understanding the Biology of Sex and Gender Differences; Wizemann TM, Pardue ML, editors. *Exploring the Biological Contributions to Human Health: Does Sex Matter?* Washington (DC): National Academies Press (US); 2001. doi:10.17226/10028.
2. Moore KL, Dalley AF, Agur AMR. *Clinically Oriented Anatomy.* 8th ed. Wolters Kluwer; 2018.
3. Standring S, ed. *Gray's Anatomy: The Anatomical Basis of Clinical Practice.* 42nd ed. Elsevier; 2020.
4. Blumenfeld H. *Neuroanatomy Through Clinical Cases.* 3rd ed. Sinauer Associates; 2019.
5. Ellis H, Logan BM, Dixon AK. *Human Sectional Anatomy.* 5th ed. CRC Press; 2018.
6. Netter FH. *Atlas of Human Anatomy.* 7th ed. Elsevier; 2019.
7. Ingerslev CH, Solow B. Sex differences in craniofacial morphology. Acta Odontol Scand. 1975;33(2):85–94. doi:10.3109/00016357509026347
8. Vasavada AN, Li S, Delp SL. Three-dimensional isometric strength of neck muscles in humans. Spine (Phila Pa 1976). 2001;26(17):1904–9. doi:10.1097/00007632-200109010-00018
9. Inamoto Y, Saitoh E, Okada S, et al. Anatomy of the larynx and pharynx: Effects of age, gender and height revealed by multidetector computed tomography. J Oral Rehabil. 2015;42(9):670–7. doi:10.1111/joor.12298
10. Ruigrok AN, Salimi-Khorshidi G, Lai MC, Baron-Cohen S, Lombardo MV, Tait RJ, Suckling J. A meta-analysis of sex differences in human brain structure. Neurosci Biobehav Rev. 2014;39(100):34–50. doi:10.1016/j.neubiorev.2013.12.004
11. Craft RM. Modulation of pain by estrogens. Pain. 2007;132(Suppl 1):S3–S12. doi:10.1016/j.pain.2007.09.028
12. Fillingim RB, King CD, Ribeiro-Dasilva MC, Rahim-Williams B, Riley JL 3rd. Sex, gender, and pain: A review of recent clinical and experimental findings. J Pain. 2009;10(5):447–485. doi:10.1016/j.jpain.2008.12.001
13. Aaron RV, Ravyts SG, Carnahan ND, et al. Prevalence of depression and anxiety among adults with chronic pain: A systematic review and meta-analysis. JAMA Netw Open. 2025;8(3):e250268. doi:10.1001/jamanetworkopen.2025.0268

8
Migraine and Headache Disorders in Women

Niranjana Bienkowska and Anita Gupta

Introduction

Migraine is the world's sixth most disabling disorder and one of the 10 most common diseases. Women are affected three times more often than men due to hormonal changes brought on by menarche, reproductive cycles, and menopause.[1–5] Because of the intricacy of hormonal fluctuations in women, it is essential to understand the pathophysiology of headaches and migraines and to develop a plan for treatment options.

Background

Biopsychosocial factors are huge contributors to the cause of migraines in women. This is further exacerbated by the constantly changing hormonal effects in a woman's life. Past research had presented the lifestyle of women affected by migraines, and there has been a great deal of work in studying the biological underpinnings to further explain and formulate treatment/management strategies. A female's age and cycle are large contributing factors to migraines that arise during menstrual cycles, pregnancy, and menopause.[6]

Epidemiology and Risk Factors

Migraine (episodic and chronic) is most common among females, with 75% of all cases affecting women.[2,7] It has been hypothesized that the reason for this gender disparity in headaches and migraines lies in the inequity of household labor. These chore-related burdens are generally compounded by menstrual migraines, which are especially prevalent in women of childbearing age.[8] However, what causes alarm is the link of migraine with pregnancy that can have the potential to cause unfavorable outcomes, affecting both the mother and fetus through conditions like diabetes, hypertensive disorders in pregnancy, preterm birth, and low birth weight.[9]

Pathophysiology

The trigeminovascular system, the brainstem nuclei, and calcitonin gene-related peptide (CGRP) are other key biological players in migraine pathophysiology. The trigeminovascular pain pathway of the trigeminal system specifically plays a key role in the regulation of cranial vasculature and pain signaling.[10] Triggering migraine involves a critical release of neuropeptides by the trigeminal system, primarily CGRP and pituitary adenylate cyclase-activating polypeptide.[5]

CGRP is highly expressed in trigeminal neurons and is a powerful dilator of cranial vasculature in addition to activating the trigeminovascular system. This vasodilator activity, especially in the cerebral arteriole, results in increased cerebral blood flow, which in turn leads to migraine symptoms.[10] It is important to note that CGRP is a well-known biological mediator in both sexes. However, its function and effect become more significant in the female brain. Animal models have found that dural CGRP leads to hyperalgesia in female but not male rats.[11]

The sex difference is believed to be due to the increased vasodilation induced by CGRP during migraine onset, which is driven by estradiol and found in meningeal vessels.[12] The estradiol receptor agonist appears to increase CGRP sensory innervation as well as induce CGRP release from meningeal artery nerve terminals to produce pain. Concurrently, prolactin also plays a significant role in female migraine induction. Animal models show that an increase in prolactin only leads to hyperalgesia in female rats and not in males, possibly due to the presence of prolactin receptors on the dural nerves of female and not male rats. This prolactin then leads to CGRP release and dural trigeminal ganglion neuronal activation to induce pain.[13,14] Additional biological mechanisms that are likely responsible for the higher prevalence of migraines in women are differences in neurotransmitter and hormone systems. Serotonin is thought to be elevated during migraine onset.

The primary enzyme that metabolizes serotonin is monoamine oxidase (MAO). In women, the introduction of estrogen downregulates MAO activity. This results in less serotonin degradation, ultimately leading to a net increase in serotonin, which can induce more pain.[15] In addition, estrogen is also believed to increase serotonin production by activation of tryptophan hydroxylase and decrease serotonin reuptake by downregulating serotonin reuptake transporter (SERT) activity.[16]

In men, testosterone activates transient receptor potential melastatin 8 (TRPM8), which has channels located on trigeminal neurons that cause a decrease in nociception. This remains true even when female rat models were supplemented with testosterone. Male rats always show an increase in antinociceptive activity.[14,17] Therefore, the different levels and mechanisms of action of sex hormones are the fundamental reasons for the observed sex dimorphism of migraines.

Diagnosis and Assessment

Because of the heterogeneity of headaches in women, neurologists have established the International Classification of Headache Disorders (ICHD-3) criteria, which have formed the backbone for the diagnosis of migraine. ICHD-3 criteria dictate that the clinician should inquire about and establish a person's medical history including headache duration, age of onset, frequency, associated symptoms, aura symptoms, and history of medication use.

Additionally, diagnostic aids such as headache diaries, the three-item ID-Migraine questionnaire, and the five-item Migraine Screen Questionnaire may be used to further support such inquiries. The clinician should also make a differential diagnosis to exclude the possibility of primary headaches being secondary to head trauma. As any red flag associated with secondary headaches could be a harbinger of a life-threatening condition, the presence of these red flags should be verified by neuroimaging.[18] MRI is preferred over CT because it has a higher resolution and does not have the ionizing radiation of CT.

Treatment Considerations

Since migraines in women are heavily influenced by hormonal factors, it is crucial to assess the patient's age and phase of the menstrual cycle. If the patient is experiencing perimenopause or menopause, it is beneficial to assess that before providing a treatment plan (Table 8.1).

To counteract menstrual migraines, pharmacologic options include triptans, nonsteroidal anti-inflammatory drugs (NSAIDs), hormonal therapies, and CGRP antagonists. However, for women experiencing migraines with auras, hormonal therapies may elevate the risk of a potential for ischemic stroke, making nonhormonal methods a safer alternative in such cases where risk may be higher.[19]

Treatment options become more complex for pregnant and nursing women. Since most triptans and NSAIDs require caution due to potential fetal risks, it is recommended that pregnant women prioritize lifestyle management, acupuncture, and relaxation techniques. If migraines are still not managed, a careful assessment of risks versus benefits is essential before prescribing NSAIDs and triptans.

As the transition into menopause involves a decline and fluctuation in estrogen levels, hormonal replacement therapies can be beneficial, especially for women with auras. If hormonal therapies are contraindicated, nonhormonal alternatives like selective serotonin reuptake inhibitors (SSRIs) or serotonin-norepinephrine reuptake inhibitors (SNRIs) may show success rates for women postmenopause.

Ultimately, each patient's requirements differ, which means it is crucial to assess an individual's needs before providing a plan. In cases where pain persists after trying various methods, a multidisciplinary approach may be most effective. Nonpharmacologic options such as mindfulness and meditation can offer promising benefits. Additionally, neuromodulation devices like transcutaneous electrical nerve stimulation (TENS) and noninvasive vagus nerve stimulators could provide relief.[20]

Comorbid Conditions

Migraines tend to be comorbid with several psychiatric or neurological conditions. Common comorbidities include depression, anxiety, premenstrual syndrome (PMS), premenstrual dysphoric syndrome (PMDD), and sleep disorders. Epilepsy patients also exhibit a higher incidence of migraines, and the risk of a stroke goes up with the onset of migraines.[21–23] Women suffering from endometriosis also appear to experience migraines more frequently.[24] These comorbidities are crucial to consider when guiding a more comprehensive diagnosis and management plan.

Table 8.1 Summary of treatment for migraine and headache disorders

Treatment	Indication/Use	Notes	References
Triptans	Acute migraine attacks, menstrual migraines	Effective but use caution in pregnancy; contraindicated with migraine aura and hormonal therapies due to stroke risk.	21, 22
Nonsteroidal anti-inflammatory drugs (NSAIDs)	Acute migraine, menstrual migraines	Used with caution in pregnancy; potential fetal risks.	21, 22
Hormonal therapies	Menstrual migraines, perimenopause, menopause	Useful but increase ischemic stroke risk in migraine with aura; beneficial in menopause with careful assessment.	21, 22
CGRP antagonists	Preventive migraine treatment	Target CGRP pathway; effective especially in hormonal migraine pathophysiology.	11, 12
SSRIs and SNRIs	Post-menopause migraine management	Nonhormonal alternative for women contraindicated for hormone therapies.	22
Lifestyle management	Pregnancy, general prevention	First-line for pregnant women; includes sleep hygiene, diet, stress reduction, exercise.	21, 22
Acupuncture and relaxation	Pregnancy, general management	Nonpharmacologic, low risk approaches suitable for pregnancy.	21, 22
Neuromodulation devices (TENS, VNS)	Resistant migraine or adjunct therapy	Nonpharmacologic, potentially useful for refractory cases.	22
Mindfulness and meditation	Adjunctive treatment for chronic migraine	Supports stress management and overall well-being.	22

CGRP, calcitonin gene-related peptide; SNRIs, serotonin-norepinephrine reuptake inhibitors; SSRIs, selective serotonin reuptake inhibitors; TENS, transcutaneous electrical nerve stimulation; VNS, vagus nerve stimulator.

Patient-Centered Approaches

A patient-centered approach is necessary in helping the patient make informed medical decisions about their migraine and headache management. It is also crucial to note if the patient is experiencing menstruation, perimenopause, or menopause to assess their specific needs. Since some of the leading causes of migraines seem to emerge from women bearing more responsibilities, including childbirth, household chores, and professional pursuits, it is important to consider each patient's biopsychosocial factors.

It is critical to approach migraines and headaches in female patients from the standpoint of recognizing their hormonal and biopsychosocial factors, which are the key underlying reasons for higher rates of migraines in women. Having conversations with patients about their lifestyle, which will differ from those of men, may be necessary to fully assess their unique condition and provide a solution.

Emerging Trends and Current Research

The expanding realm of neurology has been involved in new ventures aimed at assisting women with their headaches and migraines. Researchers have more often been including in their studies the three critical headache precipitants for women: hormones, menstruation, and pregnancy.[25] The literature is also identifying artificial intelligence and virtual reality as tools that may help with diagnosis, classification, and pain management.[26]

Clinical Pearls

- Sex differences in hormones and biopsychosocial factors explain most of the reasons as per latest literature. The solution might require looking beyond the symptom to understand the patient's unique psychosocial and biological situation.
- Therapeutic approaches might involve homing in on wide-ranging factors such as proper medication, lifestyle and nutrition awareness, and stress management.

Conclusion

Delineating the biological causes behind migraines and headaches in women is important in treating one of their most common disabilities. Providers may have to tackle migraines and headaches from a "whole patient" approach to ultimately help their patient gain control over their pain. There is still further work to be done and research to be collected in seeking remedies in the expanding field of women's pain management.

References

1. Vetvik KG, MacGregor EA. Sex differences in the epidemiology, clinical features, and pathophysiology of migraine. Lancet Neurol. 2017;16(1):76–87.

2. Simmonds L, Mehta D, Cheema S, Matharu M. Epidemiology of migraine. In: Swanson JW, Matharu M, eds. *Handbook of Clinical Neurology* (vol. 198). Elsevier: 2023; 31–38.
3. Burch R. Migraine and tension-type headache: Diagnosis and treatment. Med Clin North Am. 2019;103(2):215–233.
4. Goadsby PJ, Holland PR, Martins-Oliveira M, Hoffmann J, Schankin C, Akerman S. Pathophysiology of migraine: A disorder of sensory processing. Physiol Rev. 2017;97(2):553–622.
5. Puledda F, Shields KGE, Goadsby PJ. Migraine: From pathophysiology to treatment. J Neurol. 2023;270(7):3654–3666.
6. Amiri P, Kazemnejad A, Emami H, et al. Migraine: A review on its history, global epidemiology, risk factors, and comorbidities. Front Neurol. 2022;12:800605.
7. Maddahi A, Edvinsson L, Goadsby PJ. Progesterone distribution in the trigeminal system and its role to modulate sensory neurotransmission: influence of sex. J Headache Pain. 2023;24(1):154.
8. Ahmad SR, Rosendale N. Sex and gender considerations in episodic migraine. Curr Pain Headache Rep. 2022;26(7):505–516.
9. Cen J, Yu Y, Shen Y, et al. Global, regional, and national burden and trends of migraine among women of childbearing age from 1990 to 2021: Insights from the Global Burden of Disease Study 2021. J Headache Pain. 2024;25(1):96.
10. Edvinsson L. The trigeminovascular pathway: Role of CGRP and CGRP receptors in migraine. Headache. 2017;57(Suppl 2):47–55.
11. Avona A, Burgos-Vega C, Burton MD, Akopian AN, Price TJ, Dussor G. Dural calcitonin gene-related peptide produces female-specific responses in rodent migraine models. J Neurosci. 2019;39(22):4323–4331.
12. Russo AF, Hay DL. CGRP physiology, pharmacology, and therapeutic targets: Migraine and beyond. Physiol Rev. 2023;103(4):1565–1644.
13. Avona A, Mason BN, Burgos-Vega C, et al. Meningeal CGRP-prolactin interaction evokes female-specific migraine behavior. Ann Neurol. 2021;89(6):1129–1144.
14. Kim S, Park JW. Migraines in women: A focus on reproductive events and hormonal milestones. Headache Pain Res. 2024;25(1):3–15.
15. Bethea CL, Lu NZ, Gundlah C, Streicher JM. Diverse actions of ovarian steroids in the serotonin neural system. Front Neuroendocrinol. 2002;23(1):41–100.
16. Pecins-Thompson M, Brown NA, Kohama SG, Bethea CL. Ovarian steroid regulation of tryptophan hydroxylase mRNA expression in rhesus macaques. J Neurosci. 1996;16(21):7021–7029.
17. Alarcón-Alarcón D, Cabañero D, de Andrés-López J, et al. TRPM8 contributes to sex dimorphism by promoting recovery of normal sensitivity in a mouse model of chronic migraine. Nat Commun. 2022;13:6304.
18. Eigenbrodt AK, Ashina S, Khan S, et al. Diagnosis and management of migraine in ten steps. Nat Rev Neurol. 2021;17(8):501–514.
19. Tepper NK, Curtis KM, Nanda K, Jamieson DJ. Safety of hormonal contraceptives among women with migraine: A systematic review. Contraception. 2016;94(6):630–640.
20. Barbanti P, Nappi RE. Framing and management of migraines in women: An expert opinion on challenges, current approaches, and future multidisciplinary perspectives. Healthcare (Basel). 2025;13(2):e1234.
21. Pelzer N, de Vries Lentsch S, Ferrari MD, Terwindt GM. Neurological and psychiatric comorbidities of migraine: Concepts and future perspectives. Cephalalgia. 2023;43(6):03331024231180564.

22. McCracken, H. T., Thaxter, L. Y., & Smitherman, T. A. (2024). Psychiatric comorbidities of migraine. In J. W. Swanson & M. Matharu (Eds.), *Handbook of Clinical Neurology* (Vol. 199, pp. 505–516). Elsevier. https://doi.org/10.1016/B978-0-12-823357-3.00013-6
23. Borończyk, M., Zduńska, A., Węgrzynek-Gallina, J., Grodzka, O., Lasek-Bal, A., & Domitrz, I. (2025). Migraine and stroke: correlation, coexistence, dependence—a modern perspective. *The Journal of Headache and Pain, 26*, 1973. https://doi.org/10.1186/s10194-025-01973-w
24. Colombo, G. E., Barcellona, D., Buggio, L., et al. (2025). The association between endometriosis and migraine: A systematic review and meta-analysis of observational studies. *The Journal of Headache and Pain, 26*(1), 82. https://doi.org/10.1186/s10194-025-01874-y
25. Ghadiri-Sani, M. (2025). Migraine in women: A review. *Current Opinion in Neurology, 38*(3), 271–276. https://doi.org/10.1097/WCO.0000000000001372
26. Cerda, I. H., Dominguez, D., Salazar, C., et al. (2024). Artificial Intelligence and virtual reality in headache disorder diagnosis, classification, and management. *Current Pain and Headache Reports, 28*(9), 869–880. https://doi.org/10.1007/s11916-024-01279-7

9

Nonpharmacologic Treatments for Migraine and Headache Disorders in Women

Anand Prem, Anesh Rugnath, and Suwarna Anand

Introduction

Headaches are among the commonest pain conditions, with more than 95% Americans experiencing one during their lifetime.[1] Barring cluster headaches, most headaches, including migraines, have an increased incidence in women. As physicians, pain control is challenging in these patients, leading to chronicity, disability, and poor quality of life. Despite significant advances in the pharmacologic treatment of headaches recently, treatment failures with this approach alone are frequent due to cost, lack of insurance coverage, adverse effects, and the emergence of overuse headache. There is growing evidence that nonpharmacologic approaches such as biofeedback, cognitive behavioral therapy (CBT), acupuncture, and lifestyle modifications can be useful complementary modalities in the management of headaches. This chapter provides a brief overview of the various nonpharmacologic interventions that should be considered in any comprehensive multimodal treatment plan of patients with headaches.

Background

Headaches, particularly migraines, are associated with a variety of comorbidities and triggers such as anxiety, depression, sleep disorders, and amplified pain syndromes, thus leading to dissatisfaction in current medication-based treatment plans.[2] In one survey, two out of three patients were neutral or unsatisfied with their medication regimen, and a quarter discontinued their preventive medications due to adverse effects, lack of efficacy, or increased rebound headaches.[1] Hence, there is an unmet need for alternative treatment strategies, with more than 50% of Americans with headaches having tried alternative and complementary approaches.[3,4]

Lifestyle Modification

Stress and sleep disorders have long been identified as triggers for various headaches. Improving patient awareness of this correlation and motivating them to adopt strategies to manage stress and establish good sleep hygiene can make a positive impact on headaches and quality of life. Graded aerobic activity, resistance training, and yoga in the setting of a balanced diet and proper hydration have been shown to reduce medication intake and the frequency and intensity of headaches.[1,2] Nutrition counseling to help avoid common headache triggers and the avoidance of smoking and excess alcohol and caffeine consumption while adding dietary supplements such as magnesium, riboflavin, coenzyme Q, omega-3 fatty acids, alpha lipoic acid, and vitamin D have all proved beneficial. Avoidance of one to three food triggers for 12 weeks led to complete headache resolution in 87% children in one study.[1,3]

Herbal Supplements and Nutraceuticals

Ginger, feverfew (*Tanacetum parthenium*), butterbur (*Petasites hybridus*), cannabinoids, cinnamon, curcumin, citron, and ginkgo biloba show promise in headaches but need further validation.

Mind–Body Techniques and Behavioral Pain Management

Mind–body techniques and behavioral pain management encompass a wide variety of evidence-based techniques including biofeedback, relaxation training, and CBT, often offered by psychologists with expertise in pain management, particularly headaches.[1,5] While these modalities are more effective when administered in conjunction with pharmacologic management, barriers to treatment exist in the form of inadequate providers of such therapy, lack of insurance coverage, and a patient's lack of knowledge and reluctance to seek such treatment. The overall effectiveness of these therapies is endorsed by US Headache Consortium, World Health Organization, National Institutes of Health, American Medical Association, American Academy of Neurology, and American Headache Society. Success depends on early referral and patient education on the rationale and benefits of such treatment not only on headaches but on functioning and quality of life. There is Level A evidence for their use in posttraumatic headaches in children and adolescents.[6]

Biofeedback

As one of the most researched non-pharmacologic treatment approaches in headache management, biofeedback involves raising awareness of the patient's own physiological parameters (muscle tone, heart rate variability, galvanic skin conductance, temperature, and breathing) and incorporating techniques to control and optimize the same. Electromyographic (EMG) and thermal biofeedback devices monitor and provide "feedback" to the patient about the physical response to headache and their ability to control them. Initial clinic-based sessions followed by individualized home-based sessions have shown the most sustained benefit, giving the patient a sense of control and facilitating buy-in to the overall treatment plan.[1,7,8] In metanalyses, biofeedback has shown benefit in both migraine and TTH, also improving the response to pharmacotherapy. In a systematic review of 29 studies with more than 1,300 participants, 10 reported significant improvement in headache intensity in the biofeedback group compared to the control group. Meta-analysis of four of these studies revealed a reduction in the intensity but not the duration or frequency of headaches in patients subjected to biofeedback.[7]

Relaxation Training

An extension of biofeedback therapy, relaxation techniques help patients achieve a relaxed state through controlled diaphragmatic breathing and progressive muscle relaxation to minimize the physiological response to headache, thus reducing neural excitation and muscle tension and increasing the patient's awareness and control of biological responses to headaches.

Cognitive Behavioral Therapy

CBT is a form of stress management training that allows the patient to identify their own unique trigger factors for their headaches such as sleep disturbance, anxiety, stress, or poor eating habits and then develop coping strategies to minimize their adverse impact on quality of life. It equips the patient with a sense of self-control, preventing headaches and their associated disability. There is ample evidence to support this in refractory headache, particularly in children.[9]

Mindfulness and Meditation

The beneficial effects of meditation or mindfulness in improving sleep, pain, anxiety, and mood have long been recognized and extend to treatment of headaches as well, especially migraine and TTH.[10]

Other mind–body techniques that have proved beneficial but need more research in headaches include guided imagery and hypnosis. A review of eight studies examining hypnosis either alone or in combination with visual imagery and relaxation demonstrated the effectiveness of hypnotherapy and relaxation techniques in reducing headache episodes.[11]

Biomechanical Therapies

Refractory headaches, particularly of cervicogenic origin, respond well to physical therapy, with overall improvement in conditioning, function, and quality of life.

Spinal Manipulation

Chiropractic and osteopathic manipulation of the spine can improve headaches by altering alignment of the spine, reducing myofascial spasm and increasing release of endogenous opioids.[1,12] However, the potential for serious adverse effects from spinal and vascular injury, particularly in patients with severe degenerative cervical disease and vascular disorders, limits their widespread use.[12]

Dry Needling

This technique of using fine needles to address trigger points in tight cervical musculature to decrease muscle spasm, increase blood flow, and reduce pain, known as "dry needling," has risen in popularity as more physical therapists offer it in conjunction with deep tissue massage and myofascial release. In a meta-analysis of 10 randomized controlled trials, dry needling was associated with a significant decrease in disability and headache intensity compared to controls at 1- and 3-month follow-up.[13]

Electrical Stimulation and Neuromodulation

Transcutaneous electrical nerve stimulation (TENS) is often used as a modality during physical therapy, particularly in the treatment of cervicogenic headaches. More recently, the US Food and Drug Administration (FDA) has approved several neuromodulation devices (Gammacore, Cefaly, Nerivio) for transcutaneous vagal or trigeminal stimulation, transcutaneous magnetic stimulation, and remote electrical neuromodulation (REN), and these have had success in the management of migraine headaches, giving the patient more control and choice with minimal adverse effects.[1]

Acupuncture

Acupuncture has been extensively studied as a complementary treatment modality for headaches. Proposed mechanisms of action include endogenous endorphin release and modulation of calcitonin gene-related peptide and the cyclooxygenase-2 pathways implicated in headache pathophysiology. Acupuncture was found to be more effective than sham and at least as effective as standard pharmacotherapy in a Cochrane review of 22 trials involving almost 5,000 participants. Its role in preventing headaches makes it an attractive option, though at least 8–12 treatments may be required, often not covered by insurance.[1]

Gender-Specific Considerations

Despite headache's significant adverse impact on maternal quality of life, the use of nonpharmacologic therapies is especially preferred in pregnant women with headache to avoid fetal exposure to medications. However, scientific evidence is limited, leading to inadequate treatment, delayed diagnosis, and worsening headaches in pregnant women with deleterious impact on the mother and fetus.[14]

Emerging Trends and Current Research

Neuromodulation, both invasive and noninvasive, appears to be a rapidly emerging option in the treatment of headaches and is likely to see the most growth in the next decade. This could particularly be helpful in pregnant and breastfeeding mothers with medication-refractory headaches motivated to avoiding fetal exposure to potentially harmful drugs.[15]

Conclusion

Complementary medicine has seen an explosion in popularity in the past few decades due to a variety of factors that include patient dissatisfaction with the overdependence on medicines and technology in modern medicine, pressure on physicians contributing to erosion of the patient–physician relationship, the failure of conventional pharmaceuticals to treat chronic ailments, and the search for less toxic, safer, less invasive, and more holistic approaches to treating disease. The flip side of this is the lack of supporting scientific data, less regulation leading to dubious marketing practices, lack of consistency in quality and technique among providers of alternative therapies, and the potential for harm. The recognition that patients want a variety of different treatment approaches available to them should prompt us as physicians to further research complementary therapies, educate ourselves and patients about all these varied therapies, and allow patients to make their informed care decisions based on available evidence.

References

1. Rakel D, Minichiello VJ, eds. *Integrative Medicine*. Fifth edition. Elsevier; 2023. Accessed July 8, 2025. https://www.clinicalkey.com/dura/browse/bookChapter/3-s2.0-C20190013313
2. Buse DC, Reed ML, Fanning KM, et al. Comorbid and co-occurring conditions in migraine and associated risk of increasing headache pain intensity and headache frequency: Results of the migraine in America symptoms and treatment (MAST) study. J Headache Pain. 2020;21(1):1–16.
3. Ng JY, Hanna C. Headache and migraine clinical practice guidelines: A systematic review and assessment of complementary and alternative medicine recommendations. BMC Complement Med Ther. 2021;21(1):236. doi:10.1186/s12906–021-03401–3
4. Tepper SJ. Nutraceutical and other modalities for the treatment of headache. Continuum (Minneap Minn). 2015;21(4 Headache):1018–1031. doi:10.1212/CON.0000000000000211
5. Grinberg AS, Damush TM, Lindsey H, et al. The headache psychologists' role in pediatric and adult headache care: A qualitative study of expert practitioners. J Clin Psychol Med Settings. 2024;31(2):359–367. doi:10.1007/s10880–023-09972–2
6. Minen M, Jinich S, Vallespir Ellett G. Behavioral therapies and mind-body interventions for posttraumatic headache and post-concussive symptoms: A systematic review. Headache. 2019;59(2):151–163. doi:10.1111/head.13455
7. Martino Cinnera A, Morone G, Bisirri A, et al. Headaches treatment with EMG biofeedback: A focused systematic review and meta-analysis. Eur J Phys Rehabil Med. 2023;59(6):697–705. doi:10.23736/S1973–9087.23.07745–6

8. Andrasik F. Biofeedback in headache: An overview of approaches and evidence. Cleve Clin J Med. 2010;77(Suppl 3):S72–S76. doi:10.3949/ccjm.77.s3.13
9. Kaczynski K. Cognitive-behavioral therapy for chronic headache disorders in children and adolescents. In: Friedberg RD, Paternostro JK, eds. *Handbook of Cognitive Behavioral Therapy for Pediatric Medical Conditions*. Springer Nature: 2019;261–277.
10. Gu Q, Hou JC, Fang XM. Mindfulness Meditation for primary headache pain: A meta-analysis. Chin Med J (Engl). 2018;131(7):829–838. doi:10.4103/0366-6999.228242
11. Flynn N. Systematic review of the effectiveness of hypnosis for the management of headache. Int J Clin Exp Hypn. 2018;66(4):343–352. doi:10.1080/00207144.2018.1494432
12. Lynge S, Dissing KB, Vach W, Christensen HW, Hestbaek L. Effectiveness of chiropractic manipulation versus sham manipulation for recurrent headaches in children aged 7–14 years: A randomised clinical trial. Chiropr Man Therap. 2021;29(1):1. Published 2021 Jan 7. doi:10.1186/s12998-020-00360-3
13. Kandeel M, Morsy MA, Al Khodair KM, Alhojaily S. Dry needling techniques as a treatment for improving disability and pain in patients with different types of headaches: A systematic review and meta-analysis. Complement Ther Med. 2024;86:103085. doi:10.1016/j.ctim.2024.103085
14. Bushman ET, Cozzi G, Sinkey RG, Smith CH, Varner MW, Digre K. Randomized controlled trials of headache treatments in pregnancy: A systematic review. Am J Perinatol. 2021;38(S 01):e102–e108. doi:10.1055/s-0040-1705180
15. American Migraine Foundation. (2025, July 2). *Inside AMF's Device Corner: A Guide to Neuromodulation for Migraine*. https://americanmigrainefoundation.org/resource-library/inside-amfs-device-corner-a-guide-to-neuromodulation-for-migraine/

10
Interventional Pain Treatments for Migraine Disorders in Women

Niranjana Bienkowska and Anita Gupta

Introduction

Migraine is a primary headache disorder that affects nearly 1 billion people worldwide, making it the second leading cause of disability globally and the most common disabling headache in patients younger than 50 years of age.[1] Migraine headache is episodic in nature, often bilateral, moderate to severe in intensity, pulsating, and associated with nausea and/or vomiting as well as light and sound sensitivity.

Although significant progress has been made in the development of acute and preventive pharmacotherapies for migraine, a substantial proportion of patients continue to suffer from chronic migraine (CM), defined as ≥15 headache days per month for at least 3 months, of which at least 8 days are migrainous.[2] Patients with CM often experience poor quality of life and functional impairment as well as limited response to or intolerance of conventional medical therapy and, as such, represent a particularly underserved patient population in need of alternative treatment options.

Interventional pain procedures represent an important tool in the management of refractory migraine and other disabling headache disorders. These approaches, which range from targeted peripheral nerve blocks and chemodenervation to neuromodulatory implants, are often rationalized through the evolving understanding of headache neuroanatomy and neurophysiology, especially in relation to the trigeminal system and its convergence with cervical afferents.

This chapter reviews the various interventional treatment strategies in headache, including mechanisms of action, clinical indications, procedural techniques, and evidence of efficacy and safety, with the aim of integrating these tools into the armamentarium of the migraine treatment provider.

Anatomy and Neurophysiology of Migraine Pain Pathways

Effective interventional management of migraine necessitates a thorough understanding of the relevant neuroanatomy. Migraine pain is primarily mediated by the trigeminal nervous system, specifically the trigeminal ganglion and its three major divisions (ophthalmic V1, maxillary V2, mandibular V3). The ophthalmic division (V1) innervates structures of the forehead, eye, and anterior scalp, while the greater occipital nerve (GON) and lesser occipital nerve (LON), derived from cervical roots C2–C3, innervate the posterior scalp.

The trigeminocervical complex (TCC), located in the dorsal horn of the upper cervical spinal cord, plays a pivotal role in migraine pathophysiology. This complex receives converging input from the trigeminal nerve and cervical afferents (C1–C3), explaining why pain originating in the neck or occipital region can be referred to the head and vice versa. Sensitization of the TCC is thought to contribute to the central sensitization observed in CM.[3]

The sphenopalatine ganglion (SPG), a parasympathetic ganglion located in the pterygopalatine fossa, also holds significance. It has connections to the trigeminal nerve and receives input from the superior salivatory nucleus, playing a role in autonomic symptoms associated with migraine (e.g., lacrimation, nasal congestion). Modulation of the SPG can influence both trigeminal and autonomic pathways.[4]

Botulinum Toxin Type A

Botulinum toxin type A (BoNTA; e.g., onabotulinumtoxinA) is a treatment approved by the US Food and Drug Administration (FDA) for CM in adults. Its mechanism of action in migraine is thought to involve inhibition of acetylcholine release at the neuromuscular junction, leading to muscle relaxation, but, more importantly, it inhibits the release of various pro-nociceptive neuropeptides (e.g., substance P, calcitonin gene-related peptide [CGRP], glutamate) from peripheral sensory nerve terminals, thereby modulating peripheral and central sensitization.[5]

Indications and Patient Selection

BoNTA is indicated for the prophylactic treatment of CM) in adults who have ≥15 headache days per month, with at least 8 days meeting migraine criteria. It is typically considered after failure or intolerance to at least two conventional oral preventive medications.[6]

Procedure

The standard protocol involves 31 injections (155 units total) into seven specific head and neck muscle areas: frontalis (bilateral), corrugator (bilateral), procerus, temporalis (bilateral), occipitalis (bilateral), cervical paraspinal muscles (bilateral), and trapezius (bilateral). The injections are typically repeated every 12 weeks.[7]

Efficacy and Safety

Clinical trials, most notably the Phase 3 Research Evaluating Migraine Prophylaxis Therapy (PREEMPT) trials, demonstrated that BoNTA significantly reduces headache frequency, severity, and associated disability in patients with CM, with sustained benefits over multiple treatment cycles.[7] Common side effects are usually mild and transient, including neck pain, muscle weakness, ptosis, and temporary injection site reactions. Serious adverse events are rare.

Nerve Blocks

Nerve blocks involve injecting a local anesthetic, with or without a corticosteroid, near specific nerves to interrupt pain signal transmission. They can be used diagnostically, acutely for pain relief, or as a bridge to other therapies.

Greater Occipital Nerve Block

The GON is a mixed sensory nerve providing innervation to the posterior scalp. Blocks target its superficial course over the occiput.

- **Mechanism:** Anesthetic interruption of nociceptive input from the GON, potentially modulating the TCC.[8]
- **Indications:** Acute and prophylactic treatment of various primary headache disorders, including migraine, cervicogenic headache, cluster headache, and occipital neuralgia.
- **Procedure:** Palpation of the GON (approximately 2 cm lateral to the occipital protuberance, inferior to the nuchal line). Injection of 1–3 mL of local anesthetic (e.g., bupivacaine, lidocaine) with or without corticosteroid. Ultrasound guidance can improve accuracy and reduce complication rates.[9]
- **Efficacy:** Provides rapid, albeit often temporary, relief for acute migraine. Can be effective as a prophylactic in some patients, potentially reducing headache frequency and severity for weeks to months.[8]
- **Safety:** Generally safe. Risks include injection site pain, bruising, temporary numbness, and rarely, infection, vascular puncture, or nerve damage.

Supraorbital and Supratrochlear Nerve Blocks

These nerves, branches of the trigeminal nerve's ophthalmic division (V1), innervate the forehead and anterior scalp.

- **Mechanism:** Local anesthetic blockade of V1 sensory input.
- **Indications:** Migraine with frontal pain, supraorbital neuralgia.
- **Procedure:** Injected at the supraorbital notch/foramen and superior to the trochlea, respectively.
- **Efficacy:** Can provide localized relief for frontal headaches.
- **Safety:** Similar to GON blocks; transient numbness in the forehead is common.

Sphenopalatine Ganglion Block

The SPG is a critical relay for parasympathetic fibers and has rich connections with the trigeminal system.

- **Mechanism:** Application of local anesthetic (e.g., lidocaine) to the SPG to disrupt autonomic and trigeminal pain pathways.
- **Indications:** Acute treatment of various headaches, including migraine, cluster headache, and trigeminal neuralgia. Can also be used for prophylaxis in select cases.[4]
- **Procedure:** Typically performed transnasally using a cotton-tipped applicator soaked in local anesthetic, advanced to the posterior nasopharynx to lie over the SPG. Image guidance (fluoroscopy or endoscopy) can be used for more precise delivery via a catheter.[10]
- **Efficacy:** Offers rapid relief for acute headache episodes. Efficacy for long-term prophylaxis is less robust but can be beneficial for some patients.
- **Safety:** Generally well tolerated. Common side effects include temporary numbness in the throat/pharynx, bitter taste, and epistaxis. Serious complications are rare.

Neuromodulation Techniques

Neuromodulation involves altering nerve activity through electrical stimulation. These techniques are typically reserved for patients with chronic, refractory migraine.

Occipital Nerve Stimulation

Occipital nerve stimulation (ONS) involves surgically implanting electrodes near the greater and/or lesser occipital nerves, delivering electrical impulses to modulate their activity.

- **Mechanism:** Thought to modulate the TCC by anti-dromic activation of the occipital nerves, thereby reducing central sensitization and inhibiting trigeminal nociceptive input.[11]
- **Indications:** CM refractory to conventional medical management and other interventional therapies. Typically follows a successful trial period.
- **Procedure:** Electrodes are surgically implanted subcutaneously in the occipital region, tunneled, and connected to an implantable pulse generator (IPG) usually placed in the chest or abdomen. A trial period with externalized leads is often performed to assess efficacy.[11]
- **Efficacy:** Studies have shown ONS to significantly reduce headache frequency, intensity, and associated disability in a subset of carefully selected patients with CM.[12] Response rates vary, but a significant number of patients report at least a 30–50% reduction in headache days.
- **Safety:** Surgical risks include infection, lead migration, lead fracture, pain at the IPG site, and rarely, neurological complications. Nonsurgical side effects include uncomfortable paresthesias. Revision surgeries are common due to lead-related issues.[12]

Supraorbital Nerve Stimulation

Supraorbital nerve stimulation (SONS) involves implanting electrodes near the supraorbital and supratrochlear nerves or using noninvasive external devices.

- **Mechanism:** Modulation of trigeminal (V1) afferent input.
- **Indications:** Migraine, particularly with frontal predominance. Noninvasive external devices (e.g., Cefaly) are FDA-cleared for acute and preventive migraine treatment.
- **Procedure:** Implantable SONS is less common than ONS due to cosmetic concerns and efficacy profile. External devices are applied to the forehead.[13]
- **Efficacy:** External SONS devices have demonstrated modest efficacy in reducing migraine frequency and acute pain.
- **Safety:** External devices are generally safe, with mild skin irritation. Implantable risks are like other neurostimulation procedures.

Vagus Nerve Stimulation

Vagus nerve stimulation (VNS) involves stimulating the vagus nerve, which has widespread connections to brain regions involved in pain processing. Both implantable and noninvasive external devices exist.

- **Mechanism:** Modulation of brainstem nuclei and cortical areas involved in pain, mood, and autonomic regulation.[14]
- **Indications:** Noninvasive VNS (nVNS) is FDA-cleared for acute and preventive treatment of episodic and chronic cluster headache and acute treatment of migraine. Implantable VNS for pain is generally investigational.
- **Procedure:** nVNS devices are held against the neck over the vagus nerve.
- **Efficacy:** Evidence suggests nVNS can be effective for acute migraine relief and as a preventive in some patients.[15]
- **Safety:** nVNS is generally well-tolerated with mild side effects such as local discomfort, cough, or voice changes.

Sphenopalatine Ganglion Stimulation

Sphenopalatine ganglion stimulation (SPGS) involves implanting a small stimulator adjacent to the SPG.

- **Mechanism:** Direct electrical stimulation of the SPG, modulating both parasympathetic outflow and trigeminal nociceptive pathways.
- **Indications:** Primarily investigated for chronic cluster headache; limited data for CM.
- **Procedure:** A small lead is implanted via a minimally invasive approach into the pterygopalatine fossa.
- **Efficacy:** Promising results in chronic cluster headache. Data for migraine are emerging but limited.[16]
- **Safety:** Surgical risks are similar to other implants; includes localized pain and numbness.

Considerations for Interventional Migraine Management

Patient Selection

Careful patient selection is paramount. Ideal candidates for interventional procedures typically have

- A confirmed diagnosis of CM or another primary headache disorder.
- Significant disability due to headache.
- Failure to respond adequately to, or intolerance of, at least two to three classes of conventional oral preventive medications.
- No contraindications to the specific procedure.
- Realistic expectations regarding outcomes and potential side effects.
- Psychological stability and engagement in a comprehensive care plan.

Multidisciplinary Approach

Interventional procedures should never be performed in isolation. They are most effective when integrated into a multimodal pain management program that includes

- Pharmacologic management (acute and preventive).
- Nonpharmacologic therapies (e.g., biofeedback, cognitive behavioral therapy, physical therapy).
- Lifestyle modifications.
- Psychological support.

Diagnostic and Therapeutic Algorithm

A common approach involves

1. **Trial of less invasive procedures:** Start with diagnostic/therapeutic nerve blocks (e.g., GON blocks) to assess response and confirm anatomical targets.
2. **Chemodenervation:** Consider BoNTA for CM meeting criteria.
3. **Advanced neuromodulation:** Reserve for severe, refractory cases after thorough workup and multidisciplinary consensus, often preceded by a trial period (for ONS).

Conclusion

Interventional pain procedures (Table 10.1) offer valuable therapeutic options for patients suffering from refractory migraine and other severe headache disorders. From BoNTA and targeted nerve blocks to advanced neuromodulation techniques, these interventions aim to disrupt nociceptive pathways, modulate central sensitization, and ultimately reduce pain burden and improve quality of life. A comprehensive understanding

Table 10.1 Summary of procedures for headaches and migraine disorders

Procedure	Anatomical target	Mechanism of action	Primary indications (refractory)
Botulinum toxin A	Targeted head/ neck muscles (31 injection sites)	Peripheral chemodenervation; inhibits pronociceptive neuropeptide release (CGRP, Sub P)	Chronic migraine ($\ge$15 days/month)
Greater occipital nerve (GON) block	Posterior scalp (C2-C3 roots)	Interrupts nociceptive input; modulates trigeminocervical complex	Acute migraine; status migrainosus; occipital neuralgia
Sphenopalatine ganglion (SPG) block	Pterygopalatine fossa	Disrupts parasympathetic outflow and trigeminal pain relay	Acute migraine; cluster headache
Occipital nerve stimulation (ONS)	Subcutaneous GON/LON	Neuromodulation; reduces central sensitization via trigeminocervical complex	Chronic migraine (refractory to medications and blocks)
Noninvasive vagus nerve stimulation (nVNS)	Cervical vagus nerve	Modulates brainstem pain processing and autonomic regulation	Acute migraine; acute/ prophylactic cluster headache

of the underlying neuroanatomy, careful patient selection, and integration within a multidisciplinary treatment paradigm are crucial for optimizing outcomes and advancing effective migraine management. Ongoing research continues to refine existing techniques and explore novel interventional targets, promising further advancements in this challenging field.

References

1. GBD 2016 Headache Collaborators. Global, regional, and national burden of migraine and tension-type headache, 1990–2016: A systematic analysis for the Global Burden of Disease Study 2016. Lancet Neurol. 2018;17(11):954–976. doi:10.1016/S1474-4422(18)30322-3
2. Headache Classification Committee of the International Headache Society (IHS). The International Classification of Headache Disorders, 3rd edition (beta version). Cephalalgia. 2013;33(9):629–808. doi:10.1177/0333102413485658
3. Goadsby PJ, Charbit AR, Andreou AP, Akerman S, Holland PR. Neurobiology of migraine. Neuroscience. 2009;161(2):323–341. doi:10.1016/j.neuroscience.2009.03.016
4. Mojica J, Mo B, Ng A. Sphenopalatine ganglion block in the management of chronic headaches. Curr Pain Headache Rep. 2017;21(6):27. doi:10.1007/s11916-017-0626-8. Erratum in: Curr Pain Headache Rep. 2017;21(12):53. doi:10.1007/s11916-017-0652-6. Mojica, Jeffery [corrected to Mojica, Jeffrey]
5. Chilson CN, Brown SJ. Role of botulinum toxin type A in the prophylactic treatment of migraine headaches. Ann Pharmacother. 2005;39(12):2081–5. doi:10.1345/aph.1G239
6. Kennis K, Kernick D, O'Flynn N. Diagnosis and management of headaches in young people and adults: NICE guideline. Br J Gen Pract. 2013;63(613):443–445. doi:10.3399/bjgp13X670895

7. Aurora SK, Dodick DW, Turkel CC, et al.; PREEMPT 1 Chronic Migraine Study Group. OnabotulinumtoxinA for treatment of chronic migraine: Results from the double-blind, randomized, placebo-controlled phase of the PREEMPT 1 trial. Cephalalgia. 2010;30(7):793–803. doi:10.1177/0333102410364676
8. Mustafa MS, Bin Amin S, Kumar A, et al. Assessing the effectiveness of greater occipital nerve block in chronic migraine: A systematic review and meta-analysis. BMC Neurol. 2024;24(1):330. doi:10.1186/s12883-024-03834-6
9. Palamar D, Uluduz D, Saip S, Erden G, Unalan H, Akarirmak U. Ultrasound-guided greater occipital nerve block: An efficient technique in chronic refractory migraine without aura? Pain Physician. 2015;18(2):153–162. PMID: 25794201
10. Candido KD, Massey ST, Sauer R, Darabad RR, Knezevic NN. A novel revision to the classical transnasal topical sphenopalatine ganglion block for the treatment of headache and facial pain. Pain Physician. 2013;16(6):E769–E778. PMID: 24284858
11. Miller S, Watkins L, Matharu M. Long-term outcomes of occipital nerve stimulation for chronic migraine: A cohort of 53 patients. J Headache Pain. 2016;17(1):68. doi:10.1186/s10194-016-0659-0
12. Silberstein SD, Dodick DW, Saper J, et al. Safety and efficacy of peripheral nerve stimulation of the occipital nerves for the management of chronic migraine: Results from a randomized, multicenter, double-blinded, controlled study. Cephalalgia. 2012;32(16):1165–1179. doi:10.1177/0333102412462642. Epub 2012 Oct 3. Erratum in: Cephalalgia. 2014;34(11):944. Vaisma, Julien [corrected to Vaisman, Julien] doi:10.1177/0333102414544419
13. Schoenen J, Vandersmissen B, Jeangette S, Herroelen L, Vandenheede M, Gérard P, Magis D. Migraine prevention with a supraorbital transcutaneous stimulator: A randomized controlled trial. Neurology. 2013;80(8):697–704. doi:10.1212/WNL.0b013e3182825055
14. Goadsby PJ. Pathophysiology of cluster headache: A trigeminal autonomic cephalgia. Lancet Neurol. 2002;1(4):251–257. doi:10.1016/s1474-4422(02)00104-7
15. Tassorelli C, Grazzi L, de Tommaso M, et al.; PRESTO Study Group. Noninvasive vagus nerve stimulation as acute therapy for migraine: The randomized PRESTO study. Neurology. 2018;91(4):e364–e373. doi:10.1212/WNL.0000000000005857
16. Schoenen J, Jensen RH, Lantéri-Minet M, et al. Stimulation of the sphenopalatine ganglion (SPG) for cluster headache treatment. Pathway CH-1: A randomized, sham-controlled study. Cephalalgia. 2013;33(10):816–830. doi:10.1177/0333102412473667

11
Acute Complex Migraine Pain Managed with Multimodal Pharmacologic and Interventional Treatment

Joanna Sung, Dhiresh Bandaru, Jay Srinivas, Sumedha Shastry, and Anita Gupta

Clinical Vignette

A 47 year old female presents to the emergency department with recurrent unilateral headaches over the right side of the head and occurring more frequently over the past few months. Pain is usually throbbing/pulsating, and the attacks last 10–12 hours in duration without treatment. She rates intensity as moderate to severe, with associated symptoms of nausea/vomiting, tinnitus, photophobia, and at times visual aura. Her history and symptoms were consistent with a diagnosis of migraine with aura per criteria of the International Classification of Headache Disorders (ICHD-3).[1] Triggers are stress, lack of sleep, missed meals, menstruation, hormones, and occasionally wine or cheese. Symptoms partially improve with rest in a dark and quiet room, cold compresses, and ibuprofen. Occasionally, she used tetrahydrocannabinol (THC), which she found relieved symptoms, though this was infrequent. No reported history of trauma, seizures, weakness, or speech disturbance.

Medical History

She had no history of chronic medical conditions, no use of medication, and no recent history of infection, trauma, or systemic illness. She was a nonsmoker and consumed alcohol socially. There was no family history of stroke or epilepsy, but her mother suffered from a similar type of headache when she was in her thirties.[2] This may have been a genetic basis for migraine.

Evaluation and Diagnosis

Neurologic exam was unremarkable. CT and MRI of the brain excluded secondary headaches. A complete blood count, thyroid function test, and metabolic panels were normal. Diagnosis of migraine with aura was made on clinical grounds. She complained of more than four migraine attacks per month that had a substantial impact on her daily activities. She was started on acute and prophylactic therapy.

Treatment Plan

For acute treatment, the patient was prescribed oral sumatriptan 50 mg at the onset of headache, with a second dose allowed after 2 hours if needed (maximum 200 mg/day), in line with current guidelines for acute migraine treatment.[3] Nonsteroidal anti-inflammatory drugs (NSAIDs) (ibuprofen 400–600 mg) were advised as adjunctive treatment, and metoclopramide 10 mg orally was prescribed for nausea. Due to the frequency of attacks and functional impairment, preventive therapy was started. Topiramate 25 mg at bedtime was initiated and up-titrated to 50–100 mg/day, with monitoring for cognitive and mood-related side effects.[4] Alternatives like propranolol or amitriptyline would be considered based on patient tolerance and comorbidities. Nonpharmacologic measures were reinforced, including sleep hygiene, regular meal patterns, stress reduction with yoga and cognitive behavioral therapy (CBT), and keeping a migraine diary. The patient was advised to avoid known dietary triggers such as wine and cheese.

Interventional Pain Management Considerations

Interventional approaches were discussed given the refractory nature of her migraines (Table 11.1). OnabotulinumtoxinA (Botox) injections were discussed for chronic migraine (≥15 headache days/month) following the PREEMPT protocol, which includes 155–195 units of onabotulinumtoxinA injected at 31–39 injection sites every 12 weeks.[5] The patient was counseled that two to three cycles are typically needed to see clinical benefit. Peripheral nerve blocks were also discussed. Greater occipital nerve blocks (with lidocaine or bupivacaine with or without a corticosteroid) were mentioned as options given the location and quality of her pain.[6] Supraorbital and supratrochlear nerve blocks were also discussed in case she experienced frontal patterns of pain. The transnasal sphenopalatine ganglion block (with or without a local anesthetic or corticosteroid) was presented as a treatment option for acute exacerbations.[7] Neuromodulation approaches were also presented to the patient. Peripheral nerve stimulation (PNS) has shown efficacy for refractory headache but is an investigational and invasive procedure requiring surgical implantation of a device to stimulate the occipital or trigeminal nerves. Transcranial magnetic stimulation (TMS) is noninvasive and approved

Table 11.1 Summary of interventional treatment interventions, indications, frequency, and setting

Intervention	Indication	Frequency	Setting
CGRP mAbs	Preventive	Monthly/quarterly	Self-injectable
Botox	Chronic migraine	q12 weeks	Clinic
GON/SPG Block	Episodic/chronic migraine	PRN or q2–4 weeks	Clinic
PNS	Refractory migraine	Permanent implant	Specialty center
TMS	Migraine with aura	PRN or scheduled	Home/Clinic

CGRP, calcitonin gene-related peptide; GON, greater occipital nerve; PNS, peripheral nerve stimulation ; SPG, sphenopalatine ganglion; TMS, transcranial magnetic stimulation.

by the US Food and Drug Administration (FDA) for acute treatment of migraine with aura. TMS can modulate cortical excitability.[8]

Outcome

At her 3-month follow-up, the patient had decreased headache frequency to 4–5 migraines per month. She also reported improved control with abortive medications, decreased missed days of work, and improved quality of life. She would continue follow-up to observe response to topiramate and consider Botox or CGRP monoclonal antibodies if no further improvement occurred.

Discussion

This case illustrates the complex and often challenging nature of migraine management in women, particularly when combined with aura and a hormonally driven pattern. The multimodal treatment approach, incorporating pharmacologic, behavioral, and interventional strategies, was key to achieving sustained improvement. Interventional pain procedures such as nerve blocks and neuromodulation can be valuable additions to treatment-resistant cases and may be considered earlier in the management algorithm when functional impairment is significant.[9] Although occipital neuralgia was in the differential, the lack of lancinating pain and normal neurologic examination made it less likely. Imaging is only indicated in the presence of red flags such as acute onset, neurologic deficits, or history of trauma.[10] This case highlights the importance of a personalized, evidence-based approach to managing complex migraine cases in women.

Clinical Pearls

- Triptans are first-line abortive therapy for moderate to severe migraine attacks, particularly when taken early during an attack.
- NSAIDs can be used in combination with triptans for better acute relief, especially if inflammation plays a role (e.g., menstrual migraines).
- Prophylactic therapy is often necessary for the following reasons:
  - Migraines occur ≥4 days/month.
  - Attacks are prolonged, disabling, or poorly responsive to acute treatment.
  - Patient prefers to reduce attack frequency/severity.
- Topiramate, propranolol, and amitriptyline are common first-line preventive medications.
- CGRP antagonists (e.g., erenumab, fremanezumab) are effective, newer options for patients who fail traditional prophylaxis or have frequent attacks.
- Medication overuse headache (MOH) should be considered when abortive meds (especially triptans, NSAIDs, caffeine-containing analgesics) are used >10–15 days/month.
- Lifestyle modification is essential: regular sleep, hydration, stress management, and trigger avoidance help improve outcomes significantly—even without pharmacotherapy.

- A headache diary is a valuable tool for identifying triggers, patterns, and treatment responses.
- Patient education and expectations matter: migraine is a chronic condition; success means improvement, not necessarily elimination. Preventive medications may take 4–8 weeks to show effect.

References

1. Headache Classification Committee of the International Headache Society (IHS). *The International Classification of Headache Disorders*, 3rd edition. Cephalalgia. 2018;38(1):1–211. doi:10.1177/0333102417738202
2. Stewart WF, Staffa J, Lipton RB, Ottman R. Familial risk of migraine: A population-based study. Ann Neurol. 1997;41(2):166–172. doi:10.1002/ana.410410205
3. Goadsby PJ, et al. Pathophysiology of migraine: A disorder of sensory processing. Physiol Rev. 2017;97(2):553–622. doi:10.1152/physrev.00034.2015
4. Silberstein SD. Preventive treatment of headaches. Curr Opin Neurol. 2005;18(3):289–292. doi:10.1097/01.wco.0000169747.67653.f3
5. Dodick DW, Turkel CC, DeGryse RE, et al. OnabotulinumtoxinA for treatment of chronic migraine: Pooled results from the double-blind, randomized, placebo-controlled phases of the PREEMPT clinical program. Headache. 2010;50(6):921–936. doi:10.1111/j.1526-4610.2010.01678.x
6. Levin M. Nerve blocks in the treatment of headache. Neurotherapeutics. 2010;7(2):197–203. doi:10.1016/j.nurt.2010.03.001
7. Bautista, A. L., Coyne, K., Bautista, A., & Abd-Elsayed, A. (2025). Sphenopalatine ganglion blocks in headache management: A review. *Brain Sciences, 15*(7), 672. https://doi.org/10.3390/brainsci15070672
8. Lipton RB, Dodick DW, Silberstein SD, et al. Single-pulse transcranial magnetic stimulation for acute treatment of migraine with aura: A randomized, double-blind, parallel-group, sham-controlled trial. Lancet Neurol. 2010;9(4):373–380. doi:10.1016/S1474-4422(10)70054-5
9. Barmherzig R, Kingston W. Occipital nerve blocks in the management of headache and cranial neuralgias: A narrative review. Headache. 2019;59(3):339–357. doi:10.1111/head.13482
10. Marmura MJ, Silberstein SD, Schwedt TJ. The acute treatment of migraine in adults: The American Headache Society evidence assessment. Headache. 2015;55(1):3–20. doi:10.1111/head.12499

PART III

THORACIC AND CHEST WALL PAIN

12
Anatomical Considerations of the Female Thorax and Chest Wall

Thanh Thanh Tran and Ahmed Alassal

Introduction

The thoracic and chest wall serve as protective and dynamic structures that enclose vital organs such as the heart and the lungs while facilitating respiration and upper body movement. In females, this region has unique anatomical considerations, particularly due to the presence of breast tissue, which is affected by hormonal influences and biomechanical adaptations related to pregnancy and posture.

The female thoracic wall demonstrates greater flexibility compared to a male, with increased rib cage elasticity that accommodates diaphragmatic movement during pregnancy but may also contribute to musculoskeletal strain,[1–3] A thorough understanding of these structures, from superficial to deep, is essential for anesthesiologists managing pain syndromes, performing regional blocks, or evaluating postoperative complications.

Boundaries of the Thoracic Wall

The thoracic cage creates a protective bony enclosure with clear borders. These boundaries show significant differences in females that affect both function and clinical care.

Superior Boundary

The thoracic inlet measures about 5 cm front to back and 10 cm side to side. It has three main borders. The anterior border is the superior margin of the manubrium. The posterior border is the first thoracic vertebra. The lateral borders are the first ribs. This tight space allows passage for the trachea, esophagus, and major blood vessels. Females have a smaller thoracic inlet than males,[3,4] which could potentially increase pressure on nearby structures. Just beyond the inlet lies the thoracic outlet—the space between the first rib and clavicle. This area is prone to pinching nerves and blood vessels, explaining why females more often develop thoracic outlet syndrome.[5]

Inferior Boundary

The diaphragm forms the floor of the thorax. It is attached to three areas. The anterior portion attaches to the xiphoid process. The lateral portions attach to the lower six ribs. The posterior portion attaches to the upper lumbar vertebrae. The central part of the diaphragm sits at the level of the eighth thoracic vertebra when breathing out.

Anterior Boundary

The sternum and costal cartilages make up the anterior thoracic wall. Females' sternums differ from males in many key ways. They are approximately 15% shorter, the sternal angles are wider, and the bone itself is thinner.[6] The costal cartilages stretch more easily. These differences help accommodate pregnancy and may lead to a decrease in fractures.[2,7]

Posterior Boundary

The posterior thoracic wall consists of 12 thoracic vertebrae and their associated ribs. Females tend to have a more curved upper back compared to males,[8] with their vertebrae being smaller[1] and their ligaments more stretchable.[9,10] This affects how weight spreads across the thoracic spine and may explain why females have more mid-back pain.[11] The costovertebral and costotransverse joints allow the ribs to move like bucket handles during respiration while keeping the spine stable.

Lateral Boundary

The lateral thoracic walls are formed by the 12 ribs, with intercostal muscles filling the spaces between them. In females, the ribs have thinner outer layers (cortical bone),[12] making them more flexible and sharply angled downward.[3] This enhances thoracic expansion during pregnancy but may also increase the risk of rib fractures.[13] Between each rib, two intercostal neurovascular bundles run along the superior and inferior margins. Each bundle contains an intercostal vein, artery, and nerve—arranged in that order from superior to inferior (Figure 12.1 and Figure 12.2).

Structures of the Thoracic Wall

The Female Breast

The breast is a defining superficial structure in females, positioned between the second and sixth ribs and extending from the sternum to the midaxillary line. It lies over the pectoralis major muscle and is anchored by Cooper's ligaments (suspensory ligaments of the breast), which are fibrous bands that provide structural support through their

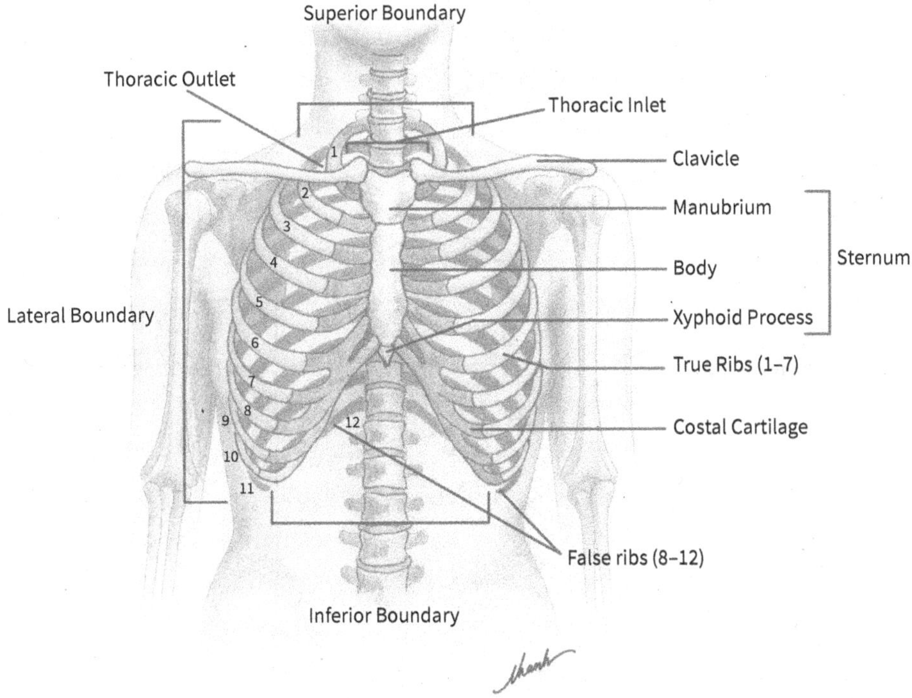

Figure 12.1 Anterior view of the female thoracic skeleton illustrating the anatomical boundaries of the thoracic wall.

attachments to both the superficial fascia and deep pectoral fascia. These ligaments can become stretched, particularly in females with macromastia or during pregnancy, leading to discomfort and chronic tension-related pain because they support breast weight against gravity.

The breast parenchyma consists of 15–20 lobes arranged radially, each containing lobules that terminate in lactiferous ducts converging at the nipple. The ductal system is embedded in adipose tissue that varies in volume with body weight and hormonal status. The nipple-areolar complex contains smooth muscle fibers that contract during lactation or stimulation, with sensory innervation primarily from the fourth intercostal nerve (T4 dermatome). The retromammary space, a potential area between the glandular breast tissue and the pectoral fascia, allows for mobility but can also serve as a site of seroma formation postoperatively following thoracic trauma.[14]

Clinical Correlation

Cyclic mastalgia, a common condition in premenopausal females, results from hormonal fluctuations and presents as diffuse breast tenderness typically peaking during the luteal phase of the menstrual cycle.

Postmastectomy pain syndrome (PMPS) can arise from injury to the intercostobrachial nerve (T2), medial pectoral nerve, or long thoracic nerve during breast surgery, as well as

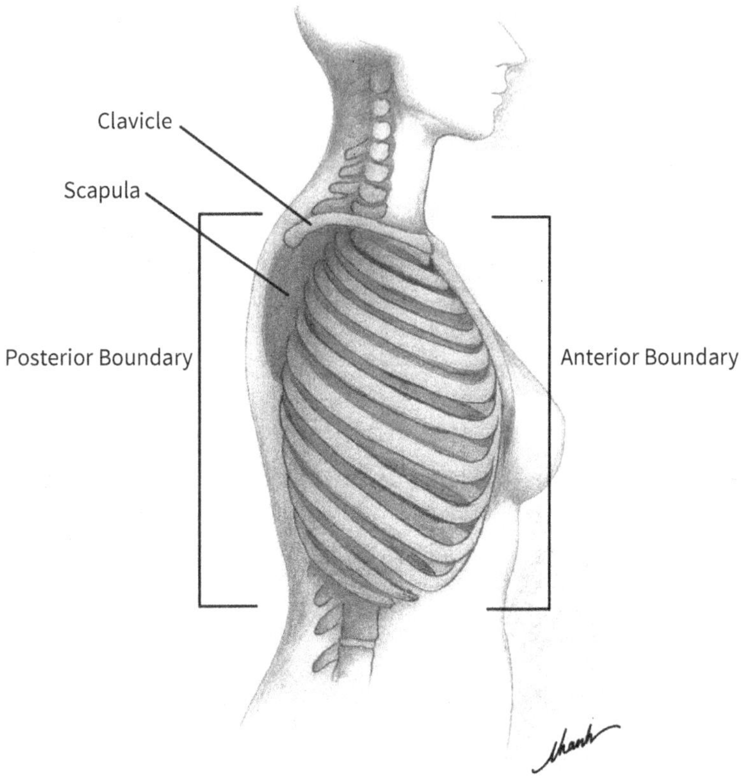

Figure 12.2 Lateral view of the female thoracic cage demonstrating the anterior and posterior boundaries.

from intercostal nerve injury due to chest tube placement. These injuries may result in persistent neuropathic pain in 20–68% of patients.[15]

The horizontal septum—a fibrous attachment between the breast tissue and the pectoral fascia—is particularly relevant in reconstructive surgery because its preservation helps maintain natural breast contour (Figure 12.3).

Fascial Layers of the Thoracic Wall

Beneath the subcutaneous tissue, the superficial fascia contains mammary glandular tissue that varies in thickness with body habitus. The pectoral fascia envelops the pectoralis major, continuing laterally as the axillary fascia. Deep to this, the clavipectoral fascia spans from the clavicle to the axilla, enclosing the pectoralis minor. The endothoracic fascia lines the inner thoracic wall, creating a potential space between intercostal muscles and parietal pleura that permits smooth respiratory movement. These fascial planes become clinically significant during breast reconstruction and thoracic regional anesthesia techniques.

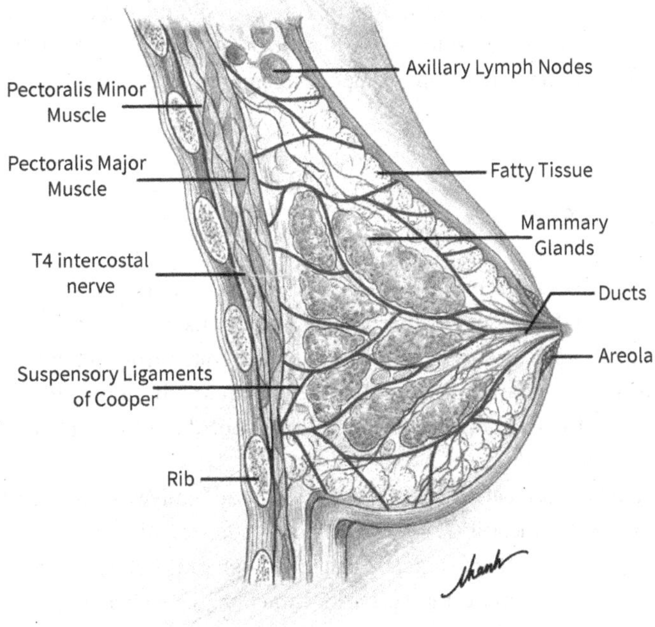

Figure 12.3 Cross-sectional anatomy of the female breast and underlying chest wall structures.

Muscles of the Thoracic Wall

The thoracic musculature is organized into superficial and deep layers, each contributing to respiration, posture, and upper limb movement.

Superficial Muscles

The pectoralis major has clavicular, sternocostal, and abdominal portions that converge into a flat tendon inserting on the intertubercular sulcus of the humerus. This arrangement allows it to act as both a respiratory accessory muscle and a prime mover for arm adduction. Overusing the arms—such as from repetitive movements at work—or having poor posture (especially in females with macromastia) can cause muscle knots called *myofascial trigger points.*[16] These trigger points can cause pain that spreads to the anterior thoracic wall and the medial aspect of the upper arm.[17]

The pectoralis minor, attaching to the coracoid process of the scapula, maintains scapular position; its tightness in thoracic outlet syndrome compresses the brachial plexus and subclavian vessels between itself and the first rib, particularly in females with narrow thoracic inlets.

The serratus anterior, innervated by the long thoracic nerve (C5–C7), originates from the first to ninth ribs and inserts along the medial border of the scapula.[18] Its lower fibers are most vulnerable to injury during prolonged recumbent positioning or improper crutch use, potentially causing scapular dyskinesis that manifests as shoulder pain and periscapular discomfort.[18,19] The latissimus dorsi forms part of the posterior axillary fold. Its connection to the thoracolumbar fascia allows lumbar paraspinal strain to refer pain to the inferolateral thoracic wall.

Respiratory Muscles

The external intercostals run inferomedially and are most active during inspiration, while the internal intercostals (oriented superomedially) dominate forced expiration. The innermost intercostal layer shares this orientation but is separated from the internal layer by the intercostal neurovascular bundle, making it a key landmark for nerve blocks. The subcostal muscles, present in the inferior thoracic cage, may contribute to postthoracotomy neuropathic pain when damaged.

The diaphragm has costal attachments to ribs 7–12 and lumbar crura extending to L3.[20] Its phrenic nerve (C3–C5) innervation[20] means cervical radiculopathy can cause referred pain to the acromial region,[21] while diaphragmatic irritation often causes referred pain to the shoulder but may also cause discomfort near its costal attachments.[20] During pregnancy, the diaphragm elevates up to 4 cm, reducing functional residual capacity while increasing subcostal angle expansion, which may strain costotransverse joints, resulting in back or rib pain[22] (Figure 12.4).

Bones and Cartilaginous Structures

The thoracic skeleton comprises the rib cage, sternum, and thoracic vertebrae (T1–T12), forming the bony framework of the chest wall.

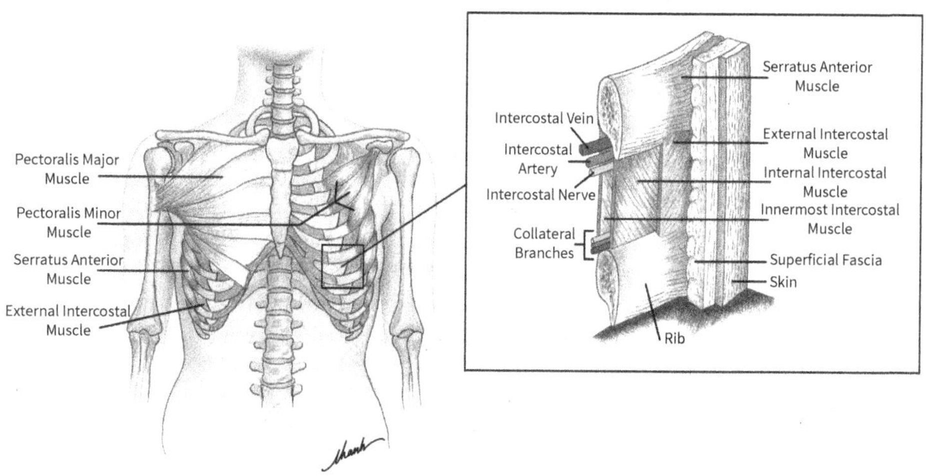

Figure 12.4 Musculature of the female chest wall and cross-sectional anatomy of the intercostal space.

Rib Cage

The first rib is the shortest and broadest, with scalene tubercle attachments that are common sites for thoracic outlet compression. Ribs 2–10 demonstrate increasing length and curvature, with the costal groove protecting the intercostal neurovascular bundle along each inferior rib margin. The costal angle (where the rib turns anterolaterally) is a key landmark for thoracentesis.

Clinical Correlation

Costochondritis typically affects the second to fifth costal cartilages, with females showing higher prevalence[23] possibly due to hormonal effects on connective tissue.[24] Rib fractures in osteoporosis most commonly occur at the posterolateral bend, where mechanical stress concentrates during breathing.[25,26]

Sternum and Thoracic Vertebrae

The sternal angle (of Louis) at vertebral levels T4–T5 demarcates the aortic arch and tracheal bifurcation. The xiphoid process, often asymmetrical, can be mistaken for an abdominal mass when prominent. Thoracic vertebrae have superior and inferior costal facets articulating with the rib head and transverse processes connecting to the tubercle, forming a dual joint system that allows the "bucket handle" rib motion during respiration. Degenerative changes in this area may cause mid-back pain radiating along the dermatomal distribution of the intercostal nerves.

Thoracic Joints and Articulations

The costovertebral joints connect rib heads to vertebral bodies through paired synovial articulations at each level, stabilized by intra-articular ligaments. Sternocostal joints demonstrate progressive mobility from the first rib's synchondrosis to the true synovial joints of ribs 2–7. The costotransverse joints between the rib tubercles and transverse processes guide rib motion during respiration while limiting excessive movement.

Innervation of the Thoracic Wall

The intercostal nerves (T1–T11) give off collateral branches that innervate the pleura before terminating as anterior cutaneous nerves emerging parasternally. The lateral cutaneous branches pierce the musculature near the midaxillary line, making these zones particularly sensitive in neuralgia. The long thoracic nerve (C5–C7) descends along the serratus anterior surface, vulnerable to traction injury during mastectomy or prolonged lateral decubitus positioning.

Thoracic Dermatomes and Pain Mapping

The thoracic dermatomes form horizontal bands with T4 at nipple level and T10 at the umbilicus. These demonstrate considerable overlap, explaining why single nerve root compression rarely causes complete anesthesia but rather produces hyperalgesia in characteristic distributions. Visceral referred pain patterns often follow these dermatomes, with cardiac ischemia typically manifesting in T1–T4 and gallbladder disease in T6–T9 regions.

Clinical Correlation

Postherpetic neuralgia most frequently involves T5–T10 dermatomes, with females older than 60 having a higher risk of chronic pain.[27] Intercostal nerve blocks require needle placement at the angle of the rib to avoid the collateral nerve branch while ensuring adequate medial spread of local anesthetic (Figure 12.5).

Blood Supply and Lymphatic Drainage

Arterial Supply

The internal thoracic artery gives off perforating branches that supply the medial breast and anterior thoracic wall, with the second intercostal space perforator often enlarged in macromastia. The lateral thoracic artery runs with the long thoracic nerve, making it susceptible to

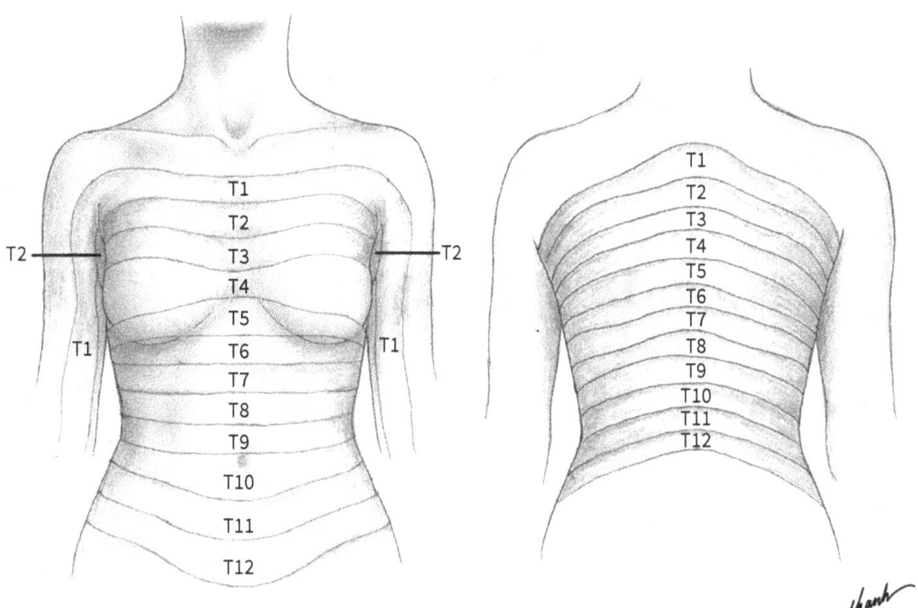

Figure 12.5 Dermatomal distribution of thoracic spinal nerves (T1–T12) in the female torso, anterior and posterior views.

injury during axillary procedures. Posterior intercostal arteries pass between the innermost and internal intercostal muscles, explaining why deep paravertebral or intercostal injections may risk vascular puncture.

Lymphatic System

The axillary lymph nodes are stratified into Level I (lateral to pectoralis minor), Level II (posterior to the muscle), and Level III (medial to the pectoralis minor). Rotter's nodes (interpectoral lymph nodes) between the pectoralis major and minor muscles represent an often-missed metastatic site. The parasternal nodes follow the internal thoracic vessels and may cause referred pain to the precordium when involved. Lymphaticovenous anastomosis in the breast explains why lymphedema can develop even with sentinel lymph node biopsy alone.

Clinical Correlation

Lymphedema risk increases when radiation follows axillary dissection, with symptoms often emerging months later as fibrosis progresses.[28] Manual lymphatic drainage techniques must account for alternative drainage pathways through the intercostal spaces to the parasternal nodes[29] (Figure 12.6).

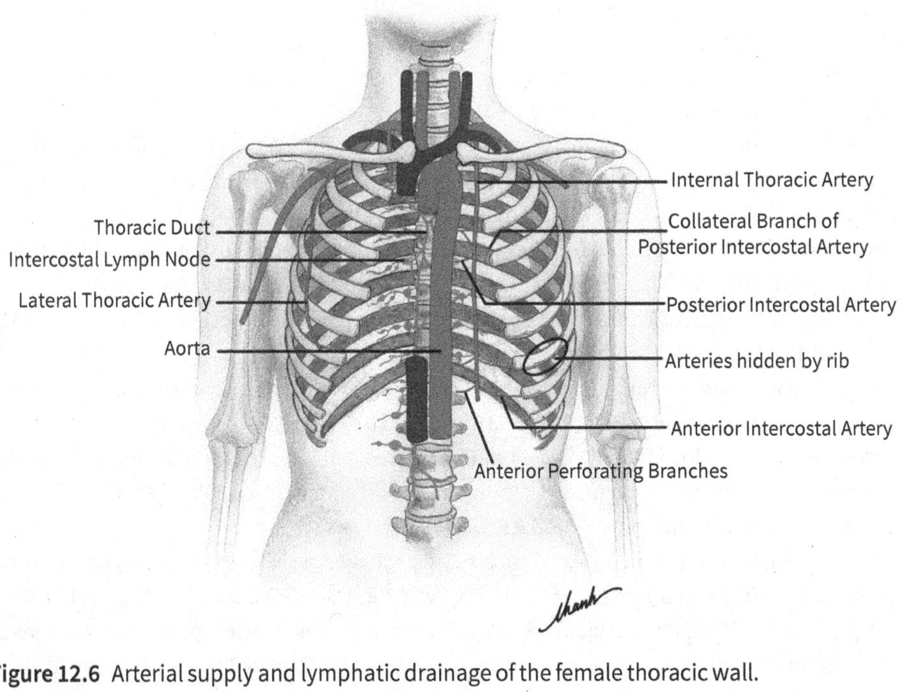

Figure 12.6 Arterial supply and lymphatic drainage of the female thoracic wall.

Conclusion

The female thoracic and chest wall demonstrates unique anatomical adaptations that influence both normal function and pain pathogenesis. From the hormonal responsiveness of breast tissue to the biomechanical stresses on the rib cage during pregnancy, these sex-specific factors require careful consideration in pain management. The subsequent chapter will apply this anatomical framework to clinical scenarios, exploring how structural relationships guide diagnostic and therapeutic interventions for thoracic pain syndromes in females.

Acknowledgments

The following standard anatomy resources were consulted for general anatomical accuracy in creating these original illustrations.

- *Grant's Dissector*, 16th edition: edited by Alan J. Detton[30]
- *Gray's Anatomy for Students*, 3rd edition; edited by Richard L. Drake, A. Wayne Vogl, Adam W. M. Mitchell[31]
- *Gray's Atlas of Anatomy*, 3rd edition: edited by Richard L. Drake, A. Wayne Vogl, Adam W. M. Mitchell, Richard M. Tibbitts, Paul E. Richardson[32]
- *Netter's Anatomy Coloring Book*, 2nd edition: edited by John T. Hansen
- *The Anatomy Coloring Book*, 4th edition: Wynn Kapit, Lawrence M. Elson
- Complete Anatomy program

References

1. Gilsanz V, Boechat MI, Gilsanz R, Loro ML, Roe TF, Goodman WG. Gender differences in vertebral sizes in adults: Biomechanical implications. Radiology. 1994;190(3):678–682. doi:10.1148/radiology.190.3.8115610
2. Goh MH, Anderson DE. Bending properties of human cartilaginous ribs and costal cartilage material vary with age, sex, and calcification. JBMR Plus. 2024;9(1):ziae153. doi:10.1093/jbmrpl/ziae153
3. Bellemare F, Jeanneret A, Couture J. Sex differences in thoracic dimensions and configuration. Am J Respir Crit Care Med. 2003;168(3):305–312. doi:10.1164/rccm.200208-876OC
4. LoMauro A, Aliverti A. Sex differences in respiratory function. Breathe (Sheff). 2018;14(2):131–140. doi:10.1183/20734735.000318
5. Illig KA, Rodriguez-Zoppi E, Bland T, Muftah M, Jospitre E. The incidence of thoracic outlet syndrome. Ann Vasc Surg. 2021;70:263–272. doi:10.1016/j.avsg.2020.07.029
6. Ateşoğlu S, Deniz M, Uslu AI. Evaluation of the morphological characteristic and sex differences of sternum by multi-detector computed tomography. Folia Morphol (Warsz). 2018;77(3):489–497. doi:10.5603/FM.a2018.0002
7. Di Napoli M, DeVoe WB, Leon S, et al. Decreased incidence of rib fractures in pregnant patients after motor vehicle collisions. Am J Crit Care. 2021;30(5):385–390. doi:10.4037/ajcc2021505
8. Ohlendorf D, Avaniadi I, Adjami F, et al. Standard values of the upper body posture in healthy adults with special regard to age, sex and BMI. Sci Rep. 2023;13(1):873. doi:10.1038/s41598-023-27976-8

9. Birt KM, McCarthy HE. The effect of estrogen on anterior cruciate ligament structure and function: A systematic review. J Musculoskelet Disord Treat. 2023;9:127. doi:10.23937/2572-3243.1510127
10. Östh, J., Brolin, K., Svensson, M. Y., & Linder, A. (2016). A female ligamentous cervical spine finite element model validated for physiological loads. *Journal of Biomechanical Engineering, 138*(6), 061005. https://doi.org/10.1115/1.4032966
11. Leboeuf-Yde C, Nielsen J, Kyvik KO, Fejer R, Hartvigsen J. Pain in the lumbar, thoracic or cervical regions: Do age and gender matter? A population-based study of 34,902 Danish twins 20–71 years of age. BMC Musculoskelet Disord. 2009;10:39. doi:10.1186/1471-2474-10-39
12. Holcombe SA, Derstine BA. Rib cortical bone thickness variation in adults by age and sex. J Anat. 2022;241(6):1344–1356. doi:10.1111/joa.13751
13. Sajjan SG, Barrett-Connor E, McHorney CA, et al. Rib fracture as a predictor of future fractures in young and older postmenopausal women: National Osteoporosis Risk Assessment (NORA). Osteoporos Int. 2012;23(3):821–828. doi:10.1007/s00198-011-1757-0
14. Srivastava V, Basu S, Shukla VK. Seroma formation after breast cancer surgery: What we have learned in the last two decades. J Breast Cancer. 2012;15(4):373–380. doi:10.4048/jbc.2012.15.4.373
15. Salati SA, Alsulaim L, Alharbi MH, et al. Postmastectomy pain syndrome: A narrative review. Cureus. 2023;15(10):e47384. doi:10.7759/cureus.47384
16. Alvarez DJ, Rockwell PG. Trigger points: Diagnosis and management. Am Fam Physician. 2002;65(4):653–660.
17. Bautista A, Webb C, Rosenquist R. Serratus anterior muscle pain syndrome: A diagnostic conundrum. Pain Med. 2017;18(8):1600–1602. doi:10.1093/pm/pnw350
18. Martin RM, Fish DE. Scapular winging: Anatomical review, diagnosis, and treatments. Curr Rev Musculoskelet Med. 2008;1(1):1–11. doi:10.1007/s12178-007-9000-5
19. Panagiotopoulos AC, Crowther IM. Scapular dyskinesia, the forgotten culprit of shoulder pain and how to rehabilitate. SICOT J. 2019;5:29. doi:10.1051/sicotj/2019029
20. Bordoni B, Kotha R, Escher AR. Symptoms arising from the diaphragm muscle: Function and dysfunction. Cureus. 2024;16(1):e53143. doi:10.7759/cureus.53143
21. Mimori K, Muneta T, Komori H, Okawa A, Shinomiya K. Relation between the painful shoulder and the cervical spine with narrow canal in patients without obvious radiculopathy. J Shoulder Elbow Surg. 1999;8(4):303–306. doi:10.1016/s1058-2746(99)90150-7
22. Jha S, Nagargoje DA. Pulmonary function in third trimester: A cross-sectional study. VIMS J Phys Ther. 2021;3(1):4–9. doi:10.46858.VIMSJPT.3101
23. Mott T, Jones G, Roman K. Costochondritis: Rapid evidence review. Am Fam Physician. 2021;104(1):73–78.
24. Samimi K. *An Overview of Costochondral Disorders.* Master's thesis. Boston University; 2023. Accessed June 2025. https://open.bu.edu/handle/2144/43727
25. Tang Y, Hong W, Xu X, Li M, Jin L. Traumatic rib fracture patterns associated with bone mineral density statuses derived from CT images. Front Endocrinol (Lausanne). 2023;14:1304219. doi:10.3389/fendo.2023.1304219
26. Liebsch C, Seiffert T, Vlcek M, et al. Patterns of serial rib fractures after blunt chest trauma: An analysis of 380 cases. PLoS One. 2019;14(12):e0224105. doi:10.1371/journal.pone.0224105
27. Forbes HJ, Thomas SL, Smeeth L, et al. A systematic review and meta-analysis of risk factors for postherpetic neuralgia. Pain. 2016;157(1):30–54. doi:10.1097/j.pain.0000000000000307
28. Allam O, Park KE, Chandler L, et al. The impact of radiation on lymphedema: A review of the literature. Gland Surg. 2020;9(2):596–602. doi:10.21037/gs.2020.03.20

29. Overall B, Langley K, Douglass J. Manual lymph drainage for post-COVID-19 related cough, breathlessness, and fatigue: Two case reports. Healthcare (Basel). 2023;11(23):3085. doi:10.3390/healthcare11233085
30. Detton AJ. *Grant's Dissector*. 16th ed. Wolters Kluwer; 2017.
31. Drake RL, Vogl AW, Mitchell AWM. *Gray's Anatomy for Students*. 3rd ed. Elsevier; 2015.
32. Drake RL, Vogl AW, Mitchell AWM, Tibbitts RM, Richardson PE. *Gray's Atlas of Anatomy*. 3rd ed. Elsevier; 2015.

13
Common Thoracic Pain Conditions in Women

Joseph A. McGuire and Richard Vaglienti

Introduction

Thoracic pain conditions can arise from a wide range of etiologies, including musculoskeletal, infectious, cardiovascular, pulmonary, neuropathic origins. While many of these conditions affect both sexes, certain disorders disproportionately impact women due to hormonal influences, anatomical differences, lifestyle factors. This chapter explores thoracic pain conditions commonly seen in women, discussing their pathophysiology, clinical presentation, implications for management.

Costochondritis

Epidemiology and Pathophysiology

Costochondritis, an inflammatory condition affecting the costosternal junctions, is a common cause of anterior chest pain. It is often idiopathic but can result from repetitive strain, poor posture, or systemic inflammatory diseases such as rheumatoid arthritis and other autoimmune disorders. Women, particularly those older than 40, experience costochondritis more frequently than do men.[1] Hormonal fluctuations, particularly estrogen levels, have been suggested as a contributing factor in the higher prevalence of this condition in women.

Clinical Presentation

Patients typically present with localized pain and tenderness over the costosternal joints, often exacerbated by movement, deep breathing, or palpation. Unlike cardiac pain, costochondritis pain does not radiate and is not relieved by nitrates. Some women report an association with stress and hormonal changes, indicating a possible interaction between inflammatory pathways and the endocrine system.

Management

Treatment includes nonsteroidal anti-inflammatory drugs (NSAIDs), heat therapy, stretching, postural correction. Patients are encouraged to modify activities that exacerbate symptoms, physical therapy may be beneficial. In resistant cases, local corticosteroid injections may provide relief. Emerging research suggests that dietary modifications, such as reducing inflammatory foods, may play a role in symptom management.

Mastitis and Breast Pain (Mastalgia)

Epidemiology and Pathophysiology

Mastitis, an infection of the breast tissue, is most common in lactating women but can also occur in nonlactating individuals, particularly those with diabetes or immunosuppression.[2] It is caused by bacterial infiltration, often from *Staphylococcus aureus*, which enters the breast tissue through cracked or irritated skin, commonly occurring during breastfeeding.

Cyclical mastalgia, associated with hormonal fluctuations, is a significant source of thoracic discomfort in premenopausal women. The condition is often linked to changes in estrogen and progesterone levels during the menstrual cycle, which cause ductal and stromal tissue changes in the breast.

Clinical Presentation

Mastitis presents with localized breast pain, swelling, redness, systemic symptoms such as fever and malaise. In more severe cases, abscess formation may occur, requiring drainage.

Noninfectious mastalgia can be diffuse, cyclical, linked to the menstrual cycle. Some women report tenderness that worsens before menstruation and subsides afterward. Hormonal contraceptives and hormone replacement therapy (HRT) can also influence mastalgia symptoms.

Management

Lactational mastitis is treated with antibiotics and continued breastfeeding to prevent milk stasis. Noninfectious mastalgia may respond to dietary modifications (e.g., reducing caffeine intake), hormonal therapy adjustments, or analgesics. Evening primrose oil and vitamin E supplements have been explored as potential treatments, although evidence remains inconclusive.

Cardiac Pain and Gender Differences in Ischemic Heart Disease

Epidemiology and Pathophysiology

Women with ischemic heart disease often present with atypical symptoms, leading to underdiagnosis and delays in treatment. Microvascular dysfunction plays a more significant role in female cardiac pain compared to obstructive coronary artery disease.[3] Additionally, women are more likely to have coronary vasospasm, stress cardiomyopathy (Takotsubo syndrome), endothelial dysfunction, which contribute to thoracic pain but may not be detected using standard diagnostic tests.

Clinical Presentation

Instead of classic exertional chest pain, women may report epigastric discomfort, dyspnea, nausea, fatigue, palpitations, back pain. These symptoms often lead to misattribution to anxiety, gastrointestinal disorders, or musculoskeletal issues, delaying appropriate cardiovascular care.

Management

Risk factor modification, lifestyle changes, medical therapy (e.g., beta-blockers, aspirin, statins) are central to management. Increased awareness of sex-specific presentations is crucial for improving diagnostic accuracy and treatment outcomes. Advanced imaging techniques such as coronary microvascular function testing may help in diagnosing women with nonobstructive coronary artery disease. If true coronary artery disease is confirmed all the usual therapies are in play.

Pleurisy and Pulmonary Embolism Pain

Epidemiology and Pathophysiology

Pleuritic chest pain, caused by inflammation of the pleura, can result from infections, autoimmune conditions (such as lupus), or pulmonary embolism (PE). Women with risk factors such as oral contraceptive use, pregnancy, recent surgery, or prolonged immobilization are at heightened risk for PE.[4] The hypercoagulable state of pregnancy and postpartum increases the risk significantly, making awareness and early intervention critical.

Clinical Presentation

Pleuritic pain is sharp and worsens with inspiration or coughing. PE may also present with dyspnea, tachycardia, hemoptysis. In pregnant women, PE is a leading cause of maternal mortality, often presenting with subtle symptoms such as shortness of breath and unexplained fatigue rather than classic pleuritic pain.

Management

Pleuritic pain management involves treating the underlying cause, such as antibiotics for infectious pleuritis or anti-inflammatory medications for autoimmune causes. PE requires anticoagulation therapy, with low-molecular-weight heparin being the preferred option during pregnancy. In severe cases, thrombolytic therapy or surgical thrombectomy may be necessary.

Shingles (Herpes Zoster) and Postherpetic Neuralgia

Epidemiology and Pathophysiology

Herpes zoster, reactivation of the varicella-zoster virus, disproportionately affects postmenopausal women due to immune senescence.[5] Additionally, stress and hormonal fluctuations may influence susceptibility to viral reactivation.

Clinical Presentation

Pain precedes the rash, often localized to a unilateral thoracic dermatome. The rash consists of vesicular lesions following a nerve distribution. Persistent neuropathic pain (postherpetic neuralgia) is more common in older women, affecting quality of life and increasing the risk of depression and sleep disturbances.

Management

Antiviral therapy (acyclovir, valacyclovir) reduces severity and duration if initiated early. Postherpetic neuralgia is managed with gabapentinoids, tricyclic antidepressants, or lidocaine patches. Vaccination (Shingrix) is highly effective in preventing herpes zoster and should be recommended for women older than 50.

Postmastectomy Pain Syndrome

Epidemiology and Pathophysiology

Post-mastectomy pain syndrome (PMPS) is a chronic neuropathic pain condition that affects up to 20–60% of women following mastectomy or breast-conserving surgery.[6,7] It typically arises within the first few months after surgery and persists for >3 months. The pain is believed to result from damage or entrapment of the intercostobrachial nerve (ICBN) during axillary lymph node dissection, as well as nerve injury from retraction, radiation, or scar tissue formation.[8] Risk factors include younger age, high body mass index (BMI), axillary lymph node dissection (vs. sentinel node biopsy), preexisting pain conditions, adjuvant radiation therapy. Notably, women with a history of anxiety or depression, or those undergoing more extensive surgery, report higher rates of PMPS, underscoring the biopsychosocial complexity of the condition.[9]

Clinical Presentation

Patients with PMPS commonly describe a burning, shooting, or stabbing pain localized to the anterior chest wall, axilla, /or upper arm. Hypoesthesia, allodynia, or paresthesia in the distribution of the ICBN is frequently reported. The pain can be spontaneous or provoked by movement, touch, or clothing pressure and often leads to functional limitations, sleep disturbances, psychological distress. Many patients also experience pain-related body image disturbances or fear of cancer recurrence, compounding emotional distress.

Management

Management of PMPS requires a multimodal approach. First-line treatments include gabapentinoids (e.g., gabapentin or pregabalin) and tricyclic antidepressants, targeting neuropathic mechanisms.[10] Topical agents like lidocaine patches or capsaicin cream may provide localized relief. Physical therapy and desensitization techniques can improve range of motion and reduce central sensitization. Psychological support, including cognitive behavioral therapy, is essential, especially in women with coexisting mood disorders. Interventional options include intercostal nerve blocks or trigger point injections in refractory cases. Prevention strategies such as nerve-sparing surgical techniques and preoperative education may reduce PMPS incidence.[11]

Conclusion

Thoracic pain in women spans a diverse spectrum of conditions, each with unique pathophysiological underpinnings and clinical implications. Awareness of sex-specific presentations and risk factors is essential to ensuring timely diagnosis and appropriate management.

References

1. Schumann JA, Sood T, Parente JJ. Costochondritis. StatPearls Publishing; 2025 Jan. https://www.ncbi.nlm.nih.gov/books/NBK532931/
2. Jahanfar S, Ng CJ, Teng CL, Ho JJ. Antibiotics for mastitis in breastfeeding women. Cochrane Database Syst Rev. 2022;2:CD005458.
3. Mehta PK, Wei J, Wenger, N. K. (2020). Ischemic heart disease in women: A focus on risk factors. Trends Cardiovasc Med. 2020;30(3):140–151.
4. Tritschler T, Kraaijpoel N, Le Gal G, Wells PS. Venous thromboembolism: Advances in diagnosis and treatment. JAMA. 2018;322(11):1037–1050.
5. Gagliardi AMZ, Andriolo BN, Torloni MR, Soares BGO, de Oliveira Gomes J. Vaccines for preventing herpes zoster in older adults. Cochrane Database Syst Rev. 2021(10):CD008858.
6. Gärtner R, Jensen MB, Nielsen J, Ewertz M, Kroman N, Kehlet H. Prevalence of and factors associated with persistent pain following breast cancer surgery. JAMA. 2009;302(18):1985–1992. https://doi.org/10.1001/jama.2009.1568

7. Andersen KG, Kehlet H. Persistent pain after breast cancer treatment: A critical review of risk factors and strategies for prevention. J Pain. 2011;12(7):725–746. https://doi.org/10.1016/j.jpain.2010.12.005
8. Juhl AA, Lund J, Andersen KG. Focal neuropathic pain after breast cancer surgery. Pain Manage. 2020;10(2):99–111. https://doi.org/10.2217/pmt-2019-0051
9. Mejdahl MK, Andersen KG, Gärtner R, Kroman N, Kehlet H. Persistent pain and sensory disturbances after treatment for breast cancer: Six-year nationwide follow-up study. BMJ. 2013;346:f1865. https://doi.org/10.1136/bmj.f1865
10. Smith, E. M. L., Pang, H., Cirrincione, C., et al. (2013). Effect of duloxetine on pain, function, and quality of life among patients with chemotherapy-induced painful peripheral neuropathy: A randomized clinical trial. *JAMA, 309*(13), 1359–1367. https://doi.org/10.1001/jama.2013.2813
11. Bruce, J., Thornton, A. J., Powell, R., et al. (2014). Psychological, surgical, and sociodemographic predictors of pain outcomes after breast cancer surgery: A population-based cohort study. *Pain, 155*(2), 232–243. https://doi.org/10.1016/j.pain.2013.09.028

14
Interventional Treatments for Thoracic and Chest Wall Pain

Loren Shamalov, Yehuda Masturov, and Gary Schwartz

Introduction

Thoracic and chest wall pain arises from a multitude of etiologies. The reported global prevalence of musculoskeletal chest pain presenting to the emergency department is 16%,[1] with women being 2.5 times as likely to experience thoracic spinal and chest pain compared to their male counterparts.[2] Breast cancer is currently the most diagnosed cancer worldwide and may cause significant chest pain in women due to invasive procedures. Chest pain in women may also arise secondary to postmastectomy pain syndrome, afflicting 25–60% of postmastectomy women.[3] Thoracic spinal pain is present in as much as 48% of the general population.[4] Although treatment largely depends on the etiology of pain, the mainstay of musculoskeletal chest pain remains conservative with nonsteroidal anti-inflammatory drugs (NSAIDs), pain control, and heat therapy.[5] However, other causes of chest pain, such as in the setting of postmastectomy pain syndrome, require step-up therapy to address pain. This chapter reviews the available interventional treatments for thoracic and chest wall pain in women.

Background

The chest wall and parietal pleura are innervated by branches of the intercostal nerves. The intercostal nerves course from the intervertebral foramen and into the paravertebral space, where they divide into ventral and dorsal branches. The anterior branches form the intercostal nerves that give off anterior and lateral cutaneous branches.[6] The T2–T6 branches supply the anterolateral chest wall, along with contributions from the pectoral, long thoracic, and supraclavicular nerves.[6] The lateral and anterior muscular branches supply the serratus superior and posterior. The dorsal branches provide innervation to the posterior chest wall.

Intraplexal nerves are also responsible for sensory and motor function of the chest wall. The supraclavicular (C3–C4) nerve supplies the upper chest wall, the thoracodorsal (C6–C8) nerve supplies the latissimus dorsi, the lateral (C5–C7) and medial (C8–T1) pectoral nerves supply the pectoralis major, with the medial pectoral nerve solely supplying the pectoralis minor.[6]

The source of thoracic spinal and referred chest pain stems from spinal facet joints.[4] The medial branches of the dorsal rami innervate the facet joints and the surrounding synovium, subchondral bone, and joint capsule at their corresponding spinal levels. These nerve roots are the targets of interventional pain management for thoracic and chest wall pain.

Overview of Interventional Techniques

Paravertebral Block

The thoracic paravertebral spinal block provides motor, sensory, and sympathetic blockade to the lateral chest and lateral abdomen. Anesthetic injection is directed into the paravertebral space where the dorsal rami, ventral rami, and sympathetic chains of the spinal nerves exit.[7] Moderate pain control to the anterolateral chest wall is achieved because the paravertebral space is continuous with the intercostal space, allowing for the anesthetic to diffuse to the intercostal nerves.[3] Both ultrasound-guided and landmark techniques can be utilized successfully to target the paravertebral space,[6] although superior analgesia with ultrasound guidance has been reported.[8]

Erector Spinae Plane Block

The erector spinae plane block is a paraspinal fascial nerve block targeting the dorsal and ventral rami of the spinal nerves. It anesthetizes the anterior, posterior, and lateral thoracic and abdominal walls, rendering it particularly useful in thoracic and abdominal surgeries.[9] The injection is performed under ultrasound guidance. The anesthetic diffuses both superiorly and inferiorly through connective tissue to provide a multidermatomal block that spans 3–4 thoracic levels.[6]

PECS I and II Blocks

Pectoralis (PECS) I and II blocks are regional anesthetic blocks that target the anterolateral chest wall. The PECS I block involves anesthetic injection into the interpectoral plane to target the medial and lateral pectoral nerves. The PECS II block involves additional injection of local anesthetic within a deeper fascial plane between the pectoralis minor and serratus anterior muscles.[6] This anesthetizes the long thoracic, intercostobrachial, and regional intercostal nerves, providing additional coverage to the anterolateral chest wall and adjacent axilla.[10] The PECS I block can be performed in conjunction with the PECS II block, with both utilized in reconstructive breast surgery.[10]

Serratus Anterior Plane Blocks

The serratus anterior plane block targets the lateral cutaneous branches of T2–T9, long thoracic nerve, thoracodorsal nerve, and intercostobrachial nerve to anesthetize the anterolateral chest wall.[11] Ultrasound-guided injection is directed into an interfascial plane either superficial or deep to the serratus anterior muscle.[12] Due to difficult ultrasound visualization, a complication is pneumothorax.

Transversus Thoracic Plane Block

The transversus thoracic plane block targets the anterior cutaneous branches of the T2–T6 intercostal nerves to provide analgesia to the anterior chest wall.[13] The anesthetic is injected under ultrasound guidance between the internal intercostal and transversus thoracic muscle at T4–T5.[6] Careful attention to avoid the internal thoracic artery between the muscle layers precludes use of this technique. Other potential complications include pneumothorax and pericardial effusion.

Intercostal Nerve Block

Intercostal nerve blocks target the intercostal nerves at the desired thoracic level to provide effective pain relief. The block is performed under ultrasound guidance between the internal and innermost intercostal muscles.[6] Complications include pneumothorax, vascular injury, and anesthetic toxicity secondary to intravascular injection.

Thoracic Facet Joint Injections

To properly utilize thoracic facet joint injections, a diagnostic thoracic medial branch injection must be performed. Diagnosis is confirmed by at least 80% pain relief and ability to perform previously painful maneuvers and concordant relief lasting longer with bupivacaine than lidocaine in accordance with the modified International Association of the Study of Pain (IASP) criteria.[14] Fluoroscopy-guided thoracic facet joint injections target the medial branches of the dorsal rami to provide adequate pain relief in patients with thoracic spinal pain.[4,14]

Botulinum Toxin Injections

Patients may experience painful muscle spasms secondary to postmastectomy pain syndrome due to surgical/reconstructive procedures or radiation. To target muscle hyperspasticity, botulinum toxin injections have been described as an effective reversible paralytic that blocks presynaptic release of acetylcholine to relax muscle fibers.[15] These blocks are also effective in the treatment of neuropathic pain, which may also contribute to muscle hyperspasticity.[3] Multiple ultrasound- or EMG-guided injections are recommended to provide adequate pain relief.

Emerging Trends and Current Research

Adjunctive therapies for thoracic and chest wall pain have become increasingly popular in place of NSAIDs and other analgesics. Stripping massage, a tissue massage technique that targets myofascial trigger points, has demonstrated significant improvements in pain and reduced need for analgesia following thoracoscopic surgery.[16] Acupuncture is an East Asian practice that interconnects the organs, body points, and associated symptoms. Although it is not widely implemented in clinical practice, it has been shown to be effective in the management of acute and postsurgery pain when compared to traditional analgesia.[17] Herbal medicines are an increasingly popular alternative pain therapy that may complement pain management regimens: however, careful consideration of adverse pharmaceutical interactions must be implemented.[18]

Clinical Pearls

- Etiology and location of pain guides appropriate interventional management
- Nerve blocks are typically performed under ultrasound guidance
- Careful consideration of neuroanatomy can target multiple cutaneous innervations due to diffusion of anesthetic

Conclusion

Interventional techniques are essential for managing thoracic and chest wall pain, especially when conservative treatments fail. Ultrasound-guided nerve blocks, tailored to the pain's location and etiology, provide targeted analgesia with minimal systemic effects. A strong understanding of chest wall neuroanatomy enhances procedural precision and outcomes. As adjunct therapies gain traction, anatomy-based interventions remain the cornerstone of effective pain management.

References

1. Mandrekar S, Venkatesan P, Nagaraja R. Prevalence of musculoskeletal chest pain in the emergency department: A systematic review and meta-analysis. Scand J Pain. 2021;21(3):434–444. doi:10.1515/sjpain-2020–0168
2. Fouquet N, Bodin J, Descatha A, et al. Prevalence of thoracic spine pain in a surveillance network. Occup Med (Lond). 2015;65(2):122–5. doi:10.1093/occmed/kqu151
3. Murugappan A, Khanna A. Interventional treatment options for post-mastectomy pain. Curr Oncol Rep. 2023;25(10):1175–1179. doi:10.1007/s11912–023-01435-z
4. Manchikanti L, Kaye A, Soin A, et al. Comprehensive evidence-based guidelines for facet joint interventions in the management of chronic spinal pain: American Society of Interventional Pain Physicians (ASIPP) guidelines facet joint interventions 2020 guidelines. Pain Physician. 2020;23:S1–S127. doi:10.36076/ppj.2020/23/S1

5. Ayloo A, Cvengros T, Marella S. Evaluation and treatment of musculoskeletal chest pain. Prim Care. 2013;40(4):863–887, viii. doi:10.1016/j.pop.2013.08.007
6. Sharma R, Louie A, Thai CP, Dizdarevic A. Chest wall nerve blocks for cardiothoracic, breast surgery, and rib-related pain. Curr Pain Headache Rep. 2022;26(1):43–56. doi:10.1007/s11916-022-01001-5
7. Zheng C, Wang J, Xie S. Ultrasound-guided thoracic paravertebral nerve block on postoperative pain, quality of life, and recovery in patients with non-small-cell lung cancer. Biomed Res Int. 2021:6692815. doi:10.1155/2021/6692815
8. Patnaik R, Chhabra A, Subramaniam R, et al. Comparison of paravertebral block by anatomic landmark technique to ultrasound-guided paravertebral block for breast surgery anesthesia: A randomized controlled trial. Reg Anesth Pain Med. 2018;43(4):385–390. doi:10.1097/aap.0000000000000746
9. Tulgar S, Ahiskalioglu A, De Cassai A, Gurkan Y. Efficacy of bilateral erector spinae plane block in the management of pain: current insights. J Pain Res. 2019;12:2597–2613. doi:10.2147/jpr.S182128
10. Kelava M, Alfirevic A, Bustamante S, Hargrave J, Marciniak D. Regional anesthesia in cardiac surgery: An overview of fascial plane chest wall blocks. Anesth Analg. 2020;131(1):127–135. doi:10.1213/ane.0000000000004682
11. Zocca JA, Chen GH, Puttanniah VG, Hung JC, Gulati A. Ultrasound-guided serratus plane block for treatment of postmastectomy pain syndromes in breast cancer patients: A case series. Pain Pract. 2017;17(1):141–146. doi:10.1111/papr.12482
12. Blanco R, Parras T, McDonnell JG, Prats-Galino A. Serratus plane block: A novel ultrasound-guided thoracic wall nerve block. Anaesthesia. 2013;68(11):1107–1113. doi:10.1111/anae.12344
13. Ueshima H, Kitamura A. Blocking of multiple anterior branches of intercostal nerves (Th2–6) using a transversus thoracic muscle plane block. Reg Anesth Pain Med. 2015;40(4):388. doi:10.1097/aap.0000000000000245
14. Manchikanti L, Singh V, Falco FJ, Cash KA, Pampati V, Fellows B. The role of thoracic medial branch blocks in managing chronic mid and upper back pain: A randomized, double-blind, active-control trial with a 2-year followup. Anesthesiol Res Pract. 2012:585806. doi:10.1155/2012/585806
15. Zehm A, Kamdar M. Palliative uses of botulinum neurotoxin #324. J Palliat Med. 2017;20(3):300–302. doi:10.1089/jpm.2016.0498
16. Hsu J, Yu S-P, Pan C-T, Huang P-M. Stripping massage and literature review in post-thoracoscopic chest pain management. Thorac Cardiovasc Surg. 2023;72(06):465–475. doi:10.1055/a-2137-9035
17. Nielsen A, Dusek JA, Taylor-Swanson L, Tick H. Acupuncture therapy as an evidence-based nonpharmacologic strategy for comprehensive acute pain care: The Academic Consortium Pain Task Force white paper update. Pain Med. 2022;23(9):1582–1612. doi:10.1093/pm/pnac056
18. Jahromi B, Pirvulescu I, Candido KD, Knezevic NN. Herbal medicine for pain management: Efficacy and drug interactions. Pharmaceutics. 2021;13(2):251. doi:10.3390/pharmaceutics13020251

15
Complex Postmastectomy Chest Wall Pain Treated with Targeted Regional Anesthesia

Huy Truong and Ioana Pasca

Clinical Vignette

A 52-year-old woman underwent a left-sided mastectomy with axillary lymph node dissection 4 months ago for invasive ductal carcinoma. She reports persistent burning, stabbing pain in the left chest wall and upper arm that began shortly after surgery and has progressively worsened. She rates the pain as 7/10 in intensity, which is aggravated by arm movement. Multiple pharmacotherapies such as gabapentin and serotonin-noradrenaline reuptake inhibitors (SNRIs) failed to provide sufficient pain relief. She also experiences intermittent tingling and numbness in the area with allodynia. The discomfort has disrupted her sleep and daily activities, leading to emotional distress and concerns about cancer recurrence.

On examination, patient weighs 180 lb. and is 5 ft, 2 in tall. A well-healed, nontender surgical scar is present on the left chest wall, consistent with previous mastectomy. Diffused tenderness on the left chest wall along dermatome 3 and 4 is evoked with light touch. The shoulder's range of motion is intact but limited by pain.

Given the patient's history and physical exam, the patient is likely to suffer chest wall pain secondary to postmastectomy pain syndrome (PMPS). Since pharmacotherapy fails to provide sufficient pain relief, the treatment plan is to perform a thoracic paravertebral (TPVB) block at T3 and T4. Postprocedure, the patient is closely monitored for signs of local anesthetic toxicity or delayed absorption to ensure her safety and optimal outcomes.

Pathophysiology

PMPS is primarily a neuropathic pain condition that develops after mastectomy due to several mechanisms. A key factor is direct injury to the intercostobrachial nerve, which innervates the breast parenchyma and overlying skin. That results in disrupted pain processing and causes abnormal sensations. Additionally, the brachial plexus, long thoracic nerve, and medial and lateral pectoral nerves may also be damaged during the procedure. Other contributing factors include chronic inflammation and fibrosis at the surgical site, as well as the formation of neuromas on pain-sensing fibers or within scar tissue. These changes lead to peripheral nerve sensitization by lowering the firing threshold of nociceptor terminals in the chest wall and their primary afferent neurons. Persistent nerve input further amplifies this process, heightening pain perception through central nervous system alterations.

Risk Factors

The risk factors for PMPS include severe acute postoperative pain, younger age, and higher body mass index. These have been consistently associated with an increased likelihood of chronic chest wall pain. Additionally, the psychosocial factors, such as anxiety, depression, and sleep disturbances, are linked to the greater risk of persistent pain and PMPS. Preoperative pain, smoking, and reduced physical activity further increase this risk. Addressing these factors through comprehensive perioperative management and preventive strategies is crucial for reducing the incidence of PMPS.

Treatment Goals

Since patients with neuropathic pain often respond poorly to standard analgesics like nonsteroidal anti-inflammatory drugs (NSAIDs) and opioids, the initial treatment for PMPS focuses on pharmacotherapy tailored to neuropathic pain. When pharmacotherapy is unsuccessful and surgical options are not viable, as seen in this patient, thoracic nerve block techniques offer a useful alternative for managing chest wall pain.

Clinical Assessment

History focuses on the characteristics of the pain (e.g., burning, tingling), its duration, location, progression, and any aggravating or alleviating factors, along with associated symptoms such as chest wall muscle pain, reduced muscle strength, and limited shoulder range of motion. The physical exam assesses sensory changes (hypersensitivity or hyposensitivity), the range of motion and strength of the ipsilateral arm, the presence of scars, and whether percussion at the scar elicits pain.

A thorough history and physical examination help identify the affected nerves, which are then targeted with perineural injections of local anesthetics, steroids, or neurolytic agents under ultrasound guidance. In situations where pain is widespread or involves multiple nerves, regional or interfascial plane blocks can be employed to achieve effective relief. Absolute contraindications for nerve block include allergy to drug and lack of consent.

Plan of Care

Performing a time-out to confirm the correct patient and procedure prior to procedure reduces medical errors. An anxiolytic with an analgesic can be administered to enhance patient comfort; however, the patient is kept awake to monitor for signs of intraneural injection, such as pain or paresthesia. The use of ultrasound guidance helps minimize complications, including nerve injury, hematoma, and secondary tissue damage. Additionally, local anesthetic systemic toxicity (LAST) can occur after anesthetic administration. Signs of LAST, such as dizziness, tinnitus, seizures, or cardiovascular instability, must be promptly recognized and addressed to ensure patient safety.

Interventional Procedures

Common thoracic nerve block techniques for treating chest wall pain due to PMPS include intercostal nerve block, thoracic paravertebral block, serratus plane block, and erector spinae plane block (ESPB). Ropivacaine or bupivacaine with epinephrine is used to prolong the block's effect. The use of ultrasound guidance significantly reduces the risk of complications, such as pneumothorax.

The intercostal nerve block provides anesthesia and analgesia in a band-like segment. Since the intercostal nerves originate from the ventral rami of thoracic spinal nerves (T1–T12), the block typically covers the dermatome corresponding to the injected level. To perform an intercostal nerve block, position the patient in the prone, lateral decubitus, or sitting position depending on comfort and access. Using ultrasound guidance, place the transducer 4 cm lateral to the spinous process in a parasagittal plane to visualize the rib, pleura, and intercostal space. Insert the needle, in-plane or out-of-plane, under the inferior border of the rib and advance it slightly beneath the rib. After confirming the absence of vascular penetration with aspiration, inject 3–5 mL of local anesthetic, observing the pleura moving away as the anesthetic is deposited. Alternatively, in the anatomic approach, palpate the rib at the mid posterior axillary line, inserting the needle under the rib and administering the local anesthetic. Multiple levels may need to be blocked for adequate coverage.

The TPVB provides unilateral pain relief at the dermatomes corresponding to the injected level and adjacent levels depending on the volume of local anesthetic injected, the anatomy of the patient, and the technique performed. To perform a TPVB, position the patient in the lateral decubitus or sitting position. This block targets the paravertebral space, where local anesthetic is injected to block spinal nerves as they emerge from the intervertebral foramina. The medial border is the vertebral body, the anterolateral border is the pleura, and the posterior border is the costotransverse ligament, with the heads of the ribs inferior and superior. Advance the needle under ultrasound guidance or using anatomic landmarks to the paravertebral space, typically at the T4 level for pain associated with breast surgery. After confirming the needle placement, inject 10–20 mL of local anesthetic to provide a unilateral somatic and sympathetic block. Compared to epidural blockade, TPVB has fewer complications, such as hypotension, urinary retention, or nausea, and it provides a unilateral block. This technique is versatile because it can serve as a supplement or alternative to general anesthesia and as a sole method for certain procedures.

Lateral chest wall pain can be effectively managed with a serratus plane block. To perform this block, position the patient and use ultrasound guidance to target the thoracic intercostal nerves, usually from T2 to T9. Place a high-frequency linear ultrasound transducer in a parasagittal plane under the mid-clavicle, rotate it 45 degrees caudally, and move it inferolateral until the fifth rib at the midaxillary line is identified. Locate the latissimus dorsi superficially and posteriorly, the teres major superiorly, and the serratus anterior muscle overlying the rib. Insert the needle in-plane from the medial side to the transducer, ensuring the needle tip is positioned either superficial or deep to the serratus muscle; a superficial injection is typically preferred. After confirming negative aspiration, inject 20 mL of local anesthetic in 5 mL increments, aspirating between injections.

The ESPB is gaining popularity as an effective method for managing acute postoperative analgesia and chronic pain conditions, including severe PMPS. This block is effective for thoracic and abdominal analgesia by targeting multiple dermatomes. To perform an ESPB, use ultrasound guidance to identify the plane between the erector spinae muscle and the transverse process of the vertebra. Position the patient in a sitting, lateral decubitus, or prone position. Using a high-frequency linear transducer, locate the desired transverse process by counting ribs or spinous processes, centering the transverse process on the ultrasound screen. Insert the needle in-plane under ultrasound visualization, advancing it to contact the transverse process. After confirming negative aspiration, inject 1–3 mL of saline to lift the erector spinae muscle off the transverse process and adjust the needle as necessary. Once positioned, inject 20–30 mL of local anesthetic in 5 mL increments, aspirating between injections, and ensure proper craniocaudal spread. For bilateral blocks or larger areas, adjust the volume and concentration of the anesthetic accordingly.

Suggested Reading

Avila F, Torres-Guzman R, Maita K, et al. A review on the management of peripheral neuropathic pain following breast cancer. Breast Cancer (Dove Med Press). 2023;15:761.

Chappell AG, Bai J, Yuksel S, Ellis MF. Post-mastectomy pain syndrome: Defining perioperative etiologies to guide new methods of prevention for plastic surgeons. World J Plast Surg. 2020;9:247.

Gong Y, Tan Q, Qin Q, Wei C. Prevalence of postmastectomy pain syndrome and associated risk factors: A large single-institution cohort study. Medicine (Baltimore). 2020;99:e19834.

Hasoon J, Urits I, Viswanath O, et al. Erector spinae plane block for the treatment of post mastectomy pain syndrome. Cureus. 2021;13:e12656.

Piracha MM, Thorp SL, Puttanniah V, Gulati A. "A tale of two planes": Deep versus superficial serratus plane block for postmastectomy pain syndrome. Reg Anesth Pain Med. 2017;42:259.

Poleshuck EL, Katz J, Andrus CH, et al. Risk factors for chronic pain following breast cancer surgery: A prospective study. J Pain. 2006;7:626.

Roth RS, Qi J, Hamill JB, et al. Is chronic postsurgical pain surgery-induced? A study of persistent postoperative pain following breast reconstruction. Breast. 2018;37:119.

Salati SA, Alsulaim L, Alharbi MH, et al. Postmastectomy pain syndrome: A narrative review. Cureus. 2023;15:e47384.

Schreiber KL, Martel MO, Shnol H, et al. Persistent pain in postmastectomy patients: Comparison of psychophysical, medical, surgical, and psychosocial characteristics between patients with and without pain. Pain. 2013;154:660.

Shah JD, Kirkpatrick K, Shah K. Post-mastectomy pain syndrome: A review article and emerging treatment modalities. Cureus. 2024;16:e56653.

Wiederhold BD, Garmon EH, Peterson E, et al. Nerve Block Anesthesia. Updated 2023 Apr 29. IStatPearls. 2024 Jan. https://www.ncbi.nlm.nih.gov/books/NBK431109/

Wisotzky EM, Saini V, Kao C. Ultrasound-guided intercostobrachial nerve block for intercostobrachial neuralgia in breast cancer patients: A case series. PMR. 2016;8:273.

Zocca JA, Chen GH, Puttanniah VG, et al. Ultrasound-guided serratus plane block for treatment of postmastectomy pain syndromes in breast cancer patients: A case series. Pain Pract. 2017;17:141.

PART IV

ABDOMINAL AND PELVIC PAIN SYNDROMES

16 Anatomical Considerations of the Female Abdominal Region

Thanh Thanh Tran and Ahmed Alassal

Introduction

The abdomen is a flexible yet protective space that houses vital organs. It adapts to changes such as pregnancy and weight fluctuations. In females, this area has unique features that affect both function and pain perception. The abdominal wall muscles and reproductive organs can create different types of pain, and anesthesiologists need to recognize these patterns. This chapter explores the anatomy above the pelvic inlet. It provides the key insights needed to understand some pain mechanisms.

Boundaries of the Abdominal Region

The abdominal cavity spans from the diaphragm at T12 superiorly to the pelvic brim at L5–S1 inferiorly. The anterior boundary comprises layered abdominal musculature, while the posterior boundary includes lumbar vertebrae and paravertebral muscles. The lateral abdominal wall arches between the costal margin and iliac crests, with neurovascular bundles traversing the flanks. The female's abdominal anatomy has special features. The wider rib cage angle makes space for the growing uterus during pregnancy.[1] Hormones also loosen ligaments to allow more spinal movement.[2,3] While helpful, these changes can reduce stability and sometimes lead to muscle strain or nerve compression issues (Figure 16.1 and Figure 16.2).

Structures of the Abdominal Wall

Superficial Layers

The subcutaneous tissue contains two distinct fascial layers: Camper's fascia forms the pliable fatty layer that varies with body composition, while the deeper Scarpa's fascia provides a sturdy membranous sheet crucial for surgical repair integrity. Between these layers runs the superficial epigastric venous network.

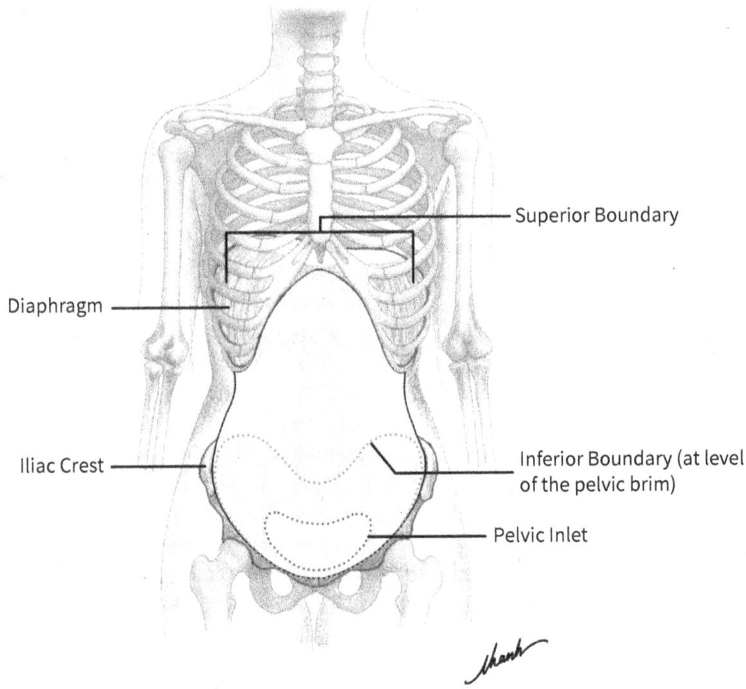

Figure 16.1 Anterior view of the female abdominal region with boundaries.

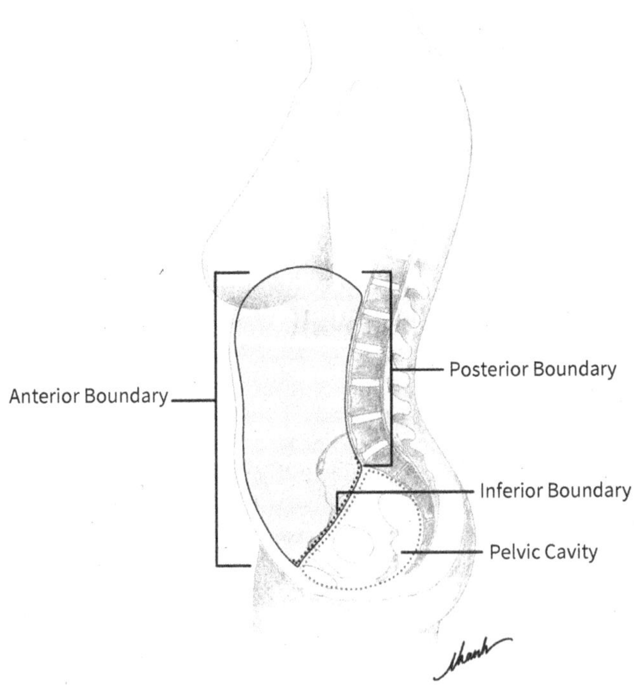

Figure 16.2 Lateral view of the female abdominal cavity illustrating anterior and posterior boundaries.

Clinical Correlation

The superficial epigastric veins can become distended due to conditions such as pregnancy or portal hypertension, reflecting altered venous return.[4] The skin undergoes distinct morphological changes, including striae gravidarum, which result from dermal collagen disruption caused by rapid abdominal expansion. Additionally, surgical scars—especially those from cesarean sections—may lead to cutaneous nerve entrapment within fibrous tissue, contributing to postoperative sensory alterations.[5]

Muscular Layers

Four muscle layers create the abdominal wall's structural framework. The external oblique muscle fibers run inferomedially like hands sliding into pockets, enabling trunk rotation. Beneath it, the internal oblique fibers course perpendicularly, providing rotational stability. The transversus abdominis forms the deepest muscular layer with horizontally oriented fibers that maintain intra-abdominal pressure. These three muscles converge medially to form the rectus sheath enclosing the vertical rectus abdominis muscles.

The linea alba, a fibrous midline raphe, stretches during pregnancy and may fail to fully recoil postpartum (diastasis recti). This avascular plane serves as the preferred incision site for many gynecologic procedures. The arcuate line at the level of the iliac crests marks the transition point where all aponeurotic layers pass anterior to the rectus muscle, altering the pattern of potential hematoma spread.

Clinical Correlation

Abdominal wall nerve entrapment syndromes commonly involve the thoracoabdominal nerves at their fascial penetration points, causing localized pain that worsens with movement.[6] Transversus abdominis plane (TAP) blocks target the neurovascular plane between the internal oblique and transversus abdominis for postoperative analgesia[7] (Figure 16.3).

Deeper Fascia and Peritoneal Layers

Supporting Structures

The transversalis fascia forms a sturdy membrane separating muscles from peritoneal contents. This layer gains surgical importance during hernia repairs and retroperitoneal approaches. The extraperitoneal fat layer cushions abdominal organs while providing an energy reserve, though excessive thickness complicates both imaging and procedural access. The preperitoneal space contains the inferior epigastric vessels, which must be avoided during abdominal wall punctures.

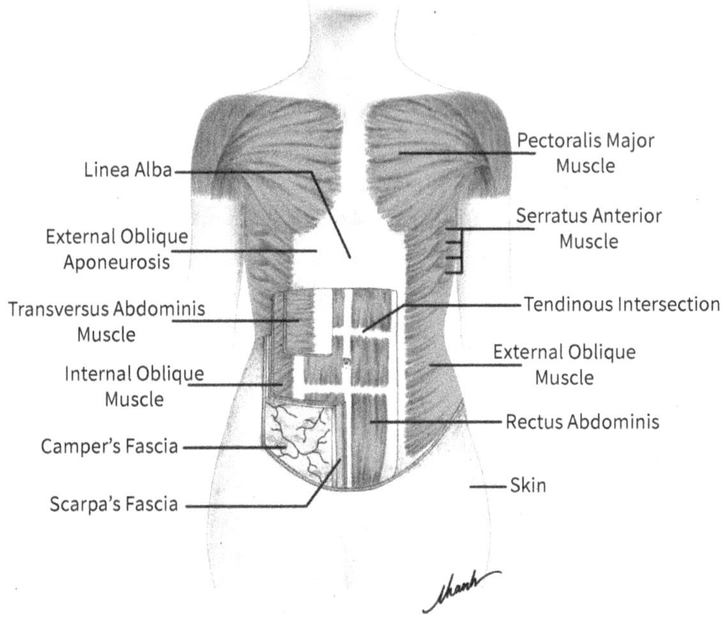

Figure 16.3 Superficial and muscular layers of the female abdominal wall.

Peritoneal Specializations

The parietal peritoneum lining the abdominal wall transmits sharp, well-localized pain through somatic nerves when irritated. In contrast, the visceral peritoneum covering organs conveys dull, poorly localized discomfort via visceral pathways. The potential space between these layers allows organ mobility while serving as a conduit for pathological fluid accumulation. The small intestine's mesentery anchors the bowel while allowing mobility, with its fan-shaped peritoneal fold containing the superior mesenteric vessels and autonomic nerves—this arrangement creates characteristic central abdominal pain when stretched or inflamed. The peritoneal reflections form clinically significant structures, including the falciform ligament (containing the obliterated umbilical vein) and the ligamentum teres hepatitis (Figure 16.4).

Clinical Correlation

The dual innervation pattern creates distinct clinical presentations. Initial visceral irritation, as seen in early appendicitis or bowel obstruction, produces diffuse periumbilical pain and nausea through autonomic pathways.[8] As inflammation progresses to involve the parietal layer, pain localizes to specific regions like McBurney's point in appendicitis, accompanied by rebound tenderness due to somatic nerve activation.[8] This same transition explains why mesenteric lymphadenitis typically maintains diffuse tenderness without precise localization. In peritonitis, parietal inflammation generates intense, localized pain upon palpation.[8] The peritoneal space also dictates pathological fluid movement, with ascites or blood

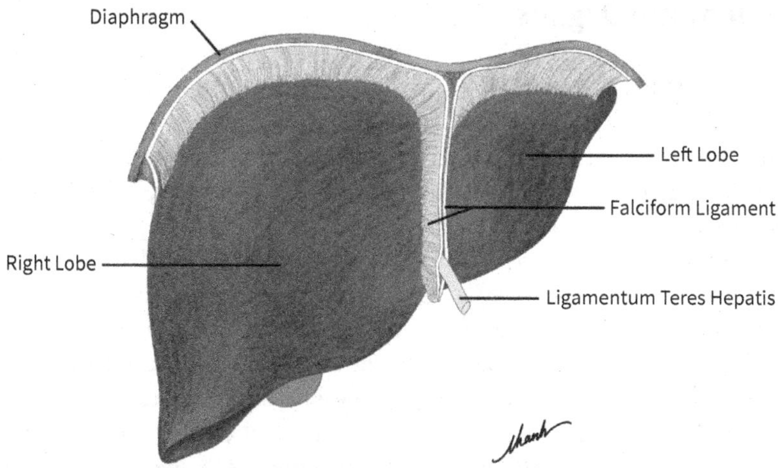

Figure 16.4 Anterior view of the liver showing peritoneal reflections and ligamentous structures.

tracking along peritoneal reflections. The falciform ligament's umbilical vein remnant may recanalize in portal hypertension, creating visible abdominal collaterals known as *caput medusae*[9,10] (Figure 16.5).

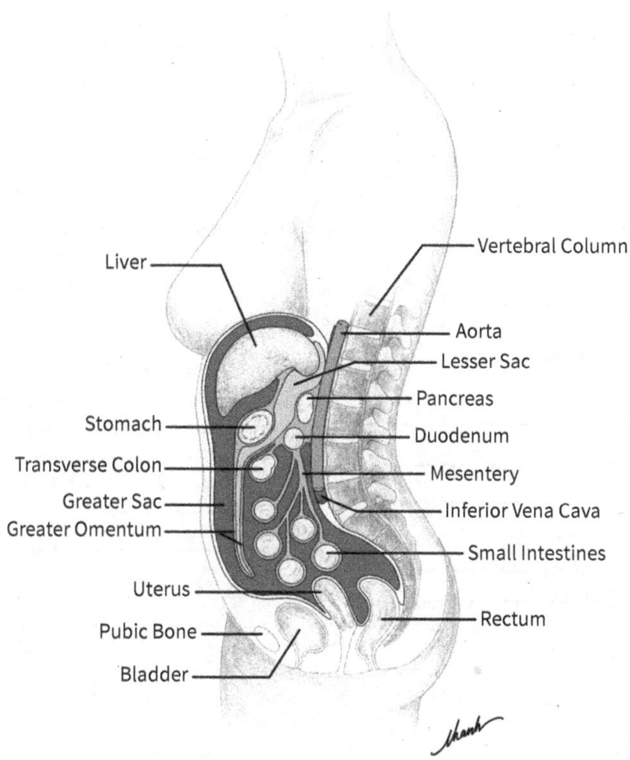

Figure 16.5 Sagittal view of the female abdominal cavity demonstrating peritoneal compartments and supporting structures.

Key Abdominal Organs

Reproductive Structures

The ovaries are dynamic endocrine and reproductive organs measuring approximately 3–5 cm in their longest axis, with size varying cyclically. They are suspended by a dual ligamentous system: the mesovarium, anchoring the ovary to the broad ligament, and the infundibulopelvic ligament, which contains the ovarian neurovascular bundle. This ligamentous suspension permits significant mobility while maintaining vascular connections.

The ovaries receive their primary blood supply from the ovarian arteries, which arise directly from the abdominal aorta just below the renal arteries (Figure 16.6). The ovarian arteries anastomose with the uterine arteries via the tubal branches, creating a collateral network. Venous drainage differs between sides, with the right ovarian vein draining directly into the inferior vena cava while the left ovarian vein terminates in the left renal vein through a longer, more tortuous pathway (Figure 16.6).

The ovaries are innervated by autonomic fibers from the ovarian plexus, a network of sympathetic and parasympathetic nerves that accompany the vessels. The fallopian tubes extend laterally from the uterine cornua, with their fimbriated ends positioned near the ovaries. The mucosal lining of the tubes consists of simple columnar epithelium containing both ciliated

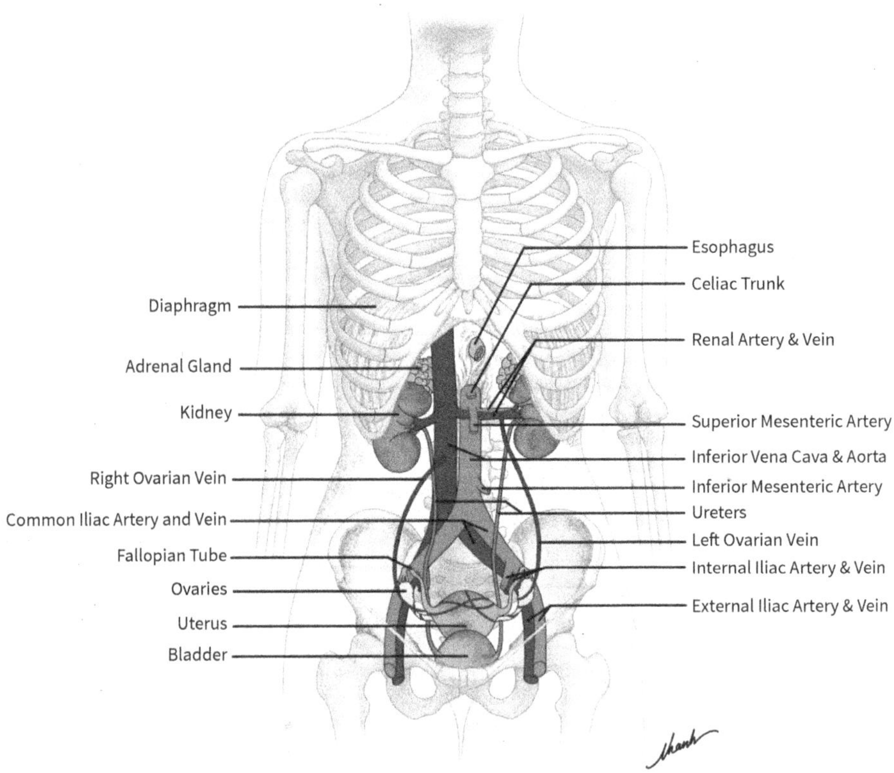

Figure 16.6 Anterior view of the female abdominal cavity highlighting reproductive, urinary, renal, and vascular structures.

and secretory (peg) cells. The cilia help facilitate ovum transport through the narrow lumens, while the muscular wall supports peristaltic movement.

Clinical Correlation

Polycystic ovary syndrome (PCOS) is a leading cause of chronic pelvic and abdominal pain in reproductive-aged females.[11,12] The pain mechanisms are multifactorial. Capsular distension occurs as multiple follicular cysts increase ovarian volume, stretching the visceral peritoneum and eliciting a dull, cyclical ache.[11] PCOS is associated with chronic low-grade inflammation and may sensitize ovarian nociceptors and lower pain thresholds.[11,12] Recurrent cyst rupture or hemorrhage may lead to adhesions, causing traction pain during movement or intercourse. Additionally, up to 17% of PCOS patients have concurrent endometriosis, compounding pain via direct invasion and neurogenic inflammation.[13]

In acute settings, ectopic pregnancy—most frequently occurring in the fallopian tubes—presents with sudden unilateral pelvic pain. Early distension of the tubal capsule causes localized discomfort, while rupture may lead to referred shoulder pain (phrenic nerve irritation) and intraperitoneal hemorrhage. The ampullary region of the tube is especially high-risk due to its vascularity.

Urinary System

The urinary bladder rises into the abdominal cavity when distended, creating suprapubic pressure. The ureters course along the psoas muscles before crossing the pelvic brim. The trigone region of the bladder demonstrates particular sensitivity due to its dense innervation, explaining the severe discomfort of cystitis in this area. The ureters pass anterior to the common iliac arteries at the pelvic brim, creating a potential compression point for ureteral obstruction.

Clinical Correlation

Clinically, colicky pain may originate in the flank and radiate toward the groin, often reflecting underlying visceral or neuropathic disturbances.[14] The intensity and pattern of radiation can provide diagnostic clues regarding the affected anatomical structures, with ureteral calculi being a common cause of this characteristic pain pattern.

Kidneys

The kidneys occupy the retroperitoneal space from T12 to L3, with the right kidney typically 1–2 cm lower than the left due to hepatic displacement. Their anterior relationships differ significantly: the right kidney contacts the liver, duodenum, and ascending colon, while the left kidney abuts the spleen, pancreas, and descending colon.

The renal capsule contains nociceptors responsive to stretch, making distension (from obstruction or edema) a potent pain generator. Three concentric tissue layers surround each kidney: the true fibrous capsule (pain-sensitive), perirenal fat (providing cushioning), and Gerota's fascia (limiting infection spread). The renal hilum transmits the ureter, renal vessels, and nerves in an anterior-to-posterior sequence of vein, artery, pelvis—a critical orientation for surgical approaches. Autonomic innervation from the renal plexus (T10–L1) mediates the classic "loin-to-groin" radiation of renal colic.

Clinical Correlation

Bladder pain from cystitis is typically suprapubic and constant,[15] while ureteral obstruction creates waxing/waning discomfort that follows embryological dermatomes (T10–L1).[16] The "ureteral jet" phenomenon seen on ultrasound demonstrates the physiological peristalsis that becomes dysrhythmic during obstruction, correlating with colicky pain episodes.[16,17]

Gastrointestinal Tract

The gastrointestinal tract's anatomical relationships help explain pain localization patterns. The appendix's variable position (retrocecal, pelvic, or subhepatic) influences pain presentation during appendiceal inflammation (appendicitis). The large intestine's fixed positions at the hepatic and splenic flexures predispose these sites to volvulus. The ligament of Treitz marks the duodenojejunal flexure, serving as a key landmark for differentiating upper and lower GI bleeding sources.

Vascular Architecture

Arterial Supply

The abdominal aorta's anterior branches provide the primary gastrointestinal blood supply through three key arteries: the celiac artery (T12–L1) feeds the foregut (stomach to duodenum), the superior mesenteric artery (SMA; L1) supplies the midgut (jejunum to proximal colon), and the inferior mesenteric artery (IMA; L3) nourishes the hindgut (distal colon to rectum). These create watershed zones at their territorial borders, particularly vulnerable to ischemic pain. Paired lateral branches include the ovarian arteries, which arise just below the renal arteries.

The marginal artery of Drummond forms a critical anastomosis between SMA and IMA systems; when underdeveloped, this collateral network predisposes to colonic ischemia. The arc of Riolan provides another potential bypass route in chronic mesenteric insufficiency. Of particular relevance to female patients is *nutcracker syndrome*, where the left renal vein becomes compressed between the SMA and aorta.[18] This vascular entrapment increases ovarian vein pressure, potentially causing pelvic congestion syndrome with chronic pelvic pain, dyspareunia, and vulvar varicosities.[18]

Venous Drainage

The left ovarian vein's longer course and insertion into the left renal vein explains its greater propensity for thrombosis compared to the right's direct IVC drainage. The portal vein forms posterior to the pancreatic neck through the confluence of the splenic and superior mesenteric veins, creating a high-pressure system susceptible to variceal formation when obstructed.

Clinical Correlation

Ovarian vein thrombosis presents with nonspecific lower abdominal pain, often postpartum.[19] Mesenteric ischemia causes severe, out-of-proportion pain as visceral nociceptors respond to hypoxia.[20] Portal hypertension manifests through dilated abdominal wall veins radiating from the umbilicus, with flow direction indicating the level of obstruction[9] (Figure 16.6).

Nervous System

Somatic Innervation

Thoracoabdominal nerves T7–T12 supply the abdominal wall in a segmental pattern, with the iliohypogastric and ilioinguinal nerves (L1) completing the inferior coverage. These pathways explain the precise localization of parietal pain and the effectiveness of regional blocks. The lateral cutaneous branches of these nerves are particularly vulnerable to entrapment as they pierce the muscular layers near the anterior axillary line (Figure 16.7).

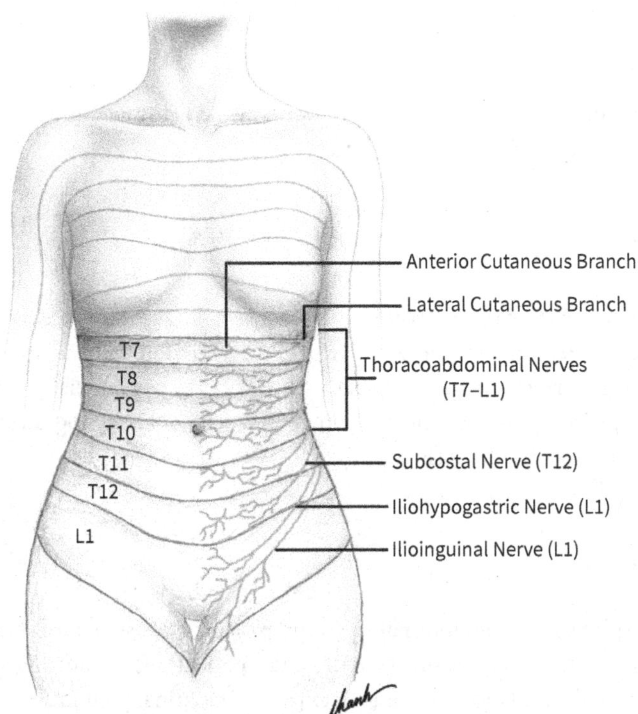

Figure 16.7 Segmental dermatomal distribution of the female abdominal wall by thoracoabdominal and pelvic nerves.

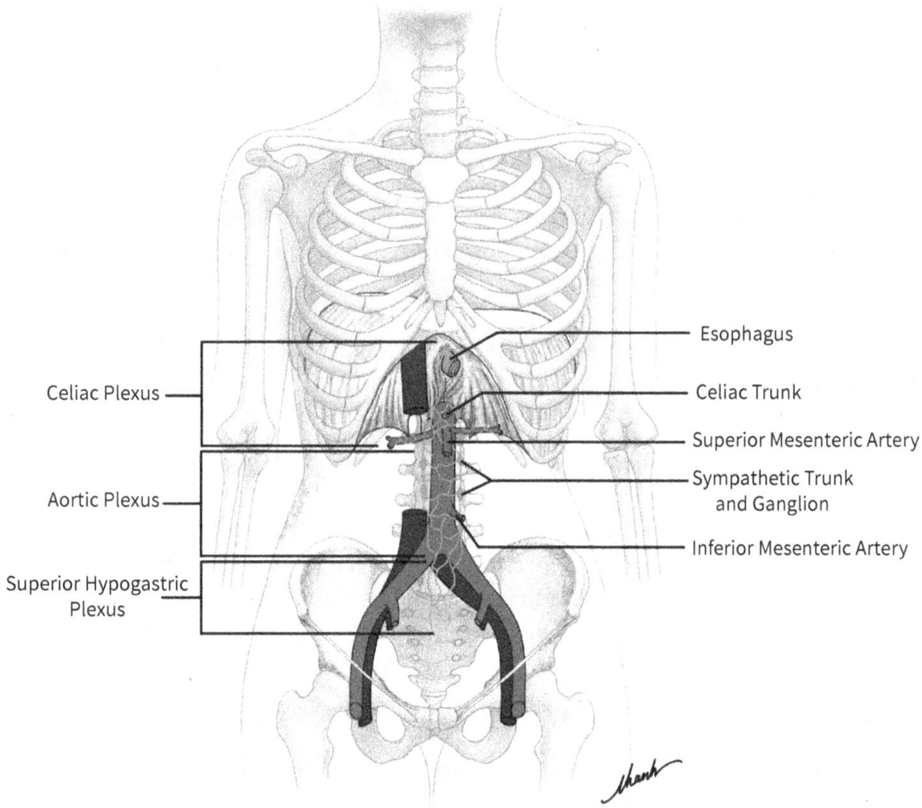

Figure 16.8 Autonomic plexuses and sympathetic pathways of the female abdominal cavity.

Autonomic

Visceral afferents travel with sympathetic fibers, referring pain to corresponding dermatomes. The celiac plexus serves as a major pain transmission pathway for upper abdominal organs. The superior hypogastric plexus (T10–L2) conveys nociceptive signals from pelvic organs, explaining why chronic pelvic pain may respond to hypogastric plexus blocks or ganglion impar interventions[21] (Figure 16.8).

Conclusion

This detailed exploration of abdominal anatomy provides the structural basis for understanding pain generation and transmission in female patients. The following sections of this volume build on this foundation, addressing chronic abdominal pain in females, diagnostic strategies, and interventional techniques for effective management.

Acknowledgments

The following standard anatomy resources were consulted for general anatomical accuracy in creating these original illustrations.

- *Grant's Dissector*,[22] 16th edition, edited by Alan J. Detton
- *Gray's Anatomy for Students*,[23] 3rd edition, edited by Richard L. Drake, A. Wayne Vogl, Adam W. M. Mitchell
- *Gray's Atlas of Anatomy*, 3rd edition,[24] edited by Richard L. Drake, A. Wayne Vogl, Adam W. M. Mitchell, Richard M. Tibbitts, Paul E. Richardson
- *Netter's Anatomy Coloring Book*, 2nd edition, edited by John T. Hansen
- *The Anatomy Coloring Book*, 4th edition, edited by Wynn Kapit, Lawrence M. Elson
- Complete Anatomy program

References

1. LoMauro A, Aliverti A. Respiratory physiology of pregnancy: Physiology masterclass. Breathe (Sheff). 2015;11(4):297–301. doi:10.1183/20734735.008615
2. Birt KM, McCarthy HE. The effect of estrogen on anterior cruciate ligament structure and function: A systematic review. J Musculoskelet Disord Treat. 2023;9:127. doi:10.23937/2572-3243.1510127
3. Östh J, Brolin K, Svensson MY, Linder A. A female ligamentous cervical spine finite element model validated for physiological loads. J Biomech Eng. 2016;138(6):061005. doi:10.1115/1.4032966
4. Blackburn P, Patel SS, Mikhail E. Abdominal wall varices in pregnancy: A case report and review of the literature. J Preg Child Health. 2016;3:266. doi:10.4172/2376-127X.1000266
5. Whiteside JL, Barber MD. Ilioinguinal/iliohypogastric neurectomy for management of intractable right lower quadrant pain after cesarean section: A case report. J Reprod Med. 2005;50(11):857–859.
6. Lam K, Vasey C. Diagnostic dilemma: Think about anterior cutaneous nerve entrapment syndrome (ACNES) in patients with atypical abdominal pain and Crohn's disease. BMJ Case Rep. 2018;2018:bcr2017224041. doi:10.1136/bcr-2017-224041
7. Mavarez AC, Hendrix JM, Ahmed AA. Transabdominal plane block. StatPearls. 2025 Jan. Updated 2023 Nov 13. Accessed June 2025. https://www.ncbi.nlm.nih.gov/books/NBK560527/
8. Schick MA, Kashyap S, Collier SA, Meseeha M. Small bowel obstruction. StatPearls. 2025 Jan 19. Accessed June 2025. https://www.ncbi.nlm.nih.gov/books/NBK448079/
9. Soni N, Israrahmed A, Singh P, Lal H. Caput medusa: A sign of portal hypertension in case of chronic Budd-Chiari syndrome. BMJ Case Rep. 2021;14(4):e242076. doi:10.1136/bcr-2021-242076
10. Garbar V, Newton BW. Anatomy, abdomen and pelvis: Falciform ligament. StatPearls. 2025 Jan. Updated 2023 Jul 24. Accessed June 2025. https://www.ncbi.nlm.nih.gov/books/NBK539858/

11. Lu KT, Ho YC, Chang CL, Lan KC, Wu CC, Su YT. Evaluation of bodily pain associated with polycystic ovary syndrome: A review of health-related quality of life and potential risk factors. Biomedicines. 2022;10(12):3197. doi:10.3390/biomedicines10123197
12. Rudnicka E, Suchta K, Grymowicz M, et al. Chronic low grade inflammation in pathogenesis of PCOS. Int J Mol Sci. 2021;22(7):3789. doi:10.3390/ijms22073789
13. Singh KB, Patel YC, Wortsman J. Coexistence of polycystic ovary syndrome and pelvic endometriosis. Obstet Gynecol. 1989;74(4):650–652.
14. Masarani M, Dinneen M. Ureteric colic: New trends in diagnosis and treatment. Postgrad Med J. 2007;83(981):469–472. doi:10.1136/pgmj.2006.055913
15. Brubaker L, Carberry C, Nardos R, Carter-Brooks C, Lowder JL. American Urogynecologic Society best-practice statement: Recurrent urinary tract infection in adult women. Female Pelvic Med Reconstr Surg. 2018;24(5):321–335. doi:10.1097/SPV.0000000000000550
16. Pérez-Aizpurua X, Cabello Benavente R, Bueno Serrano G, et al. Obstructive uropathy: Overview of the pathogenesis, etiology and management of a prevalent cause of acute kidney injury. World J Nephrol. 2024;13(2):93322. doi:10.5527/wjn.v13.i2.93322
17. Leung VY, Chu WC, Yeung CK, Metreweli C. Doppler waveforms of the ureteric jet: An overview and implications for the presence of a functional sphincter at the vesicoureteric junction. Pediatr Radiol. 2007;37(5):417–425. doi:10.1007/s00247-007-0433-1
18. Kolber MK, Cui Z, Chen CK, Habibollahi P, Kalva SP. Nutcracker syndrome: Diagnosis and therapy. Cardiovasc Diagn Ther. 2021;11(5):1140–1149. doi:10.21037/cdt-20-160
19. Alsheef M, Abuzied Y, Alosaimi M, et al. Clinical characteristics and management of ovarian vein thrombosis: A case series. Front Cardiovasc Med. 2022;9:916920. doi:10.3389/fcvm.2022.916920
20. Wu T, Nanjundappa A. Mesenteric ischemia: Recognizing an uncommon disorder and distinguishing among its causes. Cleve Clin J Med. 2024;91(9):545–550. doi:10.3949/ccjm.91a.23094
21. Urits I, Schwartz R, Herman J, et al. A comprehensive update of the superior hypogastric block for the management of chronic pelvic pain. Curr Pain Headache Rep. 2021;25(3):13. doi:10.1007/s11916-020-00933-0
22. Detton AJ. *Grant's Dissector*. 16th ed. Wolters Kluwer; 2017.
23. Drake RL, Vogl AW, Mitchell AWM. *Gray's Anatomy for Students*. 3rd ed. Elsevier; 2015.
24. Drake RL, Vogl AW, Mitchell AWM, Tibbitts RM, Richardson PE. *Gray's Atlas of Anatomy*. 3rd ed. Elsevier; 2015.

17
Common Abdominal Pain Conditions in Women

Eliot Sadik, Ankur Jain, Michael Suarez, and Jason Mizrahi

Introduction

Chronic abdominal pain (CAP) is a common, frequently distressing and functionally debilitating disorder that is often challenging for providers to accurately diagnose and treat. CAP is defined by a diverse group of gastrointestinal, gynecologic, urologic, musculoskeletal, and neuropathic conditions characterized by persistent or recurrent abdominal pain of more than 3–6 months' duration. CAP is frequently encountered by clinicians across a variety of disciplines but is disproportionately experienced by women for a variety of reasons including effects of sex hormones on immune modulation and visceral hypersensitivity and pain perception, as well as psychosocial influences and stress. In some, CAP occurs in the context of ongoing inflammation or structural disease, while in others no such pathologic findings are identified. A working knowledge of pathologic entities of the disorders of gut-brain interaction and central pain processing is critical in patients without anatomic pathologic abnormalities.

Gastrointestinal Causes

One of the most common sources of CAP includes irritable bowel syndrome (IBS), a functional gastrointestinal disorder that presents as an abdominal cramping sensation, bloating, and fluctuations of bowel habits. Women are more frequently affected by IBS, possibly due to visceral hypersensitivity. Inflammatory bowel diseases are another cause of CAP in females, most commonly Crohn's disease and ulcerative colitis. In Crohn's disease, inflammation of the digestive tract results in ongoing abdominal pain, diarrhea, fatigue, and weight loss. Similarly, the ulcers and inflammation that occur with ulcerative colitis manifest as persistent, cramping abdominal pain and rectal bleeding. Furthermore, prior abdominal surgeries such as cesarean section may lead to the formation of intestinal adhesions and subsequent CAP due to decreased bowel motility, inflammation, and potential small bowel obstructions. Last, conditions like celiac disease, chronic pancreatitis, and small intestinal bacterial overgrowth may mimic symptoms of IBS and present with CAP.

Gynecologic Causes

Endometriosis affects nearly 1 out of 10 women of reproductive age and manifests as daily or cyclical abdominal pain often worse during menstruation. Adenomyosis is another cause of CAP and may present as severe menstrual cramps, bladder or rectal pressure, and heavy, prolonged menstruation. Furthermore, nearly 80% of women may have leiomyomas by the age of 50, with 20–50% of those being symptomatic (heavy bleeding, pelvic pain, pressure symptoms). Additionally, ovarian cysts, increasingly common during the reproductive years, may cause mass effect or rupture, leading to pelvic pressure or chronic abdominal discomfort. Last, in postmenopausal women, persistent pain may be secondary to gynecological malignancy.

Urologic Causes

Interstitial cystitis can cause pain that radiates from the bladder to the lower abdomen. Small ureteral or bladder stones can also present as episodic abdominal pain; however, the pattern, location, and accompanying symptoms should help to differentiate them from other causes of abdominal pain. Furthermore, pelvic floor muscle dysfunction involves overactive, tight, or uncoordinated pelvic floor muscles, which can lead to suprapubic, perineal, or lower quadrant abdominal pain.

Musculoskeletal and Neuropathic Causes

Myofascial syndromes and nerve entrapment may often result in sharp, localized pain. The pain associated with these conditions often occurs near surgical scars or areas of prior trauma. Additionally, abdominal wall hernias affect millions of patients worldwide and can cause abdominal pain due to mechanical strain and persistent inflammation. While men may have a higher overall incidence of hernias, women have unique risk factors such as pregnancy, prior abdominal surgeries (including cesarean sections), chronic cough, and constipation.

Central Sensitization and Psychological Factors

Anxiety, depression, or history of trauma can worsen abdominal pain by altering nerve pathways through central sensitization. In conditions like fibromyalgia, normal stimuli can become painful and result in widespread discomfort. These mechanisms are common in women and may be present as CAP. Symptoms can also often overlap with IBS or pelvic pain syndromes and thus should be included in one's differential diagnoses.

Diagnostic Evaluation

The diagnostic evaluation for CAP in women should follow a stepwise, symptom-guided approach, with the dual goals of identifying harmful pathology and minimizing unnecessary testing. A comprehensive history and physical examination are foundational, serving to narrow the differential diagnosis and detect alarm features such as unintentional weight loss, gastrointestinal bleeding, or a family history of malignancy. These findings may prompt an urgent evaluation.

Clinical history should characterize pain onset, duration, location, quality, exacerbating and relieving factors, associated symptoms (including bowel, urinary, and gynecologic), psychosocial context, and any prior interventions. A thorough physical exam should include abdominal, pelvic, and musculoskeletal assessments to localize tenderness, masses, or other signs of systemic disease. Pelvic examination is essential for evaluating gynecologic causes such as endometriosis, adnexal masses, or pelvic floor dysfunction.

If no specific diagnosis or red flag features emerge from the initial evaluation, limited laboratory testing is typically appropriate. This may include a complete blood count, urinalysis, pregnancy test, and inflammatory markers (e.g., erythrocyte sedimentation rate [ESR], C-reactive protein [CRP]) to assess infection, anemia, or inflammation. Depending on the clinical scenario, renal and liver function tests, thyroid studies, or stool studies may also be warranted.

Imaging studies, though commonly ordered, should be reserved for patients with clinical findings suggestive of structural abnormalities. Pelvic ultrasonography is typically the first-line modality to evaluate uterine, ovarian, or adnexal pathology. Abdominal ultrasound or CT scanning may be indicated if gastrointestinal or urinary tract disorders are suspected. The American College of Obstetricians and Gynecologists (ACOG) recommend targeted imaging rather than routine imaging in all patients.

Endoscopic evaluation (e.g., colonoscopy, upper endoscopy) should be pursued if alarm features are present or if symptoms persist and suggest an organic gastrointestinal disease. These alarm features may include gastrointestinal bleeding (hematemesis, melena, or hematochezia), iron deficiency anemia, unintentional weight loss, persistent vomiting, dysphagia, onset of symptoms after age 50, a family history of gastrointestinal malignancy, inflammatory bowel disease, or celiac disease, and a recent or progressive change in bowel habits. The American Gastroenterological Association and the American College of Gastroenterology both highlight these features as indicators for endoscopic evaluation because they increase the likelihood of underlying organic pathology such as malignancy, inflammatory bowel disease, or other significant gastrointestinal disease. If the initial workup is unrevealing and pain continues, referral for specialized testing should be considered. While rare, laparoscopy may be indicated to evaluate for suspected endometriosis or pelvic adhesions when noninvasive evaluation is inconclusive and symptoms are severe. Urodynamic studies or cystoscopy may be required for urinary complaints, and anorectal manometry or defecography for pelvic floor dysfunction.

In some cases, pain is ultimately attributed to a functional disorder such as IBS, functional dyspepsia, or functional abdominal pain syndrome (FAPS). These are typically diagnosed only after organic disease has been excluded. A detailed history and physical examination should assess psychosocial factors, psychiatric comorbidities, and central sensitization.

Diagnosis of functional syndromes relies on symptom-based criteria, such as the Rome criteria for IBS and FAPS. Notably, FAPS is defined by constant or nearly constant abdominal pain for at least 6 months, with loss of daily function and no relationship to gut function or bowel habits. IBS is characterized by recurrent abdominal pain associated with changes in stool frequency or form, without alarm features. Further assessment should evaluate for overlapping syndromes such as fibromyalgia or bladder pain syndrome, pelvic floor dysfunction, and psychosocial contributors including trauma or mental health conditions. A biopsychosocial model of care is essential, with treatment often requiring a multidisciplinary team. Once a functional diagnosis is established, extensive repeat testing should be avoided to minimize patient harm and healthcare costs.

Conclusion

In summary, CAP in women can arise from a multitude of conditions that span multiple systems. Disorders like IBS, endometriosis, interstitial cystitis, and others of musculoskeletal or neuropathic origin contribute to its complexity. Psychological comorbidities often amplify symptoms, thus clouding diagnostic judgment. The workup for CAP in women should be anchored in a thorough history and physical examination followed by selective laboratory and imaging studies based on clinical suspicion. ACOG and the AGA emphasize a symptom-driven, judicious approach that balances timely diagnosis with avoidance of unnecessary interventions. Persistent or severe symptoms should prompt specialist referral, and, when functional pain syndromes are diagnosed, a multidisciplinary, patient-centered approach is essential for effective management.

Suggested Reading

American College of Obstetrics and Gynecology (ACOG). Chronic Pelvic Pain: ACOG Practice Bulletin Summary, Number 218. Obstet Gynecol. 2020;135(3):744–746. doi:10.1097/AOG.0000000000003717

Bulun SE. Uterine fibroids. N Engl J Med. 2013;369(14):1344–1355. doi:10.1056/NEJMra1209993

Chandler J, Wagner E, Riley K. Evaluation of female pelvic pain. Semin Reprod Med. 2018;36(2):99–106. doi:10.1055/s-0038-1676084

Chey WD, Kurlander J, Eswaran S. Irritable bowel syndrome: A clinical review. *JAMA*. 2015;313(9):949–958. doi:10.1001/jama.2015.0954

Clauw DJ. Fibromyalgia: A clinical review. JAMA. 2014;311(15):1547–1555. doi:10.1001/jama.2014.3266

Giudice LC. Clinical practice: Endometriosis. N Engl J Med. 2010;362(25):2389–2398. doi:10.1056/NEJMcp1000274

Hanno PM, Erickson D, Moldwin R, Faraday MM. Diagnosis and treatment of interstitial cystitis/bladder pain syndrome: AUA guideline amendment. J Urol. 2015;193(5):1545–1553. doi:10.1016/j.juro.2015.01.086

Lacy BE, Pimentel M, Brenner DM, et al. ACG clinical guideline: Management of irritable bowel syndrome. Am J Gastroenterol. 2021;116(1):17–44. doi:10.14309/ajg.0000000000001036

Lamvu G, Carrillo J, Ouyang C, Rapkin A. Chronic pelvic pain in women: A review. JAMA. 2021;325(23):2381–2391. doi:10.1001/jama.2021.2631

Meisenheimer ES, Carnevale AM. Chronic pelvic pain in women: Evaluation and treatment. Am Fam Physician. 2025;111(3):218–229.

Moshiree B, Drossman D, Shaukat A. AGA clinical practice update on evaluation and management of belching, abdominal bloating, and distention: Expert review. Gastroenterology. 2023;165(3):791–800.e3. doi:10.1053/j.gastro.2023.04.039

Sabo CM, Grad S, Dumitrascu DL. Chronic abdominal pain in general practice. Dig Dis. 2021;39(6):606–614. doi:10.1159/000515433

Speer LM, Mushkbar S, Erbele T. Chronic pelvic pain in women. Am Fam Physician. 2016;93(5):380–387.

Thompson WG, Longstreth GF, Drossman DA, Heaton KW, Irvine EJ, Müller-Lissner SA. Functional bowel disorders and functional abdominal pain. Gut. 1999;45(Suppl 2):II43–II47. doi:10.1136/gut.45.2008.ii43

18
Pelvic Adhesions and Pain
Integrating Surgical and Noninvasive Treatment Strategies

Rishika Voruganti, Alopi M. Patel, and Jessica Opoku-Anane

Introduction

Pelvic adhesions are bands of fibrous scar tissue that form between abdominal and pelvic organs, commonly as a result of surgery, infection, or inflammation. Typical causes include pelvic inflammatory disease (PID), the presence of foreign materials, intra-abdominal infections (i.e., appendicitis), and prior gynecologic, abdominal, or oncologic surgery. Prevention of pelvic adhesions relies on precise surgical technique that minimize peritoneal trauma and the use of chemical or physical barriers intraoperatively. This chapter explores the etiology, clinical impact, prevention, and treatment of pelvic adhesions, including both surgical and nonsurgical approaches.

Background

Pelvic adhesions occur when two separate tissue surfaces become abnormally connected by fibrous bands or thin sheets of tissue. Damage to the peritoneal surfaces activates chemical signals such as leukotriene B4 (LTB4) and prostaglandin E2 (PGE2), which increase vascular permeability and attract immune cells to the site of injury.[1,2] This inflammatory response reduces plasminogen activity, a molecule essential to fibrin breakdown, leading to fibrin accumulation by overactive fibroblasts. These fibrin-based adhesions may be identified through pelvic exams, imaging, hysterosalpingograms, or diagnostic laparoscopy and can result in chronic pelvic pain, infertility, and bowel obstruction. Emerging approaches to pelvic adhesion prevention include the use of nutritional agents aimed at reducing oxidative stress. Additionally, intraoperative materials such as adhesion barriers (i.e., oxidized regenerated cellulose, hyaluronic acid gels) have been widely studied. However, despite US Food and Drug Administration (FDA) approval, few have consistently demonstrated both safety and efficacy in preventing adhesion formation or recurrence in large, controlled clinical trials.

Epidemiology

- More than 90% of patients undergoing open procedures in the United States and 50–70% of patients undergoing laparoscopic surgery will develop pelvic adhesions.[3]
- Adhesiolysis leads to 300,000 hospitalizations annually in the United States, exceeding $1.3 billion in healthcare costs.[3]

Complications and Burden

- *Adhesion prevalence*: Following gynecological surgery, reported rates of pelvic adhesion formation are as high as 51%. Its association with chronic pelvic pain ranges from 4% to 16%.[3–5]
- *Infertility*: Adhesions involving the fallopian tubes, ovaries, and uterine cavity interfere with oocyte or sperm transport and/or embryo implantation and result in 10–20% of female infertility.[4,5] Surgical adhesiolysis improves pregnancy rates in patients with pelvic adhesions: 32% at 12 months and 45% at 24 months, compared with 11% and 16% in untreated patients.[4,5]
- *Bowel obstruction*: Abdominopelvic adhesions account for up to 65–75% of all small bowel obstructions and have a lifetime risk of 2% following any intra-abdominal surgery.[6] Incidence varies by procedure: 1–10% after appendectomy, 6.4% after cholecystectomy, 10–25% after intestinal surgery, and 17–25% after restorative proctocolectomy.[6]
- *Chronic pelvic pain*: Often multifactorial, with adhesions contributing to myofascial pain, organ tethering, and nerve entrapment. A randomized controlled trial (RCT) comparing laparoscopic adhesiolysis to diagnostic laparoscopy without adhesiolysis showed only modest pain improvement.[7]
- *Adhesion recurrence*: Recurrence rates remain high, with up to 35% of patients developing new adhesions postoperatively.[5,8,9] A 2022 systematic review including 36,178 patients demonstrated that operative management of adhesive small bowel obstruction (ASBO) was linked with a lower recurrence risk compared to conservative treatment. Up to 67–90% of patients will develop adhesions following the procedure. Multiple surgeries to remove the adhesions compound the risk, creating a cycle of adhesion formation and pelvic pain symptom recurrence.[10]

Pathophysiology

Injury to peritoneal structures prompts the infiltration of neutrophils, leukocytes, and macrophages, followed by the activation of fibroblasts, which deposit fibrin at the site of injury. Injury to the pelvic wall may result from mechanical disturbance, hypoxia, or the accumulation of reactive oxygen species (ROS). In healthy tissues, fibrolysis counteracts the activity of fibroblasts, leading to normal tissue remodeling. However, when the balance between fibrin deposition and fibrinolysis is disrupted—particularly when fibroblast activity exceeds fibrinolytic capacity—adhesions can form. If this imbalance is not corrected, the fibrin matrix stabilizes and matures into permanent adhesions.[1,2] Additional mechanisms include thermal injury, ischemia, and the presence of foreign bodies, blood, bacteria, or inflammatory drugs that provoke fibrous tissue development.[11]

Diagnosis and Assessment

Pelvic adhesions are often suspected in patients with chronic pelvic pain and confirmed via diagnostic laparoscopy. Although imaging modalities such as ultrasound, CT, or MRI can sometimes reveal distortion of pelvic anatomy suggestive of adhesions, they generally lack the sensitivity to detect adhesions as directly as laparoscopy.

Treatment Options

Medical

Anti-inflammatory agents: While glucocorticoids theoretically reduce inflammation, clinical trials have not shown consistent benefit in reducing adhesions[5] (Table 18.1).

Surgical

Adhesiolysis refers to the surgical removal of adhesions and can be performed via laparotomy or laparoscopy. However, the role of adhesiolysis in chronic pelvic pain remains debated.[12,13] Laparoscopy is generally preferred due to its lower morbidity, shorter recovery time, and lower risk of further adhesion formation.[8] Pathogenesis of adhesion formation in reproductive surgery has been well described.[2]

Although adhesiolysis can improve symptoms, especially in patients with dense stage IV adhesions, outcomes are inconsistent. Recurrence rates remain high, with some studies reporting up to 35% of patients developing new adhesions postoperatively.[5,8,9] However, adhesiolysis has been shown to improve chronic pelvic pain, especially in patients with tubal occlusion. It is also effective in treating adhesive small bowel obstruction (SBO). Studies show most selected surgical candidates show symptom resolution postoperatively.[14]

Table 18.1 Summary of nonsurgical and surgical treatment options for pelvic adhesions

Modality	Mechanism	Evidence summary	Limitations
Surgical adhesiolysis	Physical removal of adhesions	Stage IV bowel adhesions respond best; laparoscopy preferred[5]	High recurrence rate; may cause new adhesions[8,9]
Sclerotherapy	Injection of sclerosing agents into adhesion sites via percutaneous or laparoscopic approach. Localized inflammation and fibrosis to remodel or resorb existing scar tissue.	Limited experimental studies; not standard of care; minimal clinical data in pelvic adhesions[21]	Risk of worsening fibrosis, poor targeting, unclear efficacy, not routinely used
Physical therapy	Manual pressure to disrupt fibrous crosslinks	Case reports show restored tubal patency, improved bowel function, and pain relief[17]	Small sample sizes; no surgical confirmation of resolution
Pharmacologic agents	Inhibit inflammation, fibrosis, and/or pain pathways	Pregabalin shows symptom relief[20]	Limited effect; most therapies still investigational; agents do not interrupt actual adhesions

Physical Therapy

Manual therapy aims to mechanically disrupt fibrous bands through sustained, directed pressure applied to the pelvic or abdominal regions. The Clear Passage protocol and other forms of soft tissue mobilization have reported success in restoring tubal patency, restoring bowel function, and relieving pelvic pain in select retrospective and case studies.[15–17] Pelvic floor physical therapy, especially in patients with comorbid endometriosis or pelvic floor dysfunction, has shown benefits in reducing dyspareunia and improving muscle coordination.[18,19] Combined regimens often include manual techniques, guided exercises, and patient education.

Pharmacologic and Emerging Therapies

New therapies are targeting the underlying inflammatory, fibrotic, and/or pain pathways.

- *Pregabalin*: Demonstrated reduction in chronic pelvic pain in small trials but does not directly address the adhesions.[20]
- *NSAIDs and hormonal therapy*: These are often used for symptomatic relief, particularly in cases of overlapping endometriosis, but do not resolve the fibrotic pathology of adhesions.
- An experimental method, *sclerotherapy* involves injecting sclerosing agents into or near adhesion sites to induce targeted fibrosis and resorption. Preliminary studies are sparse and lack robust clinical validation.[21]

Patient-Centered Approaches

Integrative strategies focus on improving quality of life and reducing symptom burden.

- *Acupuncture*: May reduce pain through neurohormonal pathways and central desensitization.[22]
- *Dietary modifications*: Anti-inflammatory diets that reduce red meat and processed food intake while increasing fruits, vegetables, and dairy may alleviate pelvic symptoms.[23]
- *Nutritional supplements*: Omega-3 fatty acids, particularly those found in fish oil, have shown modest pain relief in small studies and may also influence systemic inflammation.[24]

Prevention

Peritoneal instillates are used intraoperatively as an adjunct therapy intended to reduce organ contact via hydroflotation, but they are rapidly absorbed. Icodextrin and hyaluronic acid (HA) gels provide more sustained separation. Cross-linked HA products like Hyalobarrier have shown efficacy in reducing postoperative adhesions, especially in hysteroscopic procedures.[5] Newer bioregenerative adhesion barriers derived from porcine or bovine extracellular matrix or human placental/amniotic tissue may also be applied intraoperatively to help separate damaged tissues. Though modest reductions in adhesion occurrence have been documented in meta-analyses, their impact on long-term fertility or pain remains unclear.[9,25] Current literature is exploring the role of NSAIDs in reducing adhesion formation by inhibiting thromboxane production.[5]

Conclusion

Pelvic adhesions are a prevalent and often underrecognized consequence of abdominal and gynecologic surgery. They contribute significantly to chronic pelvic pain, infertility, and gastrointestinal complications. While surgical adhesiolysis remains the most common treatment, emerging evidence supports the use of adjunctive and nonsurgical approaches, such as pharmacologic agents, physical therapy, and lifestyle modifications. A multidisciplinary, patient-centered approach that integrates surgical, medical, and supportive therapies is essential for effective long-term management.

References

1. Holmdahl L. The role of fibrinolysis in adhesion formation. Eur J Surg Suppl. 1997;(577):24–31.
2. Diamond MP, DeCherney AH. Pathogenesis of adhesion formation/reformation: Application to reproductive pelvic surgery. Microsurgery. 1987;8(2):103–107.
3. Kavic SM. Adhesions and adhesiolysis: The role of laparoscopy. JSLS. 2002;6(2):99–109. PMID:12113430; PMCID:PMC3043408
4. Vrijland WW, Jeekel J, van Geldorp HJ, et al. Abdominal adhesions: Intestinal obstruction, pain, and infertility. Surg Endosc. 2003;17(7):1017–1022.
5. Al-Jabri S, Tulandi T. Management and prevention of pelvic adhesions. Semin Reprod Med. 2011;29(2):130–137. doi:10.1055/s-0030-1268705
6. Attard JAP, MacLean AR. Adhesive small bowel obstruction: Epidemiology, biology and prevention. Can J Surg. 2007;50(4):291–297.
7. Cheong YC, Reading I, Bailey S, et al. Should women with chronic pelvic pain have adhesiolysis? BMC Womens Health. 2014;14:36. doi:10.1186/1472-6874-14-36
8. Wiseman DM. Adhesions and adhesiolysis: The role of laparoscopy. J Reprod Med. 1999;44(2 Suppl):180–186.
9. Ahmad G, O'Flynn H, Hindocha A, Watson A. Barrier agents for adhesion prevention after gynaecological surgery. Cochrane Database Syst Rev. 2020;4(4):CD000475.
10. Victory Srinivasan N, Khan AI, Mashat GD, et al. Recurrence of small bowel obstruction in adults after operative management of adhesive small bowel obstruction: A systematic review. Cureus. 2022;14(9):e29141. doi:10.7759/cureus.29141
11. Menzies D, Ellis H. Intestinal obstruction from adhesions: How big is the problem? Ann R Coll Surg Engl. 1990;72(1):60–63.
12. Peters AA, Trimbos-Kemper GC, Admiraal C, Trimbos JB. A randomized clinical trial of the efficacy of adhesiolysis in patients with chronic pelvic pain. Fertil Steril. 1992;57(3):533–539.
13. Mais V. Pelvic adhesions and pain: The role of adhesiolysis. Best Pract Res Clin Obstet Gynaecol. 2004;18(6):959–972.

14. Tong JWV, Lingam P, Shelat VG. Adhesive small bowel obstruction: An update. Acute Med Surg. 2020;7(1):e587. doi:10.1002/ams2.587
15. Rice M, Patterson K, Cubillos J, Rice K. The efficacy of site-specific manual therapy in women with primary and secondary infertility: A retrospective chart review. Med Sci Monit. 2015;21:1983–1992.
16. Wurn BF, Wurn LJ, King CR, et al. Treating female infertility and improving pelvic pain with a manual physical therapy technique. MedGenMed. 2004;6(2):46.
17. Rice AD, King R, Reed EDA, Patterson K, Wurn BF, Wurn LJ. Manual physical therapy for non-surgical treatment of adhesion-related small bowel obstructions: Two case reports. J Clin Med. 2013;2(1):1–12. doi:10.3390/jcm2010001
18. Del Forno S, Cofini V, Mariani ML, et al. Pelvic floor physical therapy in patients with deep infiltrating endometriosis and pelvic floor dysfunction: A prospective case-control study. Int Urogynecol J. 2024;35(2):467–475.
19. Ghaderi F, Rakhshani Z. The effect of pelvic floor muscle exercise on women with chronic pelvic pain: A randomized controlled clinical trial. J Bodyw Mov Ther. 2019;23(3):538–543.
20. Silverman, Ann MD1,*; Samuels, Qiana MS1; Gikas, Helen RN1; Nawras, Ali MD2. Pregabalin for the treatment of abdominal adhesion pain: A randomized, double-blind, placebo-controlled trial. Am J Therapeutics. 2012;19(6):419–428. doi:10.1097/MJT.0b013e318217a5f5
21. Lim HK, Cho JY, Kim SH. Sclerotherapy of peritoneal inclusion cysts: A long-term evaluation study. Abdom Imaging. 2010;35:431–436. doi:10.1007/s00261-009-9530-4
22. Sung SH, Kim YJ, Yang YS, et al. Acupuncture treatment for chronic pelvic pain in women: A systematic review and meta-analysis of randomized controlled trials. Evid Based Complement Alternat Med. 2018;2018:9415897. doi:10.1155/2018/9415897
23. Abulughod N, Valakas S, El-Assaad F. Dietary and nutritional interventions for the management of endometriosis. Nutrients. 2024;16(23):3988. doi:10.3390/nu16233988
24. Herington JL, Glore DR, Lucas JA, Osteen KG, Bruner-Tran KL. Dietary fish oil supplementation inhibits formation of endometriosis-associated adhesions in a chimeric mouse model. Fertil Steril. 2013;99(2):543–550. doi:10.1016/j.fertnstert.2012.10.007
25. Sutton C. Adhesions and their prevention. Obstet Gynaecol. 2005;7(3):168–176. doi:10.1576/toag.7.3.168.27171

Suggested Reading

ten Broek RP, Strik C, Issa Y, et al. Adhesiolysis-related morbidity in abdominal surgery. Ann Surg. 2013;258(1):98–106.

ten Broek RPG, Bakkum EA, van Laarhoven CJHM, van Goor H. Epidemiology and prevention of postsurgical adhesions revisited. Ann Surg. 2016;263(1):12–19. doi:10.1097/SLA.0000000000001286

19
Interventional Treatments for Abdominal Pain in Women

Punthitra Arpornsuksant and Vahid Grami

Introduction

Although many causes of abdominal pain can be managed conservatively with medical approaches, some women may require additional or more invasive treatments. Interventional procedures for abdominal pain range from local infiltration of the abdominal wall to more complex procedures such as peripheral nerve blockade and mechanical implants.

These techniques are used for pain refractory to conventional drug therapy or for those wanting to avoid medication side effects (e.g., opioids). This chapter covers a range of interventional procedures, indications, complications, and basic anatomy.

Regional Anesthesia

Regional anesthesia can be considered for the abdominal or truncal planes. These procedures can range from local infiltration of the abdominal wall to peripheral nerve blocks. Potential complications including nerve damage, bleeding, infection, vasovagal response, local anesthetic toxicity, scarring, and procedure failure.

Myofascial and Trigger Point Injections

Myofascial trigger point injections are considered when anterior cutaneous nerve entrapment syndrome or myofascial pain is on the differential. Abdominal pain is often worse with flexion of abdominal wall muscles. Local anesthetic is injected at the trigger points, and pain relief is anticipated within 5–10 minutes. Lidocaine, bupivacaine, mepivacaine, ropivacaine, and procaine are the most utilized local anesthetics. Steroids like methylprednisolone or triamcinolone can be added to potentially prolong pain relief and duration of local anesthesia. This modality is useful in identifying sources of pain, but rarely provides long-lasting relief.[1]

Rectus Sheath Block

A rectus sheath block is indicated if the pain is thought to be from the anterior abdominal wall, possibly from nerve entrapment or hernia surgery. The block only provides anesthesia to the anterior abdominal wall close to the midline. The rectus sheath is made of the internal oblique, external oblique, and transversus abdominis muscles. The anterior cutaneous branches of the intercostal nerves are blocked using this technique. Ultrasound is used to identify the rectus abdominis muscles, which run vertically from either side of the midline. Local anesthetic is infiltrated between the muscle and posterior rectus sheath. Complications include inadvertent intra-abdominal needle placement, viscera puncture, local anesthetic toxicity, infection, bleeding, and intravascular injection.

Transversus Abdominis Plane Block

Transversus abdominis plane blocks are indicated for pain in the anterior or lateral abdominal wall. Indications include musculoskeletal pain; neuropathic pain, including postherpetic neuralgia; nerve entrapment; or pain from hernia surgery. Local anesthetic is injected between the internal oblique muscle and the transversus abdominus muscle under ultrasound guidance.

Sympathetic Nerve Blocks

Patients suffering from pain mediated by the sympathetic nervous system are ideal candidates for sympathetic blocks. Typical sympathetic blocks for abdominal pain target either the celiac plexus or the splanchnic plexus. In upper gastrointestinal tumors, both blocks have been shown to be clinically comparable.[2]

Celiac Plexus Block

The celiac plexus is responsible for gastrointestinal tract innervation, from the distal third of the esophagus to the transverse colon. It includes the liver, biliary tract, spleen, kidneys, and adrenal glands, as well as the mesentery. The celiac plexus is located retroperitoneally over the anterolateral surface of the aorta at the L1 level. It is a network of sympathetic and parasympathetic nerve fibers receiving sympathetic transmission from the greater, lesser, and least splanchnic nerves from the T5–T12 levels. A celiac plexus block is recommended for chronic pancreatitis, pancreatic cancer, and other upper abdominal malignancies.[3,4] Techniques are typically guided by fluoroscopy, although CT and ultrasound-guided techniques are also performed. Approaches include retrocrural, transcrural, and transaortic. Celiac plexus blocks may also be safely performed endoscopically.[5]

Splanchnic Nerve Block

Splanchnic nerve blocks are indicated for pain conditions arising from the stomach, pancreas, small bowel, kidneys, proximal ureters, and proximal large bowel. They can treat both malignant and nonmalignant conditions. The splanchnic nerve block avoids the celiac artery while also interrupting pain transmission before the nerves reach the celiac plexus. The greater, lesser, and least splanchnic nerves arise between T5 and T12. Interventional approaches to the splanchnic nerves usually target T11 and T12 via a dorsal approach under fluoroscopy, where the nerves are close to the vertebral body. Local anesthetics and neurolytic agents, or a combination, have all been used to target the celiac plexus and splanchnic nerve. Common complications of celiac and splanchnic plexus blocks include orthostatic hypotension and diarrhea due to sympathetic chain block, back pain from local needle trauma, or retroperitoneal hemorrhage.

Superior Hypogastric Plexus Block

The superior hypogastric plexus contains sympathetic fibers located ventral to the L5–S1 disc space, medial to the bifurcation of the common iliac arteries. It innervates the distal colon, bladder, uterus, vagina, urethra, prostate, and testes. There are multiple approaches to the superior hypogastric plexus. One approach is posteriorly at the L5–S1 disc. A transdiscal approach can also be performed, although disadvantages include the potential for discitis or disrupting the disc architecture.

Inferior Hypogastric Plexus Block

The inferior hypogastric plexus is in the lower pelvic region, receiving input from the sacrum. It contains sympathetic and parasympathetic output from the lower pelvic organs and genitalia. Patients who have sympathetically mediated pain from pelvic malignancies are candidates for an inferior hypogastric plexus block.[6] A trans-sacral approach is used to target the inferior hypogastric plexus at the S2 foramen but can also be accessed via S1 or S3. Complications include puncture of the hollow organs or paresthesia in the sacral nerve roots.

Ganglion Impar Block

Ganglion impar blocks are indicated for nociceptive and sympathetically mediated pain in the perineum, rectum, urethra, vagina, vulva, and scrotum. In retrospective studies, it appears to be helpful in patients with coccydynia and chronic pelvic pain.[7–9] The ganglion impar is located in the pre-coccygeal space, immediately anterior to the sacrococcygeal joint. Multiple approaches to the ganglion impar have been described, the most common being the trans-sacrococcygeal technique. A spinal needle is inserted toward the sacrococcygeal ligament under fluoroscopy, just exits the anterior portion of the disc, and passes through the sacrococcygeal ligament. There is a risk of inadvertent rectal puncture and subsequent peritonitis with this technique.

Pudendal Nerve Block

A pudendal nerve block can be considered for patients with pain originating from the perineum, external genitalia, or surrounding structures.[10] Most common causes of pudendal neuralgia include microtrauma from prolonged sitting, sports activities, pelvic surgeries, or radiation therapy. There are multiple approaches to the pudendal nerve, including the transvaginal, transperineal, perirectal, and transgluteal approaches. Complications include discomfort at the injection site, bleeding, or injury to surrounding organs such as the rectum and bladder.

Neurolysis and Radiofrequency Ablation

For longer-lasting relief, neurolysis and radiofrequency ablations can be considered. Prior to these, diagnostic local anesthetic blocks are typically administered to confirm the correct target and reduce unnecessary nerve damage. If the patient achieves short-term pain relief after a diagnostic block, they could be a good candidate for neurolysis. Neurolysis involves chemical ablation using alcohol or phenols, which leads to a prolonged interruption of pain transmission through temporary or permanent nerve dysfunction. Common targets include the celiac plexus, lumbar sympathetic nerves, and peripheral nerves. Chemical neurolysis functions to denature proteins and leads to a loss of cellular fatty content in the nerves by separating the myelin sheath from the axon. The desired nerve is identified via ultrasound, nerve stimulation, or fluoroscopy.

Radiofrequency ablation uses a neurodestructive technique at the nerve plexus to cause tissue necrosis. There is a transfer of radiofrequency currents (450–1,200 kHz) through needles that are placed close to the nerve targets via image guidance. An electric field is produced through the electrodes, creating heat between the cells and causing tissue destruction. Radiofrequency currents are nonselective and disrupt all nerve transmission. Pulsed radiofrequency ablation (PRFA) utilizes brief bursts of radiofrequency energy to allow heat to dissipate through target tissues, thereby allowing less nerve damage. The goal is to modulate pain transmission rather than destroy nerve tissue. Cooled radiofrequency ablation uses electrodes cooled by a continuous flow of water.[11] However, further investigation comparing the different types of ablation is warranted to evaluate their effectiveness on abdominal pain.

Spinal Cord Stimulation

Spinal cord stimulation (SCS) is a minimally invasive technique currently used to manage conditions such as failed back surgery syndrome, complex regional pain syndrome, and peripheral neuropathy. Leads are placed in the epidural space and deliver electrical impulses along the dorsal columns of the spinal cords, which could lead to a decrease in pain. SCS is currently considered an "off-label" treatment by the US Food and Drug Administration (FDA) to treat abdominal pain, although recent studies have shown that SCS can provide durable pain relief for abdominal pain.[12] One institution trialed SCS in patients with refractory abdominal pain and found that nausea, vomiting, and abdominal pain decreased by 6 months after implementation.[13] Some studies have shown that SCS can decrease pain from chronic pancreatitis up to 1 year after implantation and also treat chronic visceral pain.[14–16] Currently, SCS may be considered when both conservative therapies and conventional interventions fail to control or decrease chronic abdominal pain. However, more studies are needed.

Conclusion

Interventional procedures are a useful adjunct to traditional pain management modalities in abdominal pain. If patients have attempted conservative therapy but still have no significant pain relief, these procedures can be considered. These therapies warrant consideration when developing a multimodal analgesia plan for many patients suffering from malignant and nonmalignant causes of abdominal pain.

References

1. Niraj G. Pathophysiology and management of abdominal myofascial pain syndrome (AMPS): A three-year prospective audit of a management pathway in 120 patients. Pain Med. Oxford Academic; 2018;19:2256–2266.
2. Shwita AH, Amr YM, Okab MI. Comparative study of the effects of the retrocrural celiac plexus block versus splanchnic nerve block, c-arm guided, for upper gastrointestinal tract tumors on pain relief and the quality of life at a six-month follow up. Korean J Pain. 2015;28:22.
3. Brown DL. A retrospective analysis of neurolytic celiac plexus block for nonpancreatic intra-abdominal cancer pain. Reg Anesth. 1989;14:63–65.
4. Eisenberg E, Carr DB, Chalmers TC. Neurolytic celiac plexus block for treatment of cancer pain: A meta-analysis. Anesth Analg. 1995;80:290–295.
5. Sey MS, Schmaltz L, Al-Haddad MA, et al. Effectiveness and safety of serial endoscopic ultrasound-guided celiac plexus block for chronic pancreatitis. Endoscopy International Open. 2015;3. https://pubmed.ncbi.nlm.nih.gov/26134773/
6. Mohamed SA-E, Ahmed DG, Mohamad MF. Chemical neurolysis of the inferior hypogastric plexus for the treatment of cancer-related pelvic and perineal pain. Pain Res Manag. 2013;18:249.
7. Gunduz OH, Sencan S, Kenis-Coskun O. Pain relief due to transsacrococcygeal ganglion impar block in chronic coccygodynia: A pilot study. Pain Med. 2015;16:1278–1281.
8. Gonnade N, Mehta N, Khera PS, Kumar D, Rajagopal R, Sharma PK. Ganglion impar block in patients with chronic coccydynia. Indian J Radiol Imaging. 2017;27:324–328.
9. Le Clerc QC, Riant T, Levesque A, et al. Repeated ganglion impar block in a cohort of 83 patients with chronic pelvic and perineal pain. Pain Physician. 2017;20. https://pubmed.ncbi.nlm.nih.gov/28934788/
10. Ghanavatian S, Leslie SW, Derian A. Pudendal nerve block. StatPearls. 2024. https://pubmed.ncbi.nlm.nih.gov/31855362/
11. Vachirakorntong B, Kawana E, Zhitny VP, et al. Radiofrequency ablation's effectiveness for treating abdominal and thoracic chronic pain syndromes: A systematic review of the current literature. Pain Physician. 2023;26. https://pubmed.ncbi.nlm.nih.gov/37976476/
12. Richter B, Novik Y, Bergman JJ, Tomycz ND. The efficacy of BurstDR spinal cord stimulation for chronic abdominal pain: A clinical series. World Neurosurg. 2020;138:77–82.
13. Kapural L, Brown BK, Harandi S, Rejeski J, Koch K. Effects of spinal cord stimulation in patients with chronic nausea, vomiting, and refractory abdominal pain. Digestive Dis Sci. 2021;67:598–605.

14. Kapural L, Gupta M, Paicius R, et al. Treatment of chronic abdominal pain with 10-khz spinal cord stimulation: Safety and efficacy results from a 12-month prospective, multicenter, feasibility study. Clin Transl Gastroenterol. 2020;11:e00133.
15. Baranidharan G, Simpson KH, Dhandapani K. *Spinal Cord Stimulation for Visceral Pain – A Novel Approach. Neuromodulation: Technology at the Neural Interface*. Wiley; 2014;17:753–758.
16. Gulisano HA, Eriksen E, Bjarkam CR, Drewes AM, Olesen SS. A sham-controlled, randomized trial of spinal cord stimulation for the treatment of pain in chronic pancreatitis. Eur J Pain. 2024;28:1627–1639.

20
Interventional Pain Strategies for Advanced Robotic-Assisted Surgical Procedures

Joanna Sung, Sumedha Shastry, Shaan Srinivas, and Anita Gupta

Introduction

Visceral pain related to advanced intra-abdominal malignancies such as metastatic colon cancer can be particularly difficult to treat and is often resistant to escalating opioid therapy.[1–3] Although opioids are a mainstay of treatment for visceral pain, their use is often limited by side effects of constipation, sedation, and respiratory depression.[1] Celiac plexus block (CPB) is a well-described interventional procedure for the management of upper abdominal visceral pain related to pancreatic and gastrointestinal cancers.[4] In this case report, we present a successful application of CPB as part of multimodal treatment for a patient with metastatic colon cancer.

Clinical Vignette

A 65-year-old woman with stage IV adenocarcinoma of the descending colon was admitted for a 3-month history of progressive upper abdominal pain. The pain was steady, deep, sharp, and burning, located in the mid-epigastric and left upper quadrant areas and radiating to the back and lower extremities. The patient's cancer was complicated by liver and bony metastases as seen on imaging studies. She was cachectic and complained of moderate distress, poor sleep, and poor appetite. Her medical history included type 2 diabetes mellitus, anemia, and hypertension. The patient was receiving palliative chemotherapy. Her pain was initially controlled with nonopioid analgesics (ibuprofen and acetaminophen), but required dose escalation to sustained-release morphine 90 mg/day with worsening pain. Opioid-related adverse effects included opioid-induced constipation, sedation, and respiratory slowing. On physical exam, the patient was tender in the mid-epigastric and left upper quadrants with no evidence of bowel obstruction or peritonitis. There were no palpable masses.

Diagnosis

The patient was diagnosed with advanced metastatic colon cancer-associated visceral pain refractory to high-dose opioid therapy.

Interventional Management

Due to intractable, opioid-refractory visceral pain, a fluoroscopically guided bilateral celiac plexus block with neurolysis was done 3 days before the scheduled robotic intra-abdominal procedure. Sterilely, CPB was administered with bupivacaine local anesthetic. A bilateral transversus abdominis plane (TAP) block was also discussed for perioperative pain management (see Table 20.1).

Table 20.1 Summary of interventional treatments for robotic and abdominal procedures

Interventional treatment	Indications	Technique/Procedure	Notes
Celiac plexus block/ Neurolysis	Chronic abdominal pain (e.g., pancreatic cancer, chronic pancreatitis)	Injection of local anesthetic ± neurolytic agent (alcohol/phenol) around celiac plexus via percutaneous (CT/ fluoroscopy-guided) approach	Can provide months of pain relief; repeat as needed
Splanchnic nerve block	Upper abdominal visceral pain	Injection of anesthetic near thoracic splanchnic nerves under imaging guidance	Alternative to celiac plexus block; useful in refractory cases
Superior hypogastric plexus block	Lower abdominal/ pelvic pain	Injection of anesthetic near superior hypogastric plexus via fluoroscopy or CT guidance	Often used for pelvic malignancy pain
Ganglion impar block	Perineal, pelvic, lower abdominal pain	Injection of anesthetic near ganglion impar (at sacrococcygeal junction)	Useful for chronic perineal pain syndromes
Intrathecal/Epidural analgesia	Severe, refractory abdominal pain	Catheter placement in epidural or intrathecal space delivering opioids/ local anesthetics	For intractable pain when systemic meds fail
Radiofrequency ablation (RFA) of celiac plexus or splanchnic nerves	Chronic visceral abdominal pain	Use of thermal energy to ablate nerve fibers under imaging guidance	Longer-lasting relief than blocks alone
Peripheral nerve blocks (ilioinguinal, iliohypogastric, etc.)	Somatic abdominal wall pain, postsurgical pain	Local anesthetic injection around specific peripheral nerves	Helpful in neuropathic or surgical site pain
Transversus abdominis plane (TAP) block	Postoperative or somatic abdominal pain	Local anesthetic injected in fascial plane between internal oblique and transversus abdominis muscles	Used mainly for acute postoperative pain control
Intraperitoneal/Visceral nerve stimulation (experimental)	Refractory abdominal pain	Implantation of neurostimulator targeting visceral nerves	Emerging therapy, limited availability

Outcome

The patient was seen in follow-up 24 hours after the procedure. At this time, the patient noted her pain had decreased from 8/10 to 3/10 on the numeric pain scale. Over the next week, the patient was able to decrease her oral morphine dose by approximately 50%. The patient also noted improvement in her appetite, sleep, and ambulation, with decrease in abdominal tenderness on exam. Follow-up 2 weeks after the block noted that the patient's quality of life had improved. The patient was then cleared for discharge. No procedural complications were noted.

Discussion

Visceral pain from advanced intra-abdominal malignancies is one of the most challenging types of pain to control. Opioids are the mainstay of treatment, but they are often associated with dose-limiting adverse effects.[5] Interventional therapies such as CPB can provide targeted pain relief by interrupting nociceptive input from the celiac plexus, which supplies the upper abdominal viscera.[6] Several studies have shown that CPB can decrease opioid consumption and improve pain control and quality of life in patients with pancreatic and gastrointestinal cancers.[2,4] Our case further supports the role of CPB in the management of advanced metastatic colon cancer with refractory visceral pain, highlighting its importance as part of a multimodal pain management approach to optimize analgesia and minimize opioid-related adverse effects.

Conclusion

This case exemplifies the positive impact of a procedural intervention such as a celiac plexus block in the management of refractory visceral pain due to advanced metastatic colon cancer. CPB was effective in providing significant pain relief, decreasing opioid requirements, and improving functional outcomes.

Clinical Pearls

- Abdominal visceral pain from colon cancer metastases can be severe and difficult to control with systemic opioids alone.
- CPB is an effective option for managing upper abdominal visceral pain, especially when pain is refractory to high-dose opioids.
- CPB can reduce opioid requirements and related side effects such as sedation, constipation, and nausea.
- The procedure is typically done under fluoroscopic, CT, or ultrasound guidance for accuracy and safety.
- Indications for CPB include pancreatic cancer, upper GI malignancies, and advanced abdominal cancers with visceral pain.

- Risks of CPB include hypotension, diarrhea, transient motor weakness, and, rarely, neurologic complications.
- Multimodal pain management with integration of procedural interventions improves patient comfort and quality of life in advanced cancer.
- Early referral to palliative care pain specialists can optimize symptom control and timely use of interventional procedures.

References

1. Ballantyne, J. C., & Mao, J. (2003). Opioid therapy for chronic pain. *The New England Journal of Medicine, 349*(20), 1943–1953. https://doi.org/10.1056/NEJMra025411
2. Kurita, G. P., Sjøgren, P., Klepstad, P., & Mercadante, S. (2019). Interventional techniques for the management of cancer-related pain: Clinical and critical aspects. *Cancers, 11*(4), Article 443. https://doi.org/10.3390/cancers11040443
3. Mercadante, S. (2010). Management of cancer pain. *Internal and Emergency Medicine, 5*(S1), 31–35. https://doi.org/10.1007/s11739-010-0448-8
4. Nagels, W., Pease, N., Bekkering, G., Cools, F., & Dobbels, P. (2013). Celiac plexus neurolysis for abdominal cancer pain: A systematic review. *Pain Medicine, 14*(8), 1140–1163. https://doi.org/10.1111/pme.12176
5. Paice, J. A., & Ferrell, B. (2011). The management of cancer pain. *CA: A Cancer Journal for Clinicians, 61*(3), 157–182. https://doi.org/10.3322/caac.20112
6. Yamamuro, M., Kusaka, K., Kato, M., & Takahashi, M. (2000). Celiac plexus block in cancer pain management. *The Tohoku Journal of Experimental Medicine, 192*(1), 1–18. https://doi.org/10.1620/tjem.192.1

PART V

PELVIC PAIN DIAGNOSIS AND ADVANCED THERAPIES

21
Anatomical Considerations of the Female Pelvis

Sophie E. Smith and Alopi M. Patel

Muscles

Pelvic Floor Muscles

The pelvic floor muscles support pelvic organs and are also critical for functions including continence, micturition, defecation, and sexual function.[1] The pelvic floor muscles are generally organized into deep and superficial layers.

The deep layer of the pelvic floor consists of the levator ani muscle group and the coccygeus muscle. The levator ani muscle group, which supports the pelvic organs, consists of the pubococcygeus, puborectalis, and the iliococcygeus muscles.[2] The coccygeus muscle provides additional support and stabilizes the sacroiliac (SI) joint.[3]

The superficial layer of the pelvic floor consists of the bulbospongiosus, ischiocavernosus, the deep transverse perineal muscle, and the superficial transverse perineal muscle.[4]

Myofascial pain of the pelvic floor muscles, which is caused by muscle hypertonicity, is one of the most common causes of chronic pelvic pain in female patients.[5] The pelvic floor muscles also commonly sustain injuries associated with childbirth.[6] Aging reduces the proportion of type II (fast) muscle fibers, leading to decreased functionality over time[6] (Figure 21.1).

Abdominal Wall Muscles

The abdominal wall muscles, especially the rectus abdominis and oblique muscles, are a common yet often overlooked component of chronic pelvic pain in females.[7,8] The median abdominal wall is primarily composed of the rectus abdominis muscle, while the lateral abdominal wall contains, from superficial to deep, the external oblique, internal oblique, and transversus abdominis muscles.[8]

The rectus abdominis muscle, which is integral for functions including postural maintenance, trunk flexion/extension, and respiration, runs along the midline of the abdominal wall and has fibers running in a superior–inferior direction.[9] The external oblique muscle forms the superficial layer of the lateral abdominal wall, and its fibers run in an inferomedial direction.[10] Deeper to that is the internal oblique muscle, with fibers running superomedially.[10]

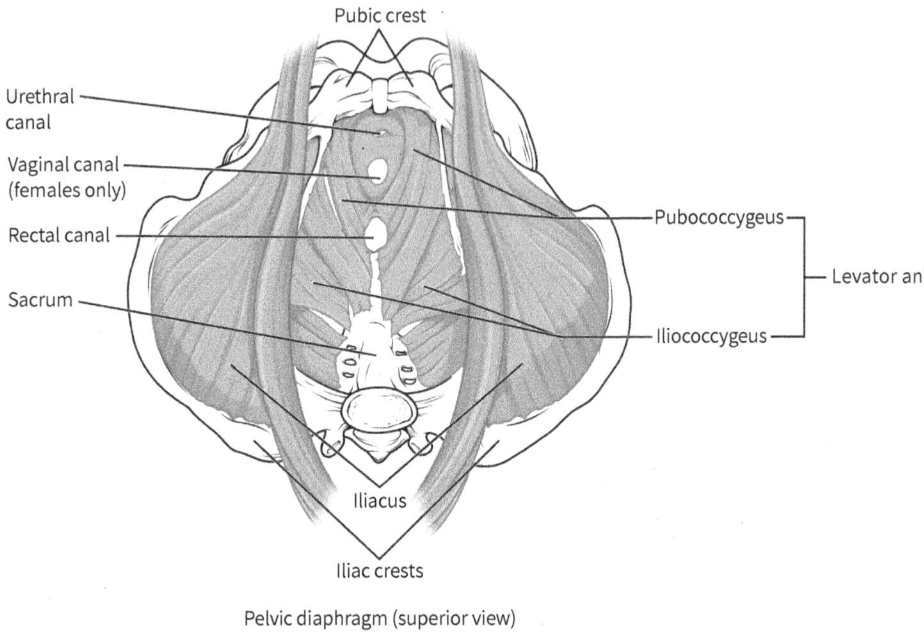

Figure 21.1 Pelvic floor muscles, superior view.

Version 8.25 from the Textbook, OpenStax Anatomy and Physiology. Source: Wikimedia Commons. Available at: https://commons.wikimedia.org/w/index.php?curid=30131690. Accessed November 21, 2025. License: CC BY 4.0.

Abdominal myofascial pain, which is caused by muscle hypertonicity, is a common contributor to chronic abdominal and pelvic pain in females.[11] Myofascial trigger points in the abdominal wall muscles, in addition to causing pain at their site of origin, may cause pain radiating to the groin and suprapubic region[11] (Figure 21.2).

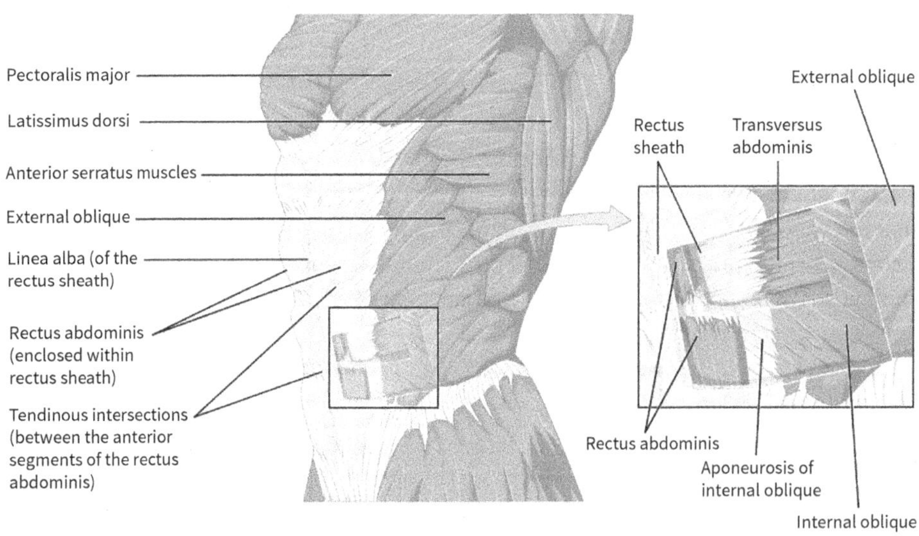

Figure 21.2 Abdominal wall muscles, anterolateral view.

Source: Wikimedia Commons. Available at: https://commons.wikimedia.org/wiki/File:1112_Muscles_of_the_Abdomen_Anterolateral.png. Accessed November 21, 2025. License: CC BY-SA 3.0.

Nerves

The autonomic innervation of the female pelvis is divided into sympathetic and parasympathetic constituents. The sympathetic nerves of the pelvis originate from T10–L2.[12] The parasympathetic nerves of the pelvis originate from S2–S4 and, occasionally, also from S1.[13] The sympathetic and parasympathetic nerves come together in inferior hypogastric plexus, which gives off branches to innervate pelvic organs including the bladder, uterus, vagina, and rectum.[13]

The pelvis receives somatic innervation primarily from the pudendal nerve, which arises from S2–S4 and innervates the external urethral and anal sphincters, perineal structures, clitoris, and labia.[14]

Pudendal neuralgia is caused by injury of the pudendal nerve and can result in perineal pain, sexual dysfunction, and bladder/bowel dysfunction.[15] Other nerve entrapment syndromes can affect the ilioinguinal, iliohypogastric, and genitofemoral nerves and can also cause pain and dysfunction affecting the pelvic region.[16] Neurogenic pelvic pain may be caused by irritation or entrapment due to anatomic variations, mechanical injuries such as childbirth, iatrogenic injury during surgery, constipation, or repetitive movements, or through nonmechanical injuries such as viral infections, tumors, radiation, multiple sclerosis, or diabetes mellitus (see Table 21.1).[13,15]

Table 21.1 Nerve innervations and nerve block options[17]

Target	Nerve root contributions	Nerve innervation	Nerve block options
Bladder	S2–S4 (parasympathetic), T10–L2 (sympathetic)	Pelvic splanchnic nerves, hypogastric nerve	Superior hypogastric plexus block, inferior hypogastric plexus block
Uterus	S2–S4 (parasympathetic), T10–L2 (sympathetic)	Pelvic splanchnic nerves, hypogastric nerve	Superior hypogastric plexus block, inferior hypogastric plexus block
Ovaries	T10–L2	Ovarian plexus, hypogastric nerve	Superior hypogastric plexus block
Rectum	S2–S4 (parasympathetic), T10–L2 (sympathetic)	Pelvic splanchnic nerves, hypogastric nerve	Ganglion impar block, superior hypogastric plexus block
Colon	S2–S4 (parasympathetic), T10–L2 (sympathetic)	Pelvic splanchnic nerves, hypogastric nerve	Superior hypogastric plexus block
Fallopian tubes	S2–S4 (parasympathetic), T10–L2 (sympathetic)	Pelvic splanchnic nerves, hypogastric nerve	Superior hypogastric plexus block
Pelvic floor muscles	S2–S4	Pudendal nerve, sacral plexus	Pudendal nerve block
Cutaneous innervation of perineum (clitoris, vulva)	S2–S4	Pudendal nerve	Pudendal nerve block

Bones

Key bony structures of the pelvic region include the lumbosacral spine, the pelvic girdle, the hip joints, and the coccyx. The pelvis contains two hip bones, also known as the pelvic girdle or os coxae, which are each made up of an ischium, ilium, and pubis.[18] Anteriorly, the pubis bones articulate with each other to form the pubic symphysis.[19] To form the posterior part of the pelvis, each ilium articulates with the sacrum to form the SI joint.[18] The coccyx articulates inferiorly to the sacrum at the sacrococcygeal joint.[19] The ilium, ischium, and pubis converge to form the acetabulum, or socket, where the femoral head articulates to form the ball-and-socket hip joint.[20]

Pelvic girdle pain is defined as pain involving the pelvic girdle bones or their articulations. Pelvic girdle pain can be caused or worsened by pregnancy, postpartum changes, trauma, repetitive use (e.g., athletics), or degenerative changes.[21] Pregnancy-related pelvic girdle pain is particularly common, affecting an estimated 1 in 5 patients in the pregnancy or postpartum period due to hormonal changes that increase the mobility of the SI joint and pubic symphysis.[22]

Coccydynia is defined as pain localized to the coccyx (tailbone), often exacerbated by sitting. Coccydynia is often caused by trauma to the coccyx, which serves as an attachment for pelvic floor muscles and is supported by ligaments.[23] Trauma or idiopathic events can result in excess mobility, subluxation, or altered curvature of the coccyx that ultimately leads to pain.[24] Coccydynia can be closely related to pelvic floor dysfunction given the close anatomical relationship between the coccyx and the pelvic floor muscles[25] (Figure 21.3).

Tissue

Visceral Organs

The visceral organs of the female pelvis include reproductive, urinary, and lower gastrointestinal organs. The female reproductive structures located in the pelvis include the uterus, ovaries, cervix, and vagina. The uterus is midline, situated with the bladder anteriorly and the sigmoid colon and rectum posteriorly.[26] The cervix is the inferior portion of the uterus, which projects into the vagina.[26] The ovaries are located laterally to the uterus and are suspended by the uteroovarian ligament medially and the infundibulopelvic ligament laterally.[26] The urinary bladder is located anterior to the uterus, with the urethra running inferiorly from the

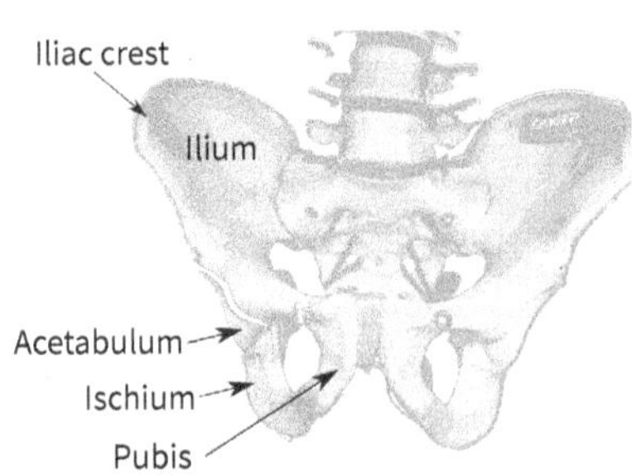

Figure 21.3 Bones of the pelvis, anterior view.

Source: Wikimedia Commons. Available at: https://commons.wikimedia.org/wiki/File:Pelvis_diagram.png. Accessed November 21, 2025. License: CC BY-SA 3.0.

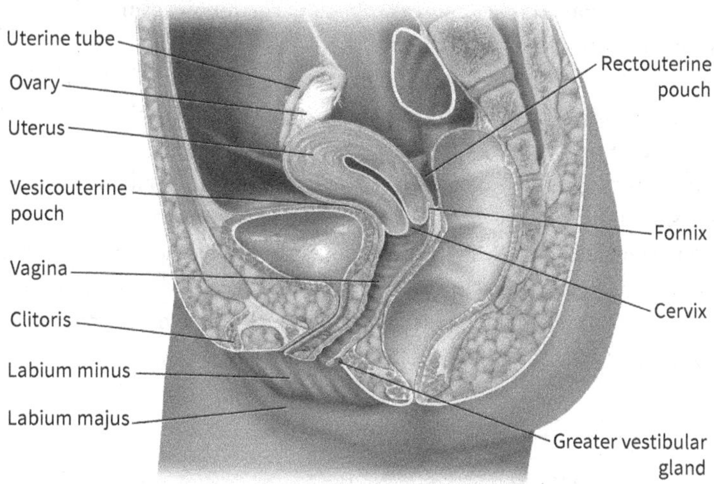

Figure 21.4 Visceral organs of the female pelvis, lateral midline view.
Source: Blausen.com staff (2014). Medical gallery of Blausen Medical 2014. WikiJournal of Medicine. 2014;1(2). doi:10.15347/wjm/2014.010. ISSN 2002-4436. Available at: https://commons.wikimedia.org/wiki/File:Blausen_0400_FemaleReproSystem_02.png. Accessed November 21, 2025. License: CC BY 3.0.

bladder across the anterior vaginal wall.[26] The sigmoid colon and rectum are located posterior to the uterus.[26]

The external anatomy of the female pelvis is comprised of the vulva, which is made up of structures including the mons pubis, labia majora, labia minora, clitoris, vestibule, urethral meatus, and vaginal introitus.[27]

Vulvodynia, defined as vulvar pain that occurs for at least 3 months without an identifiable cause, occurs in 8–10% of women.[28] The pathophysiology of vulvodynia is unclear, but it is thought to be triggered by a site-specific neuroinflammatory response.[29]

Endometriosis, defined as the presence of endometrial-like tissue outside the uterus, affects up to 10% of women.[30] These endometrial-like tissue lesions cause pelvic pain in up to 90% of affected individuals.[30]

Vaginismus, defined as involuntary muscle spasms of the muscles surrounding the vagina, can make vaginal penetration painful or impossible.[31] The etiology of vaginismus is unclear.[31]

Interstitial cystitis, also known as bladder pain syndrome, is defined as chronic bladder pain with urinary symptoms. It often co-occurs with pelvic floor dysfunction[32] (Figure 21.4).

Vasculature

The internal iliac artery provides the primary arterial blood supply to the pelvic viscera, muscles, and skin.[33] The internal iliac artery divides into an anterior and a posterior branch, which subsequently divide into additional branches that can have significant variation.[33] The posterior division of the internal iliac artery most commonly branches into the iliolumbar artery, the lateral sacral artery, and the superior gluteal artery.[33] The anterior division of the internal iliac artery gives off branches including the umbilical artery, obturator artery, inferior vesical artery, middle rectal artery, internal pudendal artery, inferior gluteal artery, uterine artery, and vaginal artery.[34] There is substantial anatomical variability in the branching patterns and origins of the pelvic arteries.[34]

Venous drainage from the pelvis has many anatomical variations and pathways for anastomosis [35] The main collecting veins of the pelvis include the internal iliac veins, the ovarian veins, and the superior rectal veins.[36]

Pelvic congestion syndrome is a cause of chronic pelvic pain resulting from incompetent (dilated and dysfunctional) pelvic veins.[37] The etiology of pelvic congestion syndrome is multifactorial and may include genetic predisposition, anatomical variation, hormonal influence, damage to the vein, valvular dysfunction, retrograde blood flow, and hypertension.[38] These factors can result in venous engorgement and varicosities with variable presentation based on the anatomical differences and multiple anastomoses within the pelvic vasculature[38] (Figure 21.5).

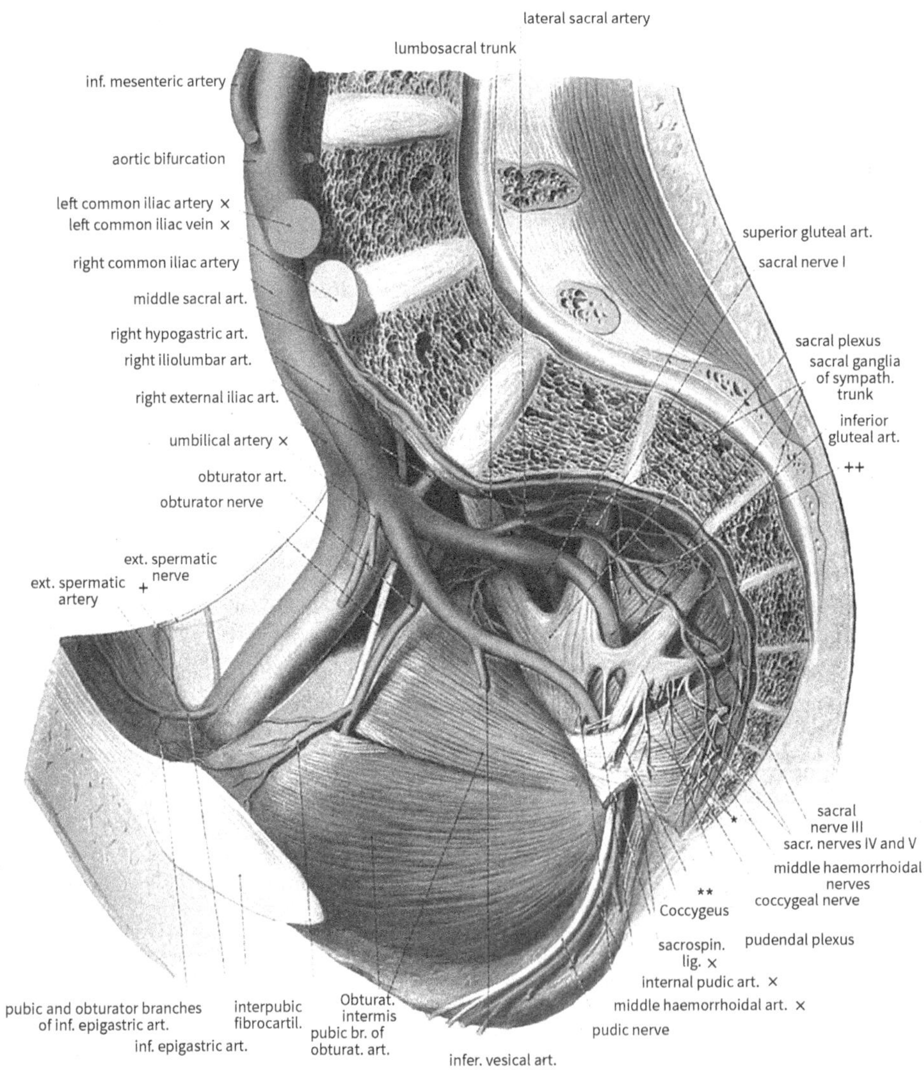

Figure 21.5 Vasculature of the pelvis, lateral midline view.

Source: Sobo. *Atlas and Text-book of Human Anatomy. Volume III: Vascular System, Lymphatic System, Nervous System and Sense Organs.* GetArchive.net. Published 1909. Accessed November 24, 2025. https://itoldya420.getarchive.net/amp/media/sobo-1909-568-09ec8b

Table 21.2 Pelvic pain diagnoses[17]

Diagnosis	Description	Treatment
Musculoskeletal		
Pudendal neuralgia	Pain due to pudendal nerve entrapment or irritation	Nerve blocks, physical therapy, neuromodulators (e.g., gabapentin)
Myofascial pelvic pain	Localized pain in pelvic floor muscles and surrounding fascia	Pelvic floor physical therapy, trigger point injections, oral neuromodulators, muscle relaxants (oral or suppository)
Pelvic floor dysfunction	Hypertonic or spastic pelvic floor muscles causing pain or urinary/gastrointestinal symptoms	Pelvic floor physical therapy, biofeedback, muscle relaxants (oral or suppository)
Levator ani syndrome	Chronic or recurrent pain in the rectum and perineum	Pelvic floor physical therapy, trigger point injections, biofeedback
Piriformis syndrome	Buttock and leg pain due to piriformis muscle compressing the sciatic nerve	Ultrasound-guided injections, physical therapy, botulinum toxin injections
Nerve entrapment syndromes	Entrapment of nerves such as ilioinguinal, iliohypogastric, and genitofemoral nerves	Ultrasound-guided nerve blocks, physical therapy, neuromodulators
Coccydynia	Pain localized to the coccyx (tailbone), often exacerbated by sitting.	Physical therapy, coccygeal manipulation, ganglion impar injection
Pelvic girdle pain	Pain involving the pelvic girdle bones (sacarum, ilium, pubic bone, coccyx)	Physical therapy, pelvic support devices, targeted injections (i.e. SI joint injection, ganglion impar block, pubic symphysis injection)
Abdominal myofascial pain	Pain from the myofascial structures of the abdominal wall	Physical therapy, muscle relaxants, trigger point injections
Gynecologic causes		
Vulvodynia	Pain condition affecting the vulva, characterized by pain without an identifiable cause	Physical therapy, Topical medications, oral neuromodulators, suppositories, pudendal nerve block, acupuncture
Endometriosis	Ectopic endometrial tissue causing pelvic pain	Hormonal therapy, surgical excision, pain management via medications and sympathetic nerve blocks
Vaginismus	Involuntary spasms of the muscles surrounding the outer third of the vagina, making vaginal penetration painful or impossible	Physical therapy, CBT, muscle relaxants (oral or suppository), trigger point injections
Urologic causes		
Interstitial cystitis/Bladder pain syndrome (IC/BPS)	Chronic bladder pain with urinary symptoms	Dietary and lifestyle modifications, bladder instillations, oral medications (e.g., amitriptyline), sympathetic nerve blocks
Vascular		
Pelvic congestion syndrome	Chronic pelvic pain due to varicosities in pelvic veins	Compressive stockings, venous embolization, pain management via medications

Skin

Dermatologic conditions are another possible etiology of pelvic pain and should not be overlooked as part of the differential diagnosis for pelvic pain. Some common dermatologic causes of pelvic pain include herpes simplex virus, contact dermatitis, intertrigo, hidradenitis suppurativa, flexural psoriasis, and lichen sclerosis.[39–44]

Rarer but important to consider dermatologic causes of pelvic pain include perineal necrotizing fasciitis and herpes zoster. Perineal necrotizing fasciitis, also known as Fournier's gangrene, is a rare but serious necrotizing infection involving the perineal or genital fascia.[45] It presents with severe pain and signs of sepsis, and urgent surgical evaluation is warranted if Fournier's gangrene is suspected.[45] Herpes zoster affecting the lumbosacral dermatomes can cause severe unilateral pelvic pain. Herpes zoster outbreaks are associated with a vesicular rash, but the pain may precede the skin findings (see Table 21.2).[46]

References

1. Quaghebeur J, Petros P, Wyndaele JJ, De Wachter S. Pelvic-floor function, dysfunction, and treatment. Eur J Obstet Gynecol Reprod Biol. 2021;265:143–149. doi:10.1016/j.ejogrb.2021.08.026
2. DeLancey JO, Mastrovito S, Masteling M, Horner W, Ashton-Miller JA, Chen L. A unified pelvic floor conceptual model for studying morphological changes with prolapse, age, and parity. Am J Obstet Gynecol. 2024;230(5):476–484.e2. doi:10.1016/j.ajog.2023.11.1247
3. Cho ST, Kim KH. Pelvic floor muscle exercise and training for coping with urinary incontinence. J Exerc Rehabil. 2021;17(6):379–387. doi:10.12965/jer.2142666.333
4. Aljuraifani R, Stafford RE, Hall LM, Van Den Hoorn W, Hodges PW. Task-specific differences in respiration-related activation of deep and superficial pelvic floor muscles. J Appl Physiol. 2019;126(5):1343–1351. doi:10.1152/japplphysiol.00704.2018
5. Torosis M, Carey E, Christensen K, et al. A treatment algorithm for high-tone pelvic floor dysfunction. Obstet Gynecol. 2024;143(4):595–602. doi:10.1097/AOG.0000000000005536
6. Tim S, Mazur-Bialy AI. The most common functional disorders and factors affecting female pelvic floor. Life. 2021;11(12):1397. doi:10.3390/life11121397
7. Mui J, Allaire C, Williams C, Yong PJ. Abdominal wall pain in women with chronic pelvic pain. J Obstet Gynaecol Can JOGC. 2016;38(2):154–159. doi:10.1016/j.jogc.2015.11.003
8. Shian B, Larson ST. Abdominal wall pain: Clinical evaluation, differential diagnosis, and treatment. Accessed May 18, 2025. https://www.aafp.org/pubs/afp/issues/2018/1001/p429.html
9. Broyles JM, Schuenke MD, Patel SR, Vail CM, Broyles HV, Dellon AL. Defining the anatomy of the tendinous intersections of the rectus abdominis muscle and their clinical implications in functional muscle neurotization. Ann Plast Surg. 2018;80(1):50. doi:10.1097/SAP.0000000000001193
10. Crommert ME, Bjerkefors A, Tarassova O, Ekblom MM. Abdominal muscle activation during common modifications of the trunk curl-up exercise. J Strength Cond Res. 2021;35(2):428. doi:10.1519/JSC.0000000000002439
11. Temel MH, Bağcıer F. Abdominal wall pain and primary dysmenorrhea: The importance of myofascial trigger points. Complement Med Res. 2023;30(4):360–361. doi:10.1159/000530035

12. Shoja MM, Sharma A, Mirzayan N, et al. Neuroanatomy of the female abdominopelvic region: A review with application to pelvic pain syndromes. Clin Anat. 2013;26(1):66–76. doi:10.1002/ca.22200
13. Aurore V, Röthlisberger R, Boemke N, et al. Anatomy of the female pelvic nerves: A macroscopic study of the hypogastric plexus and their relations and variations. J Anat. 2020;237(3):487–494. doi:10.1111/joa.13206
14. Choi BJ, Chung MS, Chung BS. Pudendal nerve identified on sectioned images of female cadaveric pelvis. Urology. 2020;142:76–80. doi:10.1016/j.urology.2020.05.007
15. Conic RRZ, Kaur P, Kohan LR. Pudendal neuralgia: A review of the current literature. Curr Pain Headache Rep. 2025;29(1):38. doi:10.1007/s11916-024-01354-z
16. Elkins N, Hunt J, Scott KM. Neurogenic pelvic pain. Phys Med Rehabil Clin N Am. 2017;28(3):551–569. doi:10.1016/j.pmr.2017.03.007
17. Patel A, Levin D, Kirpekar M, Gritsenko K. Managing musculoskeletal causes of pelvic pain. In: *Essentials of Pain Medicine*. 5th ed. Pending publication.
18. Lewis CL, Laudicina NM, Khuu A, Loverro KL. The human pelvis: Variation in structure and function during gait. Anat Rec Hoboken NJ 2007. 2017;300(4):633–642. doi:10.1002/ar.23552
19. Eickmeyer SM. Anatomy and physiology of the pelvic floor. Phys Med Rehabil Clin N Am. 2017;28(3):455–460. doi:10.1016/j.pmr.2017.03.003
20. Verbruggen SW, Nowlan NC. Ontogeny of the human pelvis. Anat Rec. 2017;300(4):643–652. doi:10.1002/ar.23541
21. Stover MD, Edelstein AI, Matta JM. Chronic anterior pelvic instability: Diagnosis and management. J Am Acad Orthop Surg. 2017;25(7):509–517. doi:10.5435/JAAOS-D-15-00338
22. Sward L, Manning N, Murchison AB, Ghahremani T, McCaulley JA, Magann EF. Pelvic girdle pain in pregnancy: A review. Obstet Gynecol Surv. 2023;78(6):349. doi:10.1097/OGX.0000000000001140
23. Woon JTK, Stringer MD. Clinical anatomy of the coccyx: A systematic review. Clin Anat. 2012;25(2):158–167. doi:10.1002/ca.21216
24. Fogel GR, Cunningham PY, Esses SI. Coccygodynia: Evaluation and management. J Am Acad Orthop Surg. 2004;12(1):49–54. doi:10.5435/00124635-200401000-00007
25. Neville CE, Carrubba AR, Li Z, Ma Y, Chen AH. Association of coccygodynia with pelvic floor symptoms in women with pelvic pain. PM&R. 2022;14(11):1351–1359. doi:10.1002/pmrj.12706
26. Roach MK, Andreotti RF. The normal female pelvis. Clin Obstet Gynecol. 2017;60(1):3. doi:10.1097/GRF.0000000000000259
27. Hill AJ, Balgobin S, Mishra K, et al. Recommended standardized anatomic terminology of the posterior female pelvis and vulva based on a structured medical literature review. Am J Obstet Gynecol. 2021;225(2):169.e1–169.e16. doi:10.1016/j.ajog.2021.02.033
28. Bergeron S, Reed BD, Wesselmann U, Bohm-Starke N. Vulvodynia. Nat Rev Dis Primer. 2020;6(1):1–21. doi:10.1038/s41572-020-0164-2
29. Bornstein J, Palzur E, Swash M, Petros P. Vulvodynia: A neuroinflammatory pain syndrome originating in pelvic visceral nerve plexuses due to mechanical factors. Arch Gynecol Obstet. 2022;306(5):1411–1415. doi:10.1007/s00404-022-06424-4
30. As-Sanie S, Mackenzie SC, Morrison L, et al. Endometriosis: A review. JAMA. Published online May 5, 2025. doi:10.1001/jama.2025.2975
31. Clinical assessment and management of vaginismus. Australian J Gen Pract. Accessed May 31, 2025. https://www1.racgp.org.au/ajgp/2024/january-february/clinical-assessment-and-management-of-vaginismus

32. Clemens JQ, Erickson DR, Varela NP, Lai HH. Diagnosis and treatment of interstitial cystitis/bladder pain syndrome. J Urol. Published online July 2022. doi:10.1097/JU.0000000000002756
33. Hajdyła P, Ostrowski P, Bonczar M, et al. Exploring the branching pattern of the posterior division of the internal iliac artery: An analysis based on 75 computed tomography angiographies. Int Urogynecology J. 2024;35(11):2171–2180. doi:10.1007/s00192-024-05944-8
34. Hajdyła P, Bonczar M, Ostrowski P, et al. The anatomy of the anterior division of the internal iliac artery: A computed tomography angiography analysis with implications for surgical and endovascular procedures. Surg Radiol Anat. 2025;47(1):68. doi:10.1007/s00276-025-03575-2
35. Zurcher KS, Staack SO, Spencer EB, et al. Venous anatomy and collateral pathways of the pelvis: An angiographic review. Radiogr Rev. 2022;42(5):1532–1545. doi:10.1148/rg.220012
36. Leiber LM, Thouveny F, Bouvier A, et al. MRI and venographic aspects of pelvic venous insufficiency. Diagn Interv Imaging. 2014;95(11):1091–1102. doi:10.1016/j.diii.2014.01.012
37. Jurga-Karwacka A, Karwacki GM, Schoetzau A, Zech CJ, Heinzelmann-Schwarz V, Schwab FD. A forgotten disease: Pelvic congestion syndrome as a cause of chronic lower abdominal pain. PLoS ONE. 2019;14(4):e0213834. doi:10.1371/journal.pone.0213834
38. Bałabuszek K, Toborek M, Pietura R. Comprehensive overview of the venous disorder known as pelvic congestion syndrome. Ann Med. 54(1):22–36. doi:10.1080/07853890.2021.2014556
39. Gnann JW, Whitley RJ. Genital herpes. N Engl J Med. 2016;375(7):666–674. doi:10.1056/NEJMcp1603178
40. Fonacier L, Bernstein DI, Pacheco K, et al. Contact dermatitis: A practice parameter–update 2015. J Allergy Clin Immunol Pract. 2015;3(3):S1–S39. doi:10.1016/j.jaip.2015.02.009
41. Kalra MG, Higgins KE, Kinney BS. Intertrigo and secondary skin infections. Am Fam Physician. 2014;89(7):569–573.
42. Sabat R, Alavi A, Wolk K, et al. Hidradenitis suppurativa. Lancet Lond Engl. 2025;405(10476):420–438. doi:10.1016/S0140-6736(24)02475-9
43. Raharja A, Mahil SK, Barker JN. Psoriasis: A brief overview. Clin Med. 2021;21(3):170–173. doi:10.7861/clinmed.2021-0257
44. Conte S, Mohamed SD, Cohen Y, et al. Clinical presentations and complications of lichen sclerosus: A systematic review. J Dtsch Dermatol Ges. 2025;23(2):143–149. doi:10.1111/ddg.15606
45. Tarasconi A, Perrone G, Davies J, et al. Anorectal emergencies: WSES-AAST guidelines. World J Emerg Surg WJES. 2021;16:48. doi:10.1186/s13017-021-00384-x
46. Dayan RR, Peleg R. Herpes zoster: Typical and atypical presentations. Postgrad Med. 2017;129(6):567–571. doi:10.1080/00325481.2017.1335574

22
Interventional Treatments for Chronic Pelvic Pain in Women

Trevor Van De Water and Stephanie Crimmel

Introduction

Chronic pelvic pain (CPP) in women is defined as persistent pain perceived to originate from the pelvis lasting for 6 months or more and not exclusively explained by menstruation, intercourse, or pregnancy. CPP in women is often associated with negative cognitive, behavioral, sexual, and emotional consequences and symptoms suggestive of lower urinary tract, sexual, bowel, myofascial, or gynecologic dysfunction.[1,2] CPP in women is often a complex and debilitating condition that affects about 15% of the female population in the United States, and the etiology is often undiagnosed.[3] Treatment of CPP in women include pharmacologic approaches, pelvic physical therapy, cognitive behavioral therapy, and interventional pain procedures. This chapter provides an overview of interventional pain procedures for women with CPP, focusing on evidence-based techniques.

Trigger Point Injections

Trigger point injections (TPIs) are a procedural option for women with CPP especially when myofascial pelvic floor or pelvic floor dysfunction is present.[4] Methodologies for TPI vary, but generally, a local anesthetic, corticosteroid, botulinum toxin, or dry needle is used to target pelvic floor muscles. The targeted muscles include the levator ani, coccygeus, obturator internus, superficial and deep transverse perinei, piriformis, or iliococcygeus. Proposed mechanism of action theories includes mechanical disruption of muscle fibers, dilution of nociceptive substances, vasodilatation removing excess metabolites, and release of nociceptive/inflammatory biochemicals.[5] Combination of TPI and physical therapy and myofascial release can enhance pain relief compared to each intervention alone.[5]

Selective Nerve Blocks

Selective nerve blocks can be both diagnostic and therapeutic in the management of CPP in women. A diagnostic block can help localize the pain generator. Treatment involves an injection performed under ultrasound or fluoroscopic guidance with local anesthetic alone or a combination of local anesthetic and corticosteroid if therapeutic results are desired. If sustained relief is achieved, these selective nerve blocks can be repeated serially every 3–4 months or longer. Additionally, ablative techniques are available to provide longer sustained relief in patients with shorter durations of relief or in those with contraindications to repeated administrations of steroids.

Pudendal Nerve Block

The pudendal nerve arises from S2–S4 nerve roots of the sacral plexus and carries sensory, motor, somatic, and sympathetic fibers to the perineum and the external genitalia.

Classical presentation of pudendal neuralgia is unilateral hyperalgesia of the external genitalia that is worsened throughout the day and with sitting.[6] Fluoroscopy can be used to identify bony landmarks such as the ischial spine and the sacrospinous ligament where the pudendal nerve is located (Figure 22.1).

Iliohypogastric and Ilioinguinal Nerve Blocks

The iliohypogastric and ilioinguinal nerves arise from T12 and L1 of the lumbar plexus. The iliohypogastric nerve innervates the skin superior to the pubis. The ilioinguinal nerves supplies sensation to the upper thigh, lateral labia, and mons pubis. Both nerves cross obliquely anterior to the quadratus lumborum and iliacus muscles and perforate the transverse abdominis muscle near the anterior part of the iliac crest where they can be selectively or

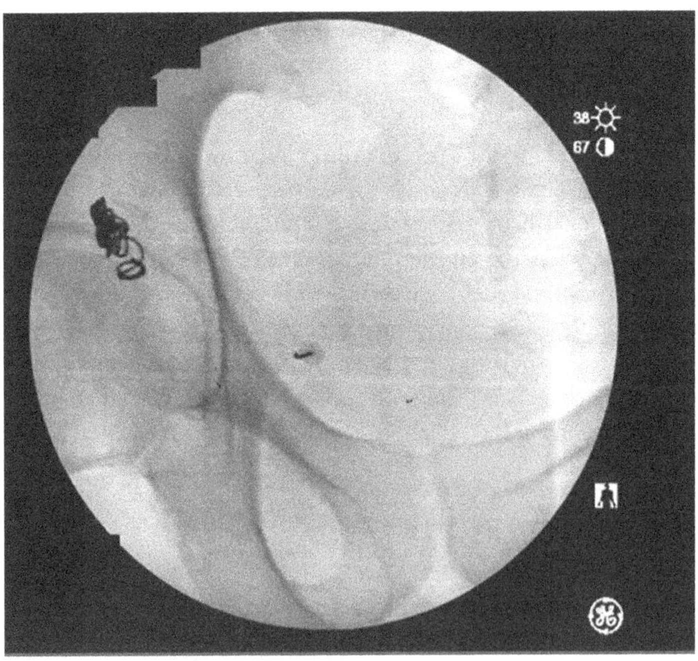

Figure 22.1 Fluoroscopic image of spinal needle targeting the pudendal nerve at the ischial spine.
Source: Courtesy of Johns Hopkins School of Medicine.

jointly blocked.[7] Arising from the L1 and L2 nerve roots, the genitofemoral nerve separates into genital and femoral branches. The landmark for blockade of the genital branch is the pubic tubercle.[7]

Sympathetic Plexus Blocks and Neurolysis

Visceral pain, often diffuse and vague, responds well to plexus-based blocks and neurolytic interventions. Sympathetic blocks can be performed with CT, fluoroscopy, or ultrasound guidance using injectates of local anesthetic, steroid, or chemical neurolytic agents such as phenol, absolute alcohol, or glycerin.[8]

Superior Hypogastric Plexus Block

The superior hypogastric plexus (SHP) is located within the retroperitoneum between vertebral levels L5 and S1. This nerve plexus is anterior and lateral to the abdominal aorta just below the aortic bifurcation. As part of autonomic abdominopelvic nervous system, the SHP contains afferent pain fibers responsible for visceral innervation of numerous pelvic structures such as the descending colon, rectum, internal sex organs, uterus, bladder, urethra, and perineum. The SHP block is performed using the traditional bilateral posterior approach to the anterolateral junction of L5–S1 under fluoroscopic guidance.[9] The SHP block was described in 1990 by Placarte et al. as a treatment for chronic pelvic pain (CPP) secondary to malignancy.[9,10]

Ganglion Impar Block

The ganglion impar (also known as the ganglion of Walther) is the final pelvic ganglion of the efferent sympathetic trunk formed by the convergence of bilateral paravertebral sympathetic chains terminating anteriorly as a single midline ganglion. It is located anterior to the sacrococcygeal ligament. The ganglion impar provides nociceptive and sympathetic innervation to the pelvic visceral, perineal region, distal rectum, distal urethra, distal third of the vagina, and vulva/scrotum.[10] The ganglion impar block was first described by Placarte et al. in 1990 for the treatment of intractable perineal cancer pain of sympathetic etiology.[9,10] Figure 22.2 shows a fluoroscopic approach targeting the ganglion impar.

Neuromodulation

Neuromodulation is well-established for treating a variety of chronic painful conditions, the most common being painful spine conditions and complex regional pain syndrome. Neuromodulation for chronic pelvic pain can be quite challenging. This is due to the extensive innervation of the pelvis encompassing spinal segments from T12 to S5.[11]

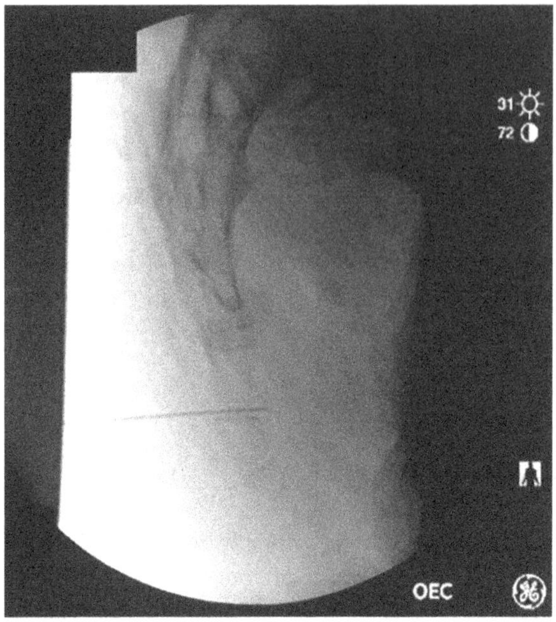

Figure 22.2 Lateral fluoroscopic image of spinal needle targeting the ganglion impar anterior to the sacrococcygeal ligament.
Source: Courtesy of Johns Hopkins School of Medicine.

Spinal Cord Stimulation and Dorsal Root Ganglia Stimulation

Spinal cord stimulation (SCS) involves the implantation of epidural-based leads connected to an internal battery generator. Paresthesia-based or paresthesia-free stimulation of the dorsal column is the basis for pain relief.[12] Dorsal root ganglia (DRG) stimulation similarly involves epidural placement with leads placed anterograde into each respective intervertebral foramen of the targeted level. The DRG intersects both sensory and sympathetic afferent fibers. Both SCS and DRG stimulation begin with a week-long percutaneous trial period with the leads attached to an external generator. If the patient has a satisfactory response to the trial, the next steps in the procedure are definitive implantation in an outpatient surgical suite.[12,13]

A novel case series by Hunter and Yang involving seven patients with CPP reported successful treatment using DRG stimulation with leads placed at bilateral L1 and S2 levels.[13] According to their anatomical rationale, the L1 DRG stimulation targets lumbar autonomic innervation through the first white communicating branch and dermatomes related to pelvic innervation from the lumbar region, including the iliohypogastric, ilioinguinal, and genitofemoral nerves. The S2 DRG stimulation addresses pelvic autonomic innervation and dermatomes associated with pelvic innervation involving the posterior femoral cutaneous, pudendal, and inferior rectal nerves.[11,13] This lead placement has shown promising results in a case series by Da Silva et al. of women with endometriosis pain. There was a significant reduction in pain scores at 12-month follow-up from the nine women who underwent permanent DRG stimulator implantation.[14]

Peripheral Nerve Stimulation

Peripheral nerve stimulation (PNS) is a neuromodulation technique that sends electrical stimulation to specific peripheral nerves to modulate pain signaling. Recent systematic reviews have suggested that PNS can be used for chronic pelvic pain in women who have not responded to other conservative therapies and when pain is localized to a specific nerve.[15] Using ultrasound or fluoroscopy guidance, PNS leads can be placed percutaneously or surgically to target the pudendal, genitofemoral, ilioinguinal, or sacral nerves, among others.[16]

References

1. American College of Obstetrics and Gynecology. Chronic pelvic pain: ACOG practice bulletin, number 218. Obstet Gynecol. 2020;135(3):e98–e109. doi:10.1097/AOG.0000000000003716
2. Lamvu G, Carrillo J, Ouyang C, Rapkin A. Chronic pelvic pain in women: A review. JAMA. 2021;325(23):2381–2391. doi:10.1001/jama.2021.2631
3. Mathias, SD, Kuppermann, M, Liberman RF, Lipschutz RC, Steege JF. Chronic pelvic pain: Prevalence, health-related quality of life, and economic correlates. Obstet Gynecol. 1996;87(3):321–327.
4. Torres JE, Nagpal AS, Iya A, McGeary D, Srinivasan M. Interventional treatment options for women with pelvic pain. Curr Phys Med Rehabil Rep. 2020;8(3):229–239.
5. Lewis GK, Chen AH, Craver EC, Crook JE, Carrubba AR. Trigger point injections followed by immediate myofascial release in the treatment of pelvic floor tension myalgia. Arch Gynecol Obstet. 2023;307(4):1027–1035. doi:10.1007/s00404-022-06880-y
6. Vancaillie T, Eggermont J, Armstrong G, Jarvis S, Liu J, Beg N. Response to pudendal nerve block in women with pudendal neuralgia. Pain Med. 2012;13(4):596–603.
7. Huntzinger J, Selassie M. Interventional pain management in the treatment of chronic pelvic pain. Curr Urol Rep. 2023;24(4):165–171.
8. Green IC, Cohen SL, Finkenzeller D, Christo PJ. Interventional therapies for controlling pelvic pain: What is the evidence? Curr Pain Headache Rep. 2010;14(1):22–32. doi:10.1007/s11916-009-0089-7
9. Khodaverdi S, Alebouyeh MR, Sadegi K, et al. Superior hypogastric plexus block as an effective treatment method for endometriosis-related chronic pelvic pain: An open-label pilot clinical trial. J Obstet Gynaecol. 2021;41(6):966–971.
10. Sousa Correia J, Silva M, Castro C, Miranda L, Agrelo A. The efficacy of the ganglion impar block in perineal and pelvic cancer pain. Support Care Cancer. 2019;27(11):4327–4330.
11. Gish B, Langford B, Sobey C, et al. Neuromodulation for the management of chronic pelvic pain syndromes: A systematic review. Pain Pract. 2024;24(2):321–340. doi:10.1111/papr.13295
12. Tate JL, Stauss T, Li S, Rotte A, Subbaroyan J. A prospective, multi-center, clinical trial of a 10-khz spinal cord stimulation system in the treatment of chronic pelvic pain. Pain Pract. 2021;21(1):45–53.
13. Hunter CW, Yang A. Dorsal root ganglion stimulation for chronic pelvic pain: A case series and technical report on a novel lead configuration. Neuromodulation. 2019;22(1):87–95.

14. Da Silva Freitas T, Barbosa de Oliveira AJ, Golovac S, Assumpcao de Monaco B. Dorsal root ganglion stimulation for chronic pelvic pain secondary to endometriosis. Neuromodulation. Published online December 24, 2024. doi: 10.1016/j.neurom.2024.11.007
15. Xu J, Sun Z, Wu J, et al. Peripheral nerve stimulation in pain management: A systematic review. Pain Physician. 2021;24(2):E131–E152.
16. Strand N, D'Souza RS, Hagedorn JM, et al. Evidence-based clinical guidelines from the American Society of Pain and Neuroscience for the use of implantable peripheral nerve stimulation in the treatment of chronic pain. J Pain Res. 2022 Aug 23;15:2483–2504. doi:10.2147/JPR.S362204

23
Uterine Fibroids and Menstrual Pain
Medical, Interventional, and Surgical Treatments

Shawana S. Moore

Introduction

Uterine fibroids, also known as *leiomyomas* or *myomas*, are benign tumors of the uterine smooth muscle. They are among the most common pelvic neoplasms in women of reproductive age, affecting up to 50–80% of women by menopause.[1] Uterine fibroids affect up to 70% of white women and 80% of black women.[2] It is estimated that at least 50% are asymptomatic; however, 20–50% of fibroids cause symptoms such as heavy menstrual bleeding, dysmenorrhea, pelvic pressure, and infertility.[3]

Menstrual pain, known as *dysmenorrhea*, may present as primary (unrelated to pathology) or secondary (linked to fibroids, endometriosis, or adenomyosis). Fibroids are a leading secondary cause of menstrual pain. This chapter reviews the pathophysiology, diagnosis, and management of fibroids with emphasis on menstrual pain, integrating medical and surgical approaches and recent advances.

Epidemiology and Risk Factors

Uterine fibroids are highly prevalent across populations, but marked disparities exist. Black women experience earlier onset, larger fibroid burden, and more severe symptoms than white women, often requiring surgical intervention at younger ages.[1] Environmental and genetic factors likely contribute. Vitamin D deficiency, obesity, and dietary patterns have been associated with increased fibroid risk, while higher parity and prolonged use of combined oral contraceptives may reduce risk.[2] Emerging research also implicates endocrine-disrupting chemicals such as phthalates and bisphenol A as possible contributors, underscoring the role of environmental exposures in fibroid development.[3]

Pathophysiology

Fibroid development is hormonally mediated, with estrogen and progesterone enhancing tumor growth. Fibroids show increased steroid hormone receptor density. Growth factors and extracellular matrix deposition contribute to pathogenesis. Genetic alterations, including MED12 mutations, are strongly implicated.[3]

Mechanisms of menstrual pain in fibroids include:

- Prostaglandin-mediated uterine hypercontractility and ischemia
- Distortion of uterine anatomy leading to abnormal contractions
- Heavy bleeding contributing to anemia and fatigue

Symptom of Uterine Fibroids

Uterine fibroid symptoms may present as abnormal uterine bleeding, pelvic pain, bulk symptoms (urinary, bowel), and reproductive dysfunction.[2] Abnormal uterine bleeding often presents as heavy or prolonged menstrual periods, sometimes accompanied by clots, which can lead to anemia and fatigue. Pelvic pain may manifest as cramping, pressure, or chronic discomfort that worsens during menstruation or intercourse. Bulk-related symptoms, such as frequent urination, constipation, or bloating, result from fibroids pressing on the bladder or bowel, while reproductive dysfunction may include infertility, recurrent pregnancy loss, or complications during pregnancy.

Diagnosis of Uterine Fibroids

Accurate diagnosis of uterine fibroids is essential for guiding appropriate management and optimizing outcomes. In addition to symptom assessment and physical examination, imaging plays a central role. Diagnostic modalities (see Table 23.1) include pelvic examination, ultrasound, MRI, sonohysterography/hysteroscopy, and laboratory studies (Table 23.1).
Ultrasound remains the most widely used modality due to its accessibility, noninvasive nature, and high sensitivity for detecting fibroids >2 cm.[3] Transvaginal ultrasound provides enhanced visualization of smaller or submucosal fibroids, while transabdominal ultrasound is often useful for mapping large or multiple fibroids. MRI is considered the gold standard for detailed characterization, offering superior accuracy in determining fibroid number,

Table 23.1 Diagnostic modalities and key features

Modality	Key features
Pelvic exam	Detects enlarged/irregular uterus; limited sensitivity
Ultrasound	First-line: >90% sensitivity for fibroids >2 cm
MRI	Gold standard for mapping and surgical planning
Sonohysterography	Good for submucosal fibroid evaluation
Hysteroscopy	Direct visualization of cavity/submucosal fibroids
Laboratory	CBC for anemia; hormone studies as indicated

size, and location, as well as differentiation from adenomyosis or other pelvic masses.[3] Sonohysterography and hysteroscopy are particularly valuable for evaluating submucosal fibroids that distort the uterine cavity, which is critical in women with infertility or recurrent pregnancy loss.[3] Laboratory evaluations, such as a complete blood count, are used to assess anemia resulting from heavy menstrual bleeding, while hormonal studies may be indicated to exclude other causes of abnormal uterine bleeding. Ultimately, a combination of clinical, imaging, and laboratory findings ensures a comprehensive diagnosis, informing treatment choices tailored to each patient's reproductive goals and symptom severity.

Management of Uterine Fibroids

Management depends on symptom severity, fibroid size/location, patient age, and fertility goals. Options span medical therapy, minimally invasive procedures, and surgery.[1] Treatment strategies are guided not only by the clinical presentation but also by the patient's preferences, commodities, and access to care.

Medical Management

Nonhormonal management strategies play an important role in reducing fibroid-related symptoms, particularly for women who prefer to avoid hormonal therapy or have contraindications to it. Nonhormonal options include:

- Nonsteroidal anti-inflammatory drugs (NSAIDs)
- Tranexamic acid

NSAIDs such as ibuprofen and naproxen are widely used as first-line agents for dysmenorrhea. These medications work by inhibiting prostaglandin synthesis, thereby decreasing uterine contractility and reducing pain. While NSAIDs are effective for pain relief, their impact on menstrual blood loss is modest, making them most suitable for women whose primary complaint is dysmenorrhea rather than heavy bleeding.[3] Tranexamic acid, an antifibrinolytic agent, offers a valuable option for reducing menstrual blood loss by 40–60%.[3] It is typically taken only during menses, providing a targeted, short-term approach without long-term hormonal exposure. Nonhormonal treatments can be used as standalone therapy in mild cases or in combination with other medical or procedural interventions when symptom control is incomplete.

Hormonal therapies provide a range of options for women with fibroid-related symptoms, offering both symptom relief and, in some cases, reduction in fibroid size. Hormonal options include the following:

- Combined oral contraceptives (COCs)
- Progestins
- Gonadotropin-releasing hormone (GnRH) agonists
- GnRH antagonists
- Selective progesterone receptor modulators (SPRMs)

Table 23.2 Medical management options

Therapy	Effects
NSAIDs	Reduce prostaglandins; relieve pain
Tranexamic acid	Reduces bleeding 40–60%
COCs	Cycle regulation; reduce bleeding/pain
Progestins (oral, injectable, LNG-IUS)	Reduce bleeding; LNG-IUS highly effective
GnRH agonists	Shrink fibroids; hypoestrogenic side effects
GnRH antagonists	Oral with add-back therapy; effective for bleeding
SPRMs	Reduce bleeding/size; safety monitoring

COC, combined oral contraceptives; GnRH, gonadotropin-releasing hormone; LNG-IUS, levonorgestrel-releasing intrauterine system; SPRM, selective progesterone receptor modulators.

COCs are commonly prescribed to regulate menstrual cycles, decrease menstrual blood loss, and alleviate dysmenorrhea, making them useful for women with moderate symptoms who also desire contraception.[3,4] Progestin-based therapies, available in oral, injectable, and intrauterine system formulations, are effective in reducing bleeding and pain; among these, the levonorgestrel-releasing intrauterine system (LNG-IUS) has demonstrated particularly strong efficacy in controlling heavy menstrual bleeding while improving quality of life.[3,4] GnRH agonists such as leuprolide act by inducing a temporary hypoestrogenic state that reduces fibroid volume and bleeding, though their use is limited by side effects including bone loss and vasomotor symptoms.[3] Recently, oral GnRH antagonists such as elagolix and relugolix have emerged as newer agents that provide rapid suppression of gonadotropins without the flare phenomenon associated with agonists.[5,6] When combined with low-dose add-back therapy, they maintain efficacy while minimizing long-term adverse effects, thereby extending their clinical utility.[1] SPRMs, including ulipristal acetate, have also shown effectiveness in reducing fibroid size and controlling bleeding; however, concerns about hepatotoxicity have led to restricted or conditional use in some regions.[5] Future research into safer SPRMs remains ongoing. Personalized medicine approaches, integrating genetic and molecular profiling of fibroids, may enable targeted treatment. Collectively, these hormonal therapies form a critical component of individualized management strategies, tailored to patient preferences, reproductive goals, and tolerance of side effects. Table 23.2 outlines each of the therapeutic options and effects.

Minimally Invasive and Novel Surgical Options

Surgical management continues to evolve toward uterus-preserving, minimally invasive strategies. Hysteroscopic myomectomy is highly effective for submucosal fibroids, improving fertility rates and reducing abnormal bleeding.[7] Laparoscopic and robotic-assisted myomectomy offer reduced recovery time and fewer complications compared with open surgery.[7] Techniques such as mini-laparotomy and single-incision laparoscopy are expanding options for patients with large or numerous fibroids.

Uterine artery embolization (UAE) remains an established option for women desiring a noninvasive option. Long-term follow-up indicates durable symptom relief, although reintervention rates range from 20% to 30% at 5 years.[8] MRI-guided focused ultrasound surgery (MRgFUS) provides a noninvasive option for carefully selected patients, though limitations include high cost, limited availability, and reduced efficacy for large or numerous fibroids.[9]

Emerging technologies, including radiofrequency ablation (RFA) via laparoscopic, transcervical, or percutaneous approaches, offer promising results with reduced hospital stay and rapid recovery.[10,11] Future comparative studies will clarify their role alongside established modalities.

Surgical Management

Surgical management of uterine fibroids remains a cornerstone of therapy, particularly for women with severe or refractory symptoms who do not respond adequately to medical or minimally invasive options.[12] Myomectomy is the primary fertility-sparing procedure and is often recommended for women who wish to maintain reproductive potential. The approach to myomectomy depends on the size, number, and location of fibroids. Hysteroscopic myomectomy is generally reserved for submucosal fibroids that distort the uterine cavity and contribute to heavy menstrual bleeding or infertility, whereas laparoscopic or open abdominal myomectomy is typically employed for larger or multiple fibroids.[12] While myomectomy can provide significant relief of symptoms and restoration of fertility, recurrence rates are reported to be between 15% and 30%, which may necessitate repeat intervention over time.[8]

For women who do not desire future fertility or who prefer a definitive solution, hysterectomy remains the most effective surgical treatment for uterine fibroids.[2] Advances in surgical techniques have made minimally invasive approaches, such as laparoscopic or robotic-assisted hysterectomy, the preferred methods whenever feasible, given their association with reduced operative morbidity, shorter hospital stays, and faster recovery compared with open procedures. Hysterectomy not only eliminates the risk of fibroid recurrence but also provides durable symptom relief, making it an important option for patients whose quality of life is significantly impacted. Careful preoperative counseling is essential to ensure that women fully understand the risks, benefits, and long-term implications of surgical management, including the loss of fertility in the case of hysterectomy. Table 23.3 outlines each of the procedures described.

Table 23.3 Surgical and minimally invasive options

Procedure	Considerations
UAE	80–90% symptom relief; recurrence risk; uncertain fertility impact
MRgFUS	Noninvasive thermoablation; effective select cases
Myomectomy	Fertility-sparing; recurrence 15–30%
Hysterectomy	Definitive; minimally invasive preferred

MRgFUS, MRI-guided focused ultrasound surgery; UAE, uterine artery embolization.

Holistic and Adjunctive Approaches

Beyond conventional therapies, lifestyle and integrative strategies may complement care. Observational studies suggest physical activity, plant-based diets, and vitamin D supplementation may reduce fibroid growth.[13] Acupuncture and herbal medicine are used in some cultural contexts, though robust clinical evidence is limited. Shared decision-making should address patient preferences for holistic care while ensuring safety and evidence-based practice.

Management of Menstrual Pain

Primary dysmenorrhea can be managed with NSAIDs, hormonal contraceptives, and lifestyle strategies (heat, exercise).[14] Secondary dysmenorrhea can be treated by treating underlying pathology (fibroids, endometriosis, adenomyosis).[14] In fibroid-related pain, use medical therapy or surgical intervention depending on fertility and severity.[1,2]

Patient-Centered Care

Shared decision-making must consider:

- Symptom burden and quality-of-life impact
- Fertility goals
- Risks, benefits, recurrence potential
- Social/cultural values regarding uterine preservation

A multidisciplinary approach is key.[2] Engaging gynecologists, interventional radiologists, reproductive endocrinologists, primary care providers, and advanced practice providers optimizes outcomes.

Quality of Life and Socioeconomic Impact

Fibroid-associated symptoms—particularly heavy menstrual bleeding and dysmenorrhea—have substantial effects on women's quality of life. Chronic anemia may result in fatigue, cognitive dysfunction, and reduced work productivity. Dysmenorrhea is linked with absenteeism and presenteeism, with estimates suggesting billions of dollars in lost productivity annually in the United States.[15] Psychological effects, including depression and anxiety, are also common in women with untreated fibroid-related pain.[16] Disparities in access to minimally invasive therapies disproportionately burden minority women, who are more likely to undergo hysterectomy as first-line treatment.[17] Addressing these inequities is critical to optimizing patient outcomes.

Fertility and Pregnancy Considerations

Fibroids can significantly affect fertility and pregnancy outcomes.[18] Submucosal fibroids distort the endometrial cavity, reducing implantation rates and increasing miscarriage risk. Intramural fibroids >4 cm may also impair fertility, though evidence remains mixed.[18] Myomectomy improves fertility in women with submucosal fibroids and selected intramural fibroids.[7]

During pregnancy, fibroids are associated with adverse outcomes such as miscarriage, preterm labor, malpresentation, cesarean delivery, postpartum hemorrhage, and intrauterine growth restriction.[7] Fibroid degeneration during pregnancy can cause severe pain and complicate obstetric management. Multidisciplinary care, including maternal–fetal medicine consultation, is recommended for pregnant patients with large or multiple fibroids.[18]

Future Directions and Research Gaps

Significant progress has been made in understanding fibroid biology and treatment, but key gaps remain. Areas of future investigation include:

- Identifying women at risk before symptom onset with use of biomarkers for early detection.
- Advanced imaging and molecular profiling for personalized treatment planning using noninvasive diagnostics.
- Comparative effectiveness trials of emerging oral GnRH antagonists, minimally invasive surgery, and UAE to guide patient-centered decisions.
- More data are needed on fertility, recurrence, and quality of life after novel therapies.
- Strategies to reduce racial and socioeconomic disparities in diagnosis and access to advanced care.

The future of fibroid management will likely integrate pharmacogenomics, precision medicine, and multidisciplinary care models to optimize outcomes for diverse patient populations. Recent advances in pharmacologic agents and minimally invasive therapies expand management options. Individualized, patient-centered care integrating medical and surgical strategies remains the cornerstone.[1,2]

Conclusion

Uterine fibroids and menstrual pain substantially affect women's health. Their impact extends beyond physical symptoms to reproductive health, mental well-being, and socioeconomic participation. Contemporary management has shifted toward individualized, minimally invasive, and fertility-sparing options. Recent pharmacologic advances, particularly oral GnRH antagonists, represent a paradigm shift in medical management. Novel procedures, including radiofrequency ablation and MRgFUS, expand the armamentarium for patients seeking alternatives to hysterectomy.

A holistic, patient-centered approach is essential, addressing not only symptom relief but also long-term reproductive goals and quality of life. Closing research gaps and reducing health disparities remain pressing priorities. Integrating advances in science, technology, and health equity within the next decade will support transformative progress in the care of women with fibroids and menstrual pain.

References

1. Stewart EA, Cookson CL, Gandolfo RA, Schulze-Rath R. Epidemiology of uterine fibroids: A systematic review. BJOG. 2017;124(10):1501–1512.
2. Giuliani E, As-Sanie S, Marsh EE. Epidemiology and management of uterine fibroids. Int J Gynecol Obstet. 2020;149(1):3–9.
3. Ahmad A, Kumar M, Bhoi NR, et al. Diagnosis and management of uterine fibroids: Current trends and future strategies. J Basic Clin Physiol Pharmacol. 2023;34(3):291–310.
4. American College of Obstetricians and Gynecologists. Practice bulletin no. 228: Management of symptomatic uterine leiomyomas. Obstet Gynecol. 2021;137(6):e100–e115.
5. Islam MS, Chen LW, Segars JH. Selective progesterone receptor modulators (SPRMs) and androgen receptor modulators (SARMs) as treatment for benign gynecologic diseases. Clin Obstet Gynecol. 2021;64(4):813–836.
6. Schlaff WD, Ackerman RT, Al-Hendy A, et al. Elagolix for heavy menstrual bleeding in women with uterine fibroids. N Engl J Med. 2020;382(4):328–340.
7. Wang P, Hughes NJ, Mehdizadeh A, Nezhat C, Nezhat F. Advances and challenges in minimally invasive myomectomy: A narrative review. J Clin Med. 2025;14(12):4313.
8. Cappelli A, Mosconi C, Cocozza MA, et al. Uterine artery embolization for the treatment of symptomatic uterine fibroids of different sizes: A single center experience. J Personalized Med. 2023;13(6):906.
9. Anneveldt KJ, Nijholt IM, Schutte JM, et al. Comparison of (cost-) effectiveness of magnetic resonance image–guided high-intensity–focused ultrasound with standard (minimally) invasive fibroid treatments: Protocol for a multicenter randomized controlled trial (MYCHOICE). JMIR Res Protocol. 2021;10(11):e29467.
10. Kwon CS, Abu-Alnadi ND. Updates on the surgical approach to fibroids: The importance of radiofrequency ablation. Semin Intervent Radiol. 2023;40(4):335–341.
11. Baxter BL, Seaman SJ, Arora C, Kim JH. (2022). Radiofrequency ablation methods for uterine sparing fibroid treatment. Curr Opin Obstet Gynecol. 2022;34(4):262–269.
12. Micić J, Radonjić M, Vujović S, et al. Currently available treatment modalities for uterine fibroids. Medicina. 2024;60(6):868.
13. Vafaei S, Yazdanpanah L, Khoshdel A, et al. Empowering strategies for Lifestyle interventions, Diet modifications, and Environmental Practices for Uterine Fibroid Prevention; unveiling the LIFE UP awareness. Nutrients. 2024;16(6):807.
14. Kho KA, Shields JK. Diagnosis and management of primary dysmenorrhea. JAMA. 2020;323(3):268–269.

15. Schoep ME, Adang EMM, Maas JW, et al. Productivity loss due to menstruation-related symptoms: A nationwide cross-sectional survey among 32 748 women. BMJ Open. 2019;9(69):e026186.
16. Chiuve SE, D'Aloisio AA, Baird DD, Wise LA. Uterine fibroids and incidence of depression, anxiety and self-directed violence: A cohort study. J Epidemiol Community Health. 2022;76(1):92–99.
17. Barnes WA, Walters MD, Wheeler TL 2nd, Ackerman AL, Flynn MK, Bradley LD. Racial and ethnic disparities in access to minimally invasive gynecologic surgery for benign pathology. Curr Opin Obstet Gynecol. 2021;33(4):279–287.
18. Alkhrait S, Malasevskaia I, Madueke-Laveaux OS. Fibroids and fertility. Obstet Gynecol Clin. 2023;50(4):663–675.

24
Endometriosis
Pathophysiology and Treatment Strategies

Insiyyah Patanwala, Farah Alvi, Laura Douglass, and O. Sandra Madueke-Laveaux

Introduction

Endometriosis is a gynecologic condition that affects 6–10% of reproductive aged women. It is a disease that is implicated in 71–87% of women with chronic pelvic pain. Pain intensity is variable and not always concordant with degree of disease.[1]

Background

Endometriosis is a chronic inflammatory condition in which endometrial-like glands or stroma implant outside the uterine cavity. Presentation can be highly variable, with symptoms ranging from dysmenorrhea, chronic pelvic pain, dyspareunia, gastrointestinal and bladder symptoms, and infertility, as well as an absence of symptoms. Endometriosis can be diagnosed based on strong clinical suspicion and confirmed surgically with visualization of lesions and histologic diagnosis with biopsies.[2] Multiple genetic, environmental, and epidemiologic factors play a role in this complex disease process with no unifying theory to explain the broad clinical and disease manifestation. Given this variability, diagnosis can often be delayed 7–8 years due to overlap of symptoms with other pain diagnoses, and treatment goals can remain challenging.[3]

Epidemiology and Risk Factors

True global burden is challenging to quantify due to significant diagnostic delays and variation in access to laparoscopy or gynecologic care.[4] Most patients are diagnosed in their reproductive years, typically between the ages of 25 and 35, although the disease can present in adolescents and, more rarely, in postmenopausal women.[5] This age distribution reflects the influence of both hormonal factors and surgical or medical histories that shape disease expression across the lifespan.[6]

Several reproductive and genetic risk factors have been consistently identified. Early menarche, shortened menstrual cycles, heavy or prolonged bleeding, nulliparity, Mullerian anomalies, and a positive family history all increase the likelihood of endometriosis. In addition, women with a low body mass index (BMI) and autoimmune conditions may be at greater risk.[7,4,8] Environmental and lifestyle exposures—including endocrine-disrupting chemicals, high dietary fat intake, and certain occupational settings—have also been implicated. No racial predisposition for endometriosis has been shown; however cultural, ethnic, and socioeconomic differences influence patterns of care. In some communities, menstruation-related symptoms may be stigmatized, leading to underrecognition and delayed treatment.[8,9]

Pathophysiology

The pathophysiology of endometriosis is multifactorial, reflecting the interplay of mechanical, hormonal, immune, and neurologic processes. No single mechanism fully accounts for the disease, and it is likely that multiple pathways act synergistically.[10]

While there is no consensus on its origin, the most enduring model is the theory of retrograde menstruation, in which viable endometrial cells reflux through the fallopian tubes and implant on peritoneal surfaces.[11] While retrograde flow occurs in most women, only a subset develop disease, suggesting that additional factors are critical.[12] Other explanations include lympho-vascular invasion, coelomic metaplasia—where peritoneal cells transform into endometrial-like tissue—and stem or progenitor cell theories, which proposes that bone marrow–derived or basalis layer stem cells contribute to ectopic lesions. These mechanisms provide plausible accounts of cases arising in extra-pelvic sites or in women without patent fallopian tubes.[11]

Additionally, immune dysregulation promotes angiogenesis and neurogenesis, driving lesion progression and the characteristic pain associated with the disorder. Hormonal imbalances further compound these effects: endometriotic tissue demonstrates heightened estrogen signaling and relative progesterone resistance, enabling proliferation and resistance to apoptosis.[11–13]

Beyond local pelvic pathology, there is growing recognition that endometriosis acts as a chronic systemic inflammatory condition. Elevated cytokines and neuroimmune interactions contribute to fatigue, mood disturbances, and overlapping gastrointestinal complaints resembling irritable bowel syndrome (IBS) or inflammatory bowel disease (IBD).[14] Central sensitization, characterized by amplification of nociceptive signaling within the spinal cord and brain initiated by peripheral sensitization, explains the disproportionate relationship between lesion burden and reported overall pain severity.[15,16] This framework underscores endometriosis as a condition not limited to the pelvis but one with widespread physiologic and psychosocial consequences (Figure 24.1).

Diagnosis and Assessment

Symptom-based questionnaires can help increase awareness of endometriosis as a potential entity, with the most predictive symptom being severe dysmenorrhea. Other common symptoms include dyspareunia, nonmenstrual pelvic pain, cyclical bloating, and dyschezia.

Both ultrasound and MRI have good sensitivity and specificity for advanced-stage endometriosis but can often miss subtle endometriosis lesions such as the superficial peritoneal (SPE) subtype. Therefore, there is a lack of evidence to replace surgical diagnosis with imaging at this time.[17]

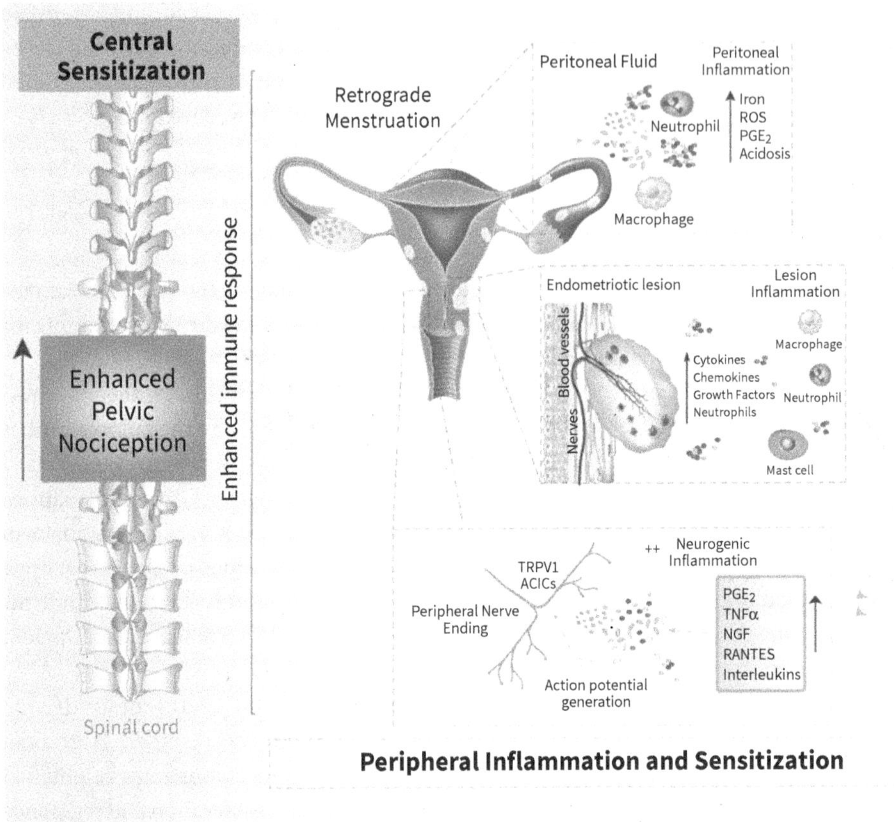

Figure 24.1 Schematic overview of an enhanced immune response leading to chronic pelvic pain in endometriosis.

Source: Maddern J, Grundy L, Castro J, Brierley SM. Pain in endometriosis. Front Cell Neurosci. 2020 Oct 6;14:590823. doi:10.3389/fncel.2020.590823. PMID: 33132854.

Definitive diagnosis requires surgical exploration with lesion biopsy and histologic confirmation. Lesion characteristics vary by appearance, size, location with histologic confirmation noting the presence of endometrial glands, stroma, and/or hemosiderin-laden macrophages. Endometriosis can be located superficially on the peritoneum, infiltrating 5 mm or more beyond the peritoneum (deep infiltrating endometriosis), or present as an ovarian cyst (endometrioma).[14] The relationship between lesions or disease burden does not correlate with symptoms with a high risk of recurrence, and empiric treatment based on a clinical suspicion is acceptable outside of histologic confirmation[18] (Figure 24.2).

Management

Management options for patients depend on their primary symptoms and fertility goals. Nonsteroidal anti-inflammatory drugs often help with dysmenorrhea and pelvic pain but will not address the underlying disease process. The mainstay of treatment is hormonal suppression, which can be started with or without a confirmed surgical diagnosis of endometriosis.

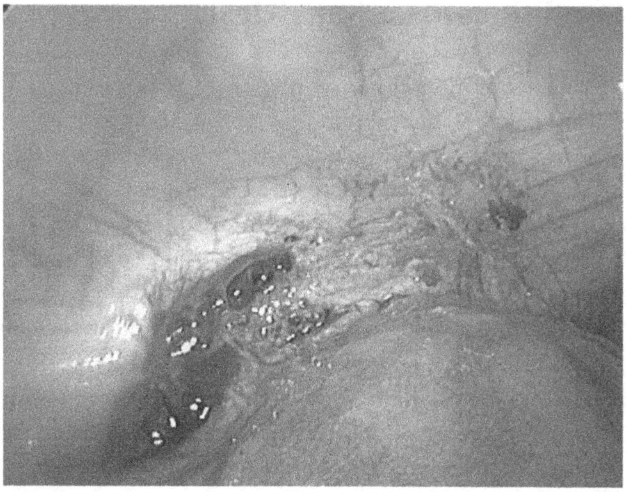

Figure 24.2 Endometriosis of the anterior cul-de-sac between the uterus and the bladder.
Source: Hic et nunc. Endometriosis on peritoneum between bladder and uterus. Wikimedia Commons. Published June 20, 2009. Accessed November 27, 2025. https://commons.wikimedia.org/wiki/File:Endometriosis1.jpg.

Estrogen is a known stimulant of disease progression, but, when combined with progesterone therapy, it can be used to help with symptoms. Common birth control methods such as the oral contraceptive pill are often used in women with endometriosis to decrease pain. Continuous use of oral contraceptive pills (skipping placebo tablets) is recommended for complete suppression of menses. Higher-dose progestins or progestin-only methods are more effective in controlling endometriosis-related symptoms, and some may regress endometriosis lesions. Gonadotropin-releasing hormone (GnRh) analogues, such as leuprolide or elagolix, which induce a menopausal state, are usually the most effective in decreasing pain and endometriosis burden medically. However, these medications have significant side effects such as hot flashes, mood swings, and decreased libido and can only be continued for 1–2 years due to their adverse effect on bone density. Aromatase inhibitors have been used off-label for endometriosis suppression as well.[9] Danazol, which is an androgenic therapy, is also very effective but is infrequently used for endometriosis due to masculinization side effects; however, it can be considered in patients who desire gender transition and also have endometriosis.[19]

Laparoscopic surgery provides definitive diagnosis of endometriosis. Surgical removal of endometriosis has been shown to improve fertility outcomes and is utilized in women actively trying to conceive since they cannot be on a form of hormonal suppression.[20] Surgically, endometriotic lesions can be excised or ablated. If a patient has an ovarian endometrioma, removal via a cystectomy is recommended rather than simple drainage because recurrence rates are high.[21]

For patients not attempting to conceive, hormonal suppression after surgery is strongly recommended to prevent recurrence of endometriosis. If fertility is not desired, hysterectomy with or without bilateral salpingoophorectomy can be considered but is not recommended as first-line management. Even after hysterectomy, up to 25% of women can experience recurrent pain and 10% will need additional surgery.[9]

Comorbid Conditions in Endometriosis

IBS is among the most common comorbidities in endometriosis patients.[22] Because bloating, bowel habit changes, and abdominal pain overlap with cyclical endometriosis symptoms, misdiagnosis is common. Similarly, IBD shares inflammatory pathways and clinical presentations with endometriosis, making it difficult to distinguish between the two conditions in clinical practice.[23] Bladder pain syndrome/interstitial cystitis (IC/BPS) is also well-documented as a comorbid condition.[24] More broadly, women with endometriosis demonstrate high rates of coexisting immune and pain conditions, consistent with a chronic overlapping pain phenotype that intensifies functional impairment.[25]

Pelvic floor musculoskeletal dysfunction is often found in patients with endometriosis due to pain sensitization and chronic adhesive disease. Muscle hypertonicity can cause dyspareunia, pelvic pain with activity, and urinary and defecatory dysfunction.

Infertility represents a particularly profound consequence of endometriosis, affecting up to 40% of women with the condition.[26] Adhesions, ovarian endometriomas, and altered peritoneal inflammation all contribute to impaired reproductive potential. Beyond physical barriers, infertility brings significant psychosocial distress, amplifying the emotional toll already imposed by chronic pain and delayed diagnosis.

The Role of a Patient-Centered Approach

Given this heterogeneity and multimorbidity, care should pivot to patient-centered shared decision-making that elicits goals (pain relief, fertility preservation, quality of life) and tailors therapy accordingly.[27,28] Implementation research shows that patient-centered care improves satisfaction and outcomes when patient values are explicitly integrated into planning.

A modern multimodal model situates patients within a coordinated, multidisciplinary team to address their physical, emotional, and social needs.[29] This team can include

- Gynecologic surgeons
- Infertility specialists
- Pain specialists
- Pelvic floor physical therapists
- Nutritionists
- Mental health professionals

For patients seeking pregnancy, individualized planning is critical. Medical therapy may control symptoms but delay conception; surgery may aid fertility in selected scenarios. Shared decision-making helps balance the chances of spontaneous conception, the roles of assisted reproductive technology (ART), and surgical risks, which reduces overtreatment, undertreatment, and value-discordant care[28] (Figure 24.3).

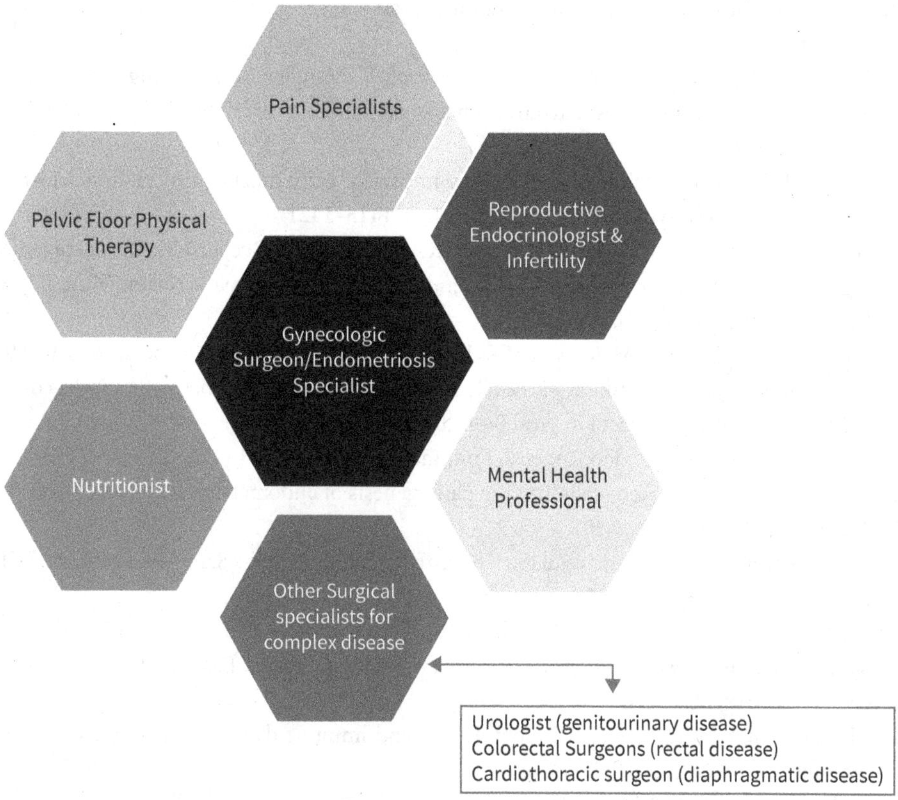

Figure 24.3 Multimodal model: Multidisciplinary team for endometriosis management.
Source: Addressing cervical cancer disparities in Texas: Expansion of a community-based prevention initiative for medically underserved populations—Scientific Figure on ResearchGate. Available from: https://www.researchgate.net/figure/Components-of-the-program-for-reducing-cervical-cancer-as-implemented-in-participating_fig2_375122071. Accessed January 3, 2026.

Conclusion

Endometriosis is a multisystem pain condition that intersects with gastrointestinal, urinary, and reproductive health. Management can and should be multidisciplinary and employ different treatment modalities. A patient-centered, shared decision-making approach grounded in clear communication and in alignment with fertility goals offers the most promising path to optimizing outcomes and restoring quality of life for women living with endometriosis.

References

1. American College of Obstetrics and Gynecology. Practice bulletin no. 114: Management of endometriosis. Obstet Gynecol. 2010;116(1).
2. Falcone T, Flyckt R. Clinical management of endometriosis. Obstet Gynecol. 2018; 131(3):557–571.

3. Begum IA. The connection between endometriosis and secondary dysmenorrhea. J Reprod Immunol. 2025;168:104425.
4. Harder E, Helbig M, Renner SP, Wenzl R, Ulrich U, Mangler M. Assessing the true prevalence of endometriosis: A narrative review of literature data. Int J Gynaecol Obstet. 2024;167(3):883–900.
5. Kaveh M, Kaveh F, Ziaei S, Akbari H. The impact of early diagnosis of endometriosis on quality of life. Arch Gynecol Obstet, 2025. 311(5): 1415–1421.
6. Gemmell LC, Webster KE, Kirtley S, Vincent K, Zondervan KT, Becker CM. The management of menopause in women with a history of endometriosis: A systematic review. Hum Reprod Update. 2017;23(4):481–500.
7. Zondervan KT, Becker CM, Missmer SA. Endometriosis. Nat Rev Dis Primers. 2018;4(1):9.
8. Parazzini F, Viganò P, Candiani M, Fedele L. Epidemiology of endometriosis and its comorbidities. Eur J Obstet Gynecol Reprod Biol. 2017;209:3–7.
9. As-Sanie S, Giudice LC, Lobo RA, et al. Endometriosis: A review. JAMA. 2025;334(1):64–78.
10. Sasson IE, Taylor HS. Stem cells and the pathogenesis of endometriosis. Ann N Y Acad Sci. 2008;1127:106–115.
11. Bulun SE. Endometriosis and ovulatory menstruation: Beyond the Sampson principle. J Clin Invest. 2025;135(13): e188787.
12. Patel BG, Lenk EE, Lebovic DI, Shu Y, Yu J, Taylor RN. Pathogenesis of endometriosis: Interaction between endocrine and inflammatory pathways. Best Pract Res Clin Obstet Gynaecol. 2018;50:50–60.
13. Ahn SH, Singh V, Tayade C. Pathophysiology and immune dysfunction in endometriosis. Biomed Res Int. 2015(2015):795976.
14. Taylor HS, Kotlyar AM, Flores VA. Endometriosis is a chronic systemic disease: Clinical challenges and novel innovations. Lancet. 2021;397(10276):839–852.
15. Stratton P, Berkley KJ. Chronic pelvic pain and endometriosis: Translational evidence of the relationship and implications. Hum Reprod Update. 2011;17(3):327–346.
16. Maddern J, Grundy L, Castro J, Brierley SM. Pain in endometriosis. Front Cell Neurosci. 2020;14:590823. doi:10.3389/fncel.2020.590823.
17. Young SL, Evans S, Johnson NP. Nonsurgical approaches to the diagnosis and evaluation of endometriosis. Fertil Steril. 2024;121(2):140–144.
18. Abrao MS, Andres MP, Miller CE, et al. Endometriosis Classification: An anatomy-based surgical complexity score. J Minim Invasive Gynecol. 2021;28(11):1941–1950.e1. doi:10.1016/j.jmig.2021.09.709
19. Scatoni A, Roberts Z, Boskey ER, et al. Danazol's use for menstrual suppression in transgender individuals: A retrospective multi-site cohort study. Womens Health (Lond). 2024;20:17455057241265081. doi:10.1177/17455057241265081
20. Jin X, Ruiz Beguerie J. Laparoscopic surgery for subfertility related to endometriosis: A meta-analysis. Taiwanese J Obstet Gynecol. 2014;53(3):303–308. doi:10.1016/j.tjog.2013.02.004
21. Alborzi S, Momtahan M, Parsanezhad ME, Dehbashi S, Zolghadri J, Alborzi S. A prospective, randomized study comparing laparoscopic ovarian cystectomy versus fenestration and coagulation in patients with endometriomas. Fertil Steril. 2004;82(6):1633–1637. doi:10.1016/j.fertnstert.2004.04.067
22. Seaman HE, Ballard KD, Wright JT, de Vries CS. Endometriosis and its coexistence with irritable bowel syndrome and pelvic inflammatory disease: Findings from a national case-control study – Part 2. BJOG. 2008;115(11):1392–1396. doi:10.1111/j.1471-0528.2008.01879.x

23. Nabi MY, Akhtar MA, Riaz M, et al. Endometriosis and irritable bowel syndrome: A systematic review and meta-analyses. Front Med (Lausanne). 2022;9:914356.
24. Wu CC, Chung SD, Lin HC. Endometriosis increased the risk of bladder pain syndrome/interstitial cystitis: A population-based study. Neurourol Urodyn. 2018;37(4):1413–1418. doi:10.1002/nau.23462
25. Sinaii N, Cleary SD, Ballweg ML, Nieman LK, Stratton P. High rates of autoimmune and endocrine disorders, fibromyalgia, chronic fatigue syndrome and atopic diseases among women with endometriosis: a survey analysis. Hum Reprod. 2002;17(10):2715–2724. doi:10.1093/humrep/17.10.2715
26. Agarwal SK, Chapron C, Giudice LC. Clinical diagnosis of endometriosis: A call to action. Am J Obstet Gynecol. 2019;220(4):354 e1–354 e12.
27. Fallon L, Lau A, Ciccia D, et al. Health-related decision-making experiences of people with endometriosis: A qualitative analysis. Psychol Health. 2025:1–26. doi:10.1080/08870446.2025.2502866
28. Montori VM, Ruissen MM, Hargraves IG, Brito JP, Kunneman M. Shared decision-making as a method of care. BMJ Evid Based Med. 2023;28(4):213–217. doi:10.1136/bmjebm-2022-112068
29. Mick I, Freger SM, van Keizerswaard J, Gholiof M, Leonardi M. Comprehensive endometriosis care: A modern multimodal approach for the treatment of pelvic pain and endometriosis. Ther Adv Reprod Health. 2024;18:26334941241277759. doi:10.1177/26334941241277759

25

Advanced Interventional Treatment of Endometriosis-Related Pain

Anuj Bapodra and Gary Schwartz

Introduction

Endometriosis is a chronic, inflammatory disease characterized by the presence of ectopic endometrial tissue outside the uterine cavity.[1] Most cases of ectopic endometrium are found in the ovaries, but it can infiltrate different areas such as the pelvic peritoneum, uterosacral ligaments, and fallopian tubes. Endometriosis is a prevalent gynecological condition, affecting approximately 10% of women in their reproductive years.[2] It is associated with heterogeneous symptoms such as chronic pelvic pain (CPP), defined as persistent pain perceived in the pelvic areas that occur over a period of 6 months.[3] While pain originates from endometrial lesions, its manifestation is often attributed to processes such as neuroinflammation, angiogenesis, and sensitization.[4]

Diagnosis

Endometriosis is difficult to diagnose, and the true prevalence remains uncertain. No biomarkers to detect or rule out endometriosis are available. The predominantly intra-abdominal location of the lesions and their small size means that laparoscopic visualization with histologic verification remains the standard for diagnosis.[5] Endometriomas can be identified reliably by transvaginal ultrasonography or MRI, with greater than 90% sensitivity and specificity.[6] A skilled specialist can identify deep endometriosis and adhesions involving pelvic organs with transvaginal ultrasonography. MRI has 94% sensitivity for detecting deep endometriosis, but the specificity is only 79%.[6]

Although most adults report that their pelvic pain began during adolescence, most young women do not receive timely treatment. Women see, on average, seven physicians before endometriosis is diagnosed because of the varied symptoms and inaccuracy in algorithmic evaluations.[7] Surgery is appropriate only when symptoms reach a level of severity to justify the risk. The complex diagnostic challenge of endometriosis includes nonspecific symptoms, lack of sensitive and specific biomarkers, and lack of awareness on the part of both the public (with symptoms discounted) and practitioners (with symptoms dismissed or inadequately investigated) resulting in diagnostic delay.[1]

Comprehensive Management

Pelvic pain can arise from common gynecological causes including endometriosis, adenomyosis, ovarian cysts, pelvic fibroids, pelvic inflammatory disease, and vulvodynia.[8] Among these origins, endometriosis is a leading cause of pelvic pain. Patients with chronic pelvic pain often undergo a comprehensive therapy involving physical therapy, psychosocial support, pharmacologic agents, and nerve blocks.

Pharmacologic Treatments

Current hormonal treatment for endometriosis-associated pain focuses on systemic or local estrogen suppression, inhibition of tissue proliferation and inflammation, or both.[1] The oral contraceptive pill is considered first-line treatment, and gonadotropin-releasing hormone (GnRH) agonists are second-line therapy.[1] Analgesia for endometriosis-associated pain consists of a combination of acetaminophen and nonsteroidal anti-inflammatory drugs. The International Association for the Study of Pain recommends opioids for severe, short-lived pain during acute events but not for chronic pain conditions.[9]

Surgical Treatments

In women with hormone-resistant pain associated with endometriosis, surgical treatment should be considered. Surgery has been shown to decrease pain in some but not all women.[5] The aim is complete destruction or removal of endometriotic tissue and adhesions; success may largely depend on surgical skill. Hysterectomy is common; endometriosis-associated pain is the leading indication for hysterectomy among women 30–34 years of age, accounting for 18% of all hysterectomies in the United States.[10] However, posthysterectomy pain is three times as likely among women with preoperative pain as among those without preoperative pain.[11] Current surgical and medical approaches to endometriosis are ineffective for a considerable proportion of women, and, when effective, they can be associated with complications and morbidity.

Nonpharmacologic Treatments

Nonpharmaceutical options, including acupuncture and local use of botulinum toxin, may ameliorate the musculoskeletal component of pelvic pain. Patients with endometriosis experience central sensitization leading to hyperalgesia when compared to healthy participants.[12] Studies show women with endometriosis have an increased prevalence of concomitant psychiatric disorders that should be managed while addressing pelvic pain.[13] Exploration of overlapping pain and mental health conditions may yield more precise individualized treatment.

Interventional Treatment

Neural Innervation of the Pelvis

Neural innervation of the pelvis is essential when addressing chronic pelvic pain. Each can be a potential target for interventional treatment. Dorsal afferent sensory roots and ventral efferent motor roots emerge from the dorsal and ventral horns of the spinal cord, respectively. The dorsal afferent sensory root travels toward the periphery, including pseudo-unipolar cell bodies that collect as a bundle and form a dorsal root ganglion (DRG).[14] Somatic innervation transmitting sensory and motor signals to and from the pelvis includes ilioinguinal-iliohypogastric nerves (L1), genitofemoral (L1–L2), and pudendal nerves (S2, S3, S4).[15] The ganglion of impar is a sympathetic ganglion located in the retroperitoneal space anterior to the sacrococcygeal joint.[16] The ganglion of impar is formed from the merging of two sacral sympathetic chains.

Interventional Targets for Refractory Pelvic Pain

When conservative management for pelvic pain fails, refractory cases are trialed with ganglion impar blocks, caudal epidural steroid injections, or superior or inferior hypogastric blocks. The central and peripheral nervous system may be targeted using neuromodulation. These interventional treatments include spinal cord stimulation (SCS), dorsal root ganglion (DRG) stimulation, and peripheral nerve stimulation (PNS).[8]

Peripheral Nerve Stimulation and Neuromodulation Techniques

PNS leads are ideally placed parallel to a peripheral nerve. The most common targets in chronic pelvic pain include the posterior tibial nerve and pudendal nerve.[15] Other targets include the genitofemoral, ilioinguinal, and iliohypogastric nerves. Common SCS and DRG stimulation targets for chronic pelvic pain are S2–S3.[15] Previous studies have shown promising results with decreased pelvic pain after SCS and DRG stimulation therapy. Sacral neuromodulation (SNM) is not currently an approved US Food and Drug Administration (FDA) indication.[17] However, a recent Finnish national study is the first to demonstrate promising long-term results in the difficult to treat group of endometriosis patients with chronic pelvic pain after surgery.[17]

Sacral Neuromodulation in Endometriosis-Related Chronic Pelvic Pain

In the recent retrospective study by Zagrea et al., a total of 16 women, with a median age of 39 (25–50) years, underwent SNM treatment for chronic pelvic pain related to endometriosis, with a median follow-up time of 73 (48–85) months.[17] All the patients had previously undergone medical management and at least one surgery due to endometriosis.

SNM was performed in two stages using standard programs. In the evaluation stage I, a tined lead was placed in the S3 or S4 foramina. After a successful trial period of 14 days, stage II was performed with implantation of an internal pulse generator (IPG). Pain numerical rating scale values dropped from median 7.4 (3.6–10) before SNM to 2.3 (0–6.5) by the end of the follow-up.[17] It was suggested that a major contributing factor for endometriosis-associated pain is not the ectopic growths themselves, but rather nerve activity from surrounding tissues, which affects the activity of neurons in the spinal cord and brain.[18] This could explain why SNM is effective.

These findings encourage the consideration of SNM as a long-term treatment option for patients with refractory CPP due to endometriosis, particularly in cases where standard surgical and hormonal therapies fail. While neuromodulation shows great potential, there is significant need for larger multicenter prospective studies.

References

1. Zondervan KT, Becker CM, Missmer SA. Endometriosis. N Engl J Med. 2020;382: 1244–1256.
2. Horne AW, Missmer A. Pathophysiology, diagnosis, and management of endometriosis. BMJ (Clin Res Ed). 2022;379:e070750.
3. Missmer SA, Tu FF, Agarwal SK, et al. Impact of endometriosis on life-course potential: A narrative review. Int J Gen Med. 2021;14:9–25.
4. Cuffaro F, Russo E, Amedei A. Endometriosis, pain, and related psychological disorders: Unveiling the interplay among the microbiome, inflammation, and oxidative stress as a common thread. Int J Mol Sci. 2024;25(12):6473. doi:10.3390/ijms25126473
5. Dunselman GA, Vermeulen N, Becker C, et al. ESHRE guideline: Management of women with endometriosis. Hum Reprod. 2014;29:400–412.
6. Nisenblat V, Bossuyt PMM, Farquhar C, Johnson N, Hull ML. Imaging modalities for the non-invasive diagnosis of endometriosis. Cochrane Database Syst Rev. 2016;2:CD009591.
7. Ballard K, Lowton K, Wright J. What's the delay? A qualitative study of women's experiences of reaching a diagnosis of endometriosis. Fertil Steril. 2006;86:1296–1301.
8. Roy H, Offiah I, Dua A. Neuromodulation for pelvic and urogenital pain. Brain Sci. 2018;8:1–16.
9. International Association for the Study of Pain. IASP statement on opioids. February 2018. https://www.iasp -pain.org/ Advocacy/Content.aspx?ItemNumber=7194
10. Whiteman MK, Hillis SD, Jamieson DJ, et al. Inpatient hysterectomy surveillance in the United States, 2000–2004. Am J Obstet Gynecol. 2008;198(1):34.e1–34.e7.
11. Brandsborg B, Nikolajsen L. Chronic pain after hysterectomy. Curr Opin Anaesthesiol. 2018;31:268–273.
12. Bajaj P, Bajaj P, Madsen H, Arendt-Nielsen L. Endometriosis is associated with central sensitization: A psychophysical controlled study. J Pain. 2003;4:372–380.
13. Casalechi M, Vieira-Lopes M, Quessada MP, Arão TC, Reis FM. Endometriosis and related pelvic pain: Association with stress, anxiety and depressive symptoms. Minerva Obstet Gynecol. 2021;73:283–289.
14. Krames E. The dorsal root ganglion in chronic pain and as a target for neuromodulation: A review. Neuromodulation. 2015;18:24–32.

15. Patel CB, Patel AA, Diwan S. The role of neuromodulation in chronic pelvic pain: A review article. Pain Physician. 2022;25(4):E531–E542.
16. Gonnade N, Mehta N, Khera PS, Kumar D, Rajagopal R, Sharma PK. Ganglion impar block in patients with chronic coccydynia. Indian J Radiol Imaging. 2017;27:324–328.
17. Zegrea A, Ojala E, Kirss J, et al. Good long-term results of sacral neuromodulation for endometriosis related chronic pelvic pain. BMC Womens Health. 2025;25(1):162. doi:10.1186/s12905-025-03699-y
18. Stratton P, Berkley KJ. Chronic pelvic pain and endometriosis: Translational evidence of the relationship and implications. Hum Reprod Update. 2011;17(3):327–346. https://doi.org/10.1093/humupd/dmq050

26
Nonsurgical Comprehensive Treatments for Pelvic Pain in Women

Hirsch K. Srivastava, Benjamin Allen Fujita-Howie, Melissa Chao, and Tanvee Singh

Introduction

Chronic pelvic pain (CPP) is a common and often disabling condition affecting up to 25% of woman globally.[1] It is defined as noncyclic pain lasting ≥6 months localized to the pelvis, anterior abdominal wall, or lower back, and severe enough to result in functional disability or require medical intervention.[2] CPP is complex and can be difficult to treat given its multifactorial etiology in gynecologic, urologic, gastrointestinal, musculoskeletal, neurologic, and psychological domains.[3,4] CPP is usually a clinical diagnosis because pain often persists without commensurate visible pathology.[1,2]

The pelvic floor musculature serve crucial functions in maintaining pelvic organ positioning, controlling continence, and equilibrating intra-abdominal pressure.[5,6] Failure of these systems due to mechanisms ranging from childbirth, overuse, or trauma can lead to myofascial dysfunction, referred pain, and organ descent.

CPP often represents a nociplastic pain state, marked by central sensitization and altered nociception.[7] Psychological factors (trauma, anxiety, and depression) exacerbate CPP through increased pelvic floor tension and dysregulation of cortical pain networks.[8] For all these reasons a comprehensive, interdisciplinary, and tailored approach is necessary to optimize effective care.

Chronic Pelvic Pain and Chronic Primary Pelvic Pain Syndrome

Chronic primary pelvic pain syndrome (CPPPS) is pelvic pain lasting 3–6 months or more in the absence of identifiable pathology and is primarily driven by central pain amplification and neuromuscular dysfunction.[9] CPPPS can be understood by using the structured UPOINTS classification system (Urinary, Psychosocial, Organ-specific, Infection, Neurologic, Tenderness, and Sexual domains) as it provides a uniform lens for both evaluation and management of CPPPS.

Within UPOINTS, "tenderness" frequently represents myofascial dysfunction of the pelvic floor, particularly trigger points in the levator ani.[7,8] A single-digit vaginal examination can detect muscle hypertonicity, trigger point referral, and reduced mobility, even in the presence of normal imaging.[4] First-line management includes pelvic floor physical therapy

(PT), which incorporates myofascial release, biofeedback, and neuromuscular retraining to reduce tension and improve coordination. Nonsurgical options for CPPPS include trigger point injections, botulinum toxin injections (onabotulinumtoxinA), nerve blocks, intravenous ketamine, or lidocaine infusions or neuromodulation.

Pudendal Neuralgia

Pudendal neuralgia is characterized by a burning, lancinating, or electric pain in the clitoris, vulva, perineum, rectum, or anus, worsened with sitting and relieved by standing. The pudendal nerve arises from the S2–S4 nerve roots and is vulnerable to entrapment and dynamic compression.

Diagnosis of PN is clinical and supported by the Nantes criteria, which includes pain in the pudendal distribution, sitting-related worsening, no sensory loss, and relief with a pudendal nerve block.[10] Physical exam may reveal tenderness at the ischial spine or obturator internus. Conservative treatment includes pelvic PT, particularly targeted release of the obturator internus and posterior pelvic musculature. Serotonin norepinephrine reuptake inhibitors (SNRIs) and gabapentinoids may also reduce neuropathic symptoms.

Interventional pudendal nerve blocks are diagnostic and therapeutic and performed via either a transgluteal (Figure 26.1) or transvaginal approach. If pelvic floor hypertonicity is a contributing factor, botulinum toxin A may be injected under image guidance. Advanced interventional options include pulsed radiofrequency ablation, peripheral nerve stimulation, and surgical decompression.[11,12]

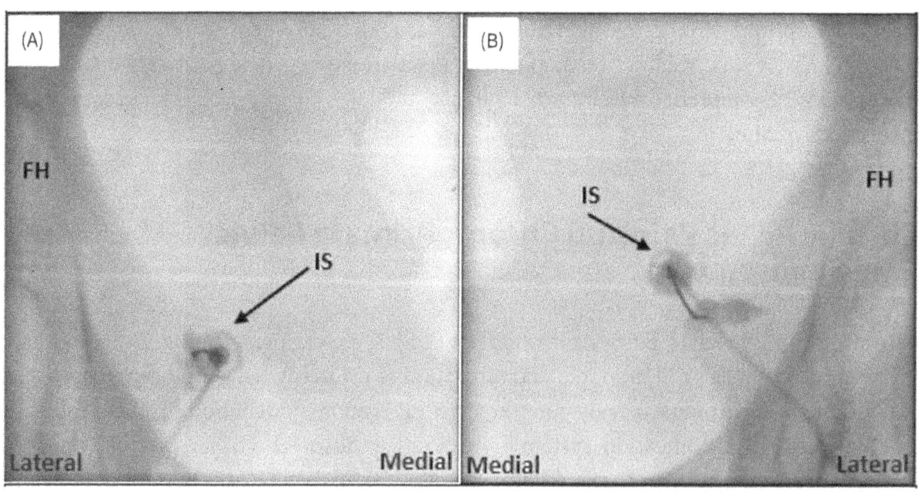

Figure 26.1 Left (A) and right (B) fluoroscopic transgluteal pudendal nerve block needle placement at the ischial spine with contrast spread. Note that the patient is placed in the prone position and contrast is used for final needle position to avoid intravascular injection of local anesthetic and/or steroid.

Source: Levin D, Van Florcke D, Schmitt M, Kendall LK, Patel A, Doan LV, Kirpekar M. Fluoroscopy-guided transgluteal pudendal nerve block for pudendal neuralgia: A retrospective case series. J Clin Med. 2024;13(9):2636. doi:10.3390/jcm13092636. PMID: 38731163; PMCID: PMC11084891.

Coccydynia

Coccydynia is pain localized to the coccyx, often exacerbated by sitting, standing from sitting, or defecation; the condition disproportionately affects women. Etiologies include trauma, coccygeal instability, and muscle-driven posterior traction, especially from hypertonic levator ani or coccygeus muscles.[6]

Physical exam involves direct coccygeal palpation and potentially a rectal exam. Imaging is reserved for cases with suspected neoplasm, infection, or failed conservative therapy.[4] Conservative treatment consists of corrective biomechanics and postural strategies, anti-inflammatory medications, and pelvic PT geared toward normalizing levator and gluteal muscle tone. Interventional measures include ganglion impar blocks (Figure 26.2) or neurolysis.[13]

Provoked Vulvodynia

Provoked vulvodynia is a localized pain syndrome around the area surrounding the vaginal opening and presents as burning pain with tampon insertion, intercourse, or pelvic exam. A positive cotton swab test localizes sensitivity to the vulvar vestibule. Contributing factors include hypertonic pelvic floor muscles (puborectalis, obturator internus), trauma, and pain-associated anxiety or posttraumatic stress disorder (PTSD).[8]

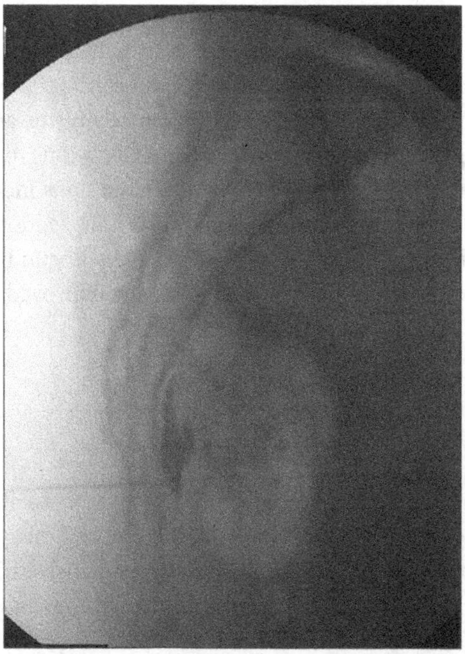

Figure 26.2 Fluoroscopic lateral view of a ganglion impar block. Note that the needle traverses through the sacrococcygeal joint and contrast is used to confirm spread up and down along the anterior surface of the sacrum. Care is taken not to advance the needle too far anterior past the junction of this joint because the rectum lies anterior to the ganglion impar.

Source: Turchan A, Fahmi A, Subianto H. Impar ganglion block with combination of neurolysis drugs and radiofrequency thermocoagulation for perineal pain. Asian J Neurosurg. 2018;13(3):838–841. doi:10.4103/ajns.AJNS_306_16. PMID: 30283560; PMCID: PMC6159014.

Treatment options include pelvic floor PT, topical lidocaine, tricyclic antidepressants, oral muscle relaxants, and intravaginal diazepam. For persistent muscular hypertonicity, onabotulinumtoxinA injections may improve outcomes when combined with PT. Cognitive behavioral therapy (CBT), mindfulness-based strategies, and sexual counseling address the emotional and behavioral components of PVD.[14]

Painful bladder syndrome or Interstitial Cystitis

Painful bladder syndrome (PBS) or interstitial cystitis (IC) is a chronic bladder disorder (>6 weeks duration) characterized by pelvic pain and dysuria that cannot be attributed to an identifiable cause. The etiology is likely multifactorial and may involve neurogenic upregulation, mast cell activation, or urothelial dysregulation. Interdisciplinary assessment is often beneficial because IC is a diagnosis of exclusion. No single test can diagnose IC, and assessment could involve urinalysis, cystoscopy, or biopsy. Multimodal treatment approach consists of lifestyle modification, PT, and pharmacotherapy.[15,16] Pudendal and superior hypogastric nerve blocks can be effective in treating medical refractory IC.

Endometriosis

Endometriosis is characterized by ectopic implantation of functional uterine tissue outside the uterine cavity that can cause dysmenorrhea, dyspareunia and dyschezia, and dysuria. Interdisciplinary assessment can be beneficial. Diagnosis can be confirmed with laparoscopy, biopsy, or noninvasive imaging modalities. Multiple mechanisms are involved in the pain physiology, including nociception, inflammation, and alterations in peripheral and central nervous system pain processing. Nonsurgical treatment options include nonsteroidal anti-inflammatory drugs (NSAIDs) or hormone therapy that limits endometrial tissue growth.[17] Targeted image-guided nerve blocks, trigger points, sympathetic blocks, and neuromodulation techniques described above can be employed for improved analgesia and reduced disability.

Conclusion

CPP is a debilitating condition that necessitates interdisciplinary treatment approaches given its multifactorial etiology. CPP spans musculoskeletal, visceral, neurologic, and psychological domains. Diagnostic workup should include comprehensive history, UPOINTS classification, internal exam, selective imaging, and surgical diagnosis and management when indicated.

A stepwise, holistic treatment approach is recommended. First-line strategies include pelvic floor PT, patient education, CBT, and pharmacologic interventions. Interventional options such as trigger point injections, nerve blocks, and onabotulinumtoxinA may be second-line treatments. Neuromodulation techniques may be considered for patients with persistent or centralized pain. Setting realistic expectations is crucial, and improvements in quality of life should be treatment benchmarks. Long-term success requires an integrated team approach.

References

1. Lamvu G, Carrillo J, Ouyang C, Rapkin A, Lokken RP, As-Sanie S. Chronic pelvic pain: A clinical review. JAMA. 2021;325(23):2381–2391. doi:10.1001/jama.2021.5196
2. American College of Obstetrics and Gynecology. ACOG Committee on Practice Bulletins – Gynecology. Practice bulletin no. 218: Chronic pelvic pain. Obstet Gynecol. 2020;135(3):e98–e109. doi:10.1097/AOG.0000000000003716
3. Petros PE. *The Female Pelvic Floor: Function, Dysfunction and Management According to the Integral Theory*. 1st ed. Springer-Verlag; 2004. doi:10.1007/978-3-662-05445-1
4. Allaire C, Yong PJ, Bajzak K, et al. Guideline no. 445: Management of chronic pelvic pain. J Obstet Gynaecol Can. 2024;46(1):102283. doi:10.1016/j.jogc.2023.102283
5. DeLancey JOL. Pelvic floor anatomy and pathology. In: Hoyte L, Damaser M, eds. *Biomechanics of the Female Pelvic Floor*. 2nd ed. Academic Press; 2016:13–51. doi:10.1016/B978-0-12-803228-2.00002-7
6. Kotarinos RK. Musculoskeletal pelvic anatomy. In: Hoyte L, Damaser M, eds. *Biomechanics of the Female Pelvic Floor*. 2nd ed. Academic Press; 2016:53–87. doi:10.1016/B978-0-12-803228-2.00003-9
7. Shi JY, Paredes Mogica JA, De EJB. Non-surgical management of chronic pelvic pain in females. Curr Urol Rep. 2022;23(10):245–254. doi:10.1007/s11934-022-01110-z
8. Namazi G, Chauhan N, Handler S. Myofascial pelvic pain: The forgotten player in chronic pelvic pain. Curr Opin Obstet Gynecol. 2024;36(4):273–281. doi:10.1097/GCO.0000000000000966
9. Parsons BA, Baranowski AP, Berghmans B, et al. Management of chronic primary pelvic pain syndromes. BJU Int. 2022;129(5):572–581. doi:10.1111/bju.15609
10. Labat JJ, Riant T, Robert R, Amarenco G, Lefaucheur JP, Rigaud J. Diagnostic criteria for pudendal neuralgia by pudendal nerve entrapment (Nantes criteria). Neurourol Urodyn. 2008;27(4):306–310. doi:10.1002/nau.20505
11. Wang CL, Song T. The clinical efficacy of high-voltage long-duration pulsed radiofrequency treatment in pudendal neuralgia: A retrospective study. Neuromodulation. 2022;25(8):1372–1377. doi:10.1111/ner.13401
12. Hao D, Yurter A, Chu R, et al. Neuromodulation for management of chronic pelvic pain: A comprehensive review. Pain Ther. 2022;11(4):1137–1177. doi:10.1007/s40122-022-00430-9
13. Usmani H, Dureja GP, Andleeb R, Tauheed N, Asif N. Conventional radiofrequency thermocoagulation vs pulsed radiofrequency neuromodulation of ganglion impar in chronic perineal pain of nononcological origin. Pain Med. 2018;19(12):2348–2356. doi:10.1093/pm/pnx244. PMID: 29329442
14. Schlaeger JM, Glayzer JE, Villegas-Downs M, et al. Evaluation and treatment of vulvodynia: State of the science. J Midwifery Womens Health. 2023;68(1):9–34. doi:10.1111/jmwh.13456
15. Lim Y, Leslie SW, O'Rourke S. Interstitial cystitis/Bladder pain syndrome. [Updated 2024 Oct 7]. StatPearls. 2025 Jan. https://www.ncbi.nlm.nih.gov/books/NBK570588/

16. Hanno P, Dmochowski R. Status of international consensus on interstitial cystitis/bladder pain syndrome/painful bladder syndrome: 2008 snapshot. Neurourol Urodyn. 2009;28(4):274–286. doi:10.1002/nau.20687
17. Tsamantioti ES, Mahdy H. Endometriosis. [Updated January 23, 2023]. StatPearls. 2025 Jan. https://www.ncbi.nlm.nih.gov/books/NBK567777/

27
Integrative and Complementary Therapies for Pelvic Pain

Anand Prem and James Sturvidant

Introduction

Chronic pelvic pain (CPP) is a term that encompasses multiple disorders of various pelvic organs, including the urinary tract, female reproductive system, and gastrointestinal organs, as well as pain of musculoskeletal, neurologic, and psychogenic origin.[1,2] Given the complex and multifactorial nature of CPP, there is no single treatment modality for this condition. Instead, an optimal approach to treatment should be multimodal in nature.[1,3] One such increasingly utilized modality is *complementary and alternative medicine* (CAM).[4] CAM refers to techniques and therapies that are not considered part of conventional medicine.[5] The purpose of this chapter is to discuss some of the most commonly utilized CAM treatments for CPP, granting the reader a basic familiarity with treatment modalities that may not be often described elsewhere in common medical literature.

Background

Most CAM therapies practiced today can be placed in one of five broad groups: alternative medical systems (including chiropractic care and acupuncture), biological-based approaches, mind–body interventions, energy therapies, and muscle and joint manipulation.[5,6] CAM therapies offer a wide range of treatment approaches that aim to address not only the physical symptoms of pain, but also its psychological, emotional, and lifestyle-related aspects. These therapies may include acupuncture, herbal remedies, mind–body practices, manual therapies, and dietary interventions. As patients become increasingly interested in CAM therapies, it is important for healthcare practitioners to have some degree of familiarity with these modalities. What follows is a review of some common CAM therapies for CPP. While not exhaustive, this chapter should serve as an overview for treatments that are often overlooked in medicine.

Chiropractic Care

"Chiropractic care" is a term that most commonly references spinal manipulation (low-amplitude, high-velocity thrusts to spinal joints), but it can include a variety of therapies designed to treat neurological or musculoskeletal disorders.[7] In recent decades,

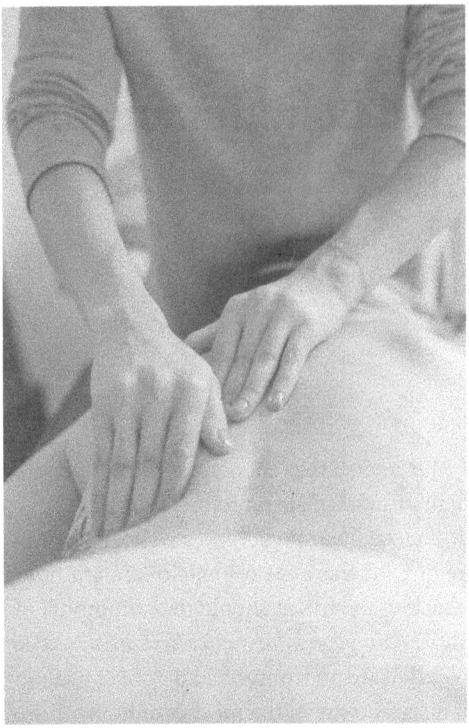

Figure 27.1 Chiropractic technique using hands for spinal adjustment on mid-lower back.
Photo by Toa Heftiba on Unsplash.

the utilization of chiropractic care for a variety of pain syndromes, most commonly low back pain, has increased. This serves as an alternative to traditional pain management therapies, including medical management. For treatment of pelvic pain, chiropractic therapies include spinal manipulation therapy (Figure 27.1), exercises, patient education and advice on strategies to reduce anxiety and pain, and use of support devices, such as belts.[7,8] Chiropractors may also provide adjunctive care, such as the use of transcutaneous electrical nerve stimulation, massage, myofascial release, stretching, and acupuncture.

Acupuncture

Acupuncture is a form of ancient Chinese therapy that involves placing needles into the skin at certain set specific points on the body (Figure 27.2). This is traditionally believed to facilitate the flow of energy through the body via channels known as *meridians*. More recently, the efficacy of acupuncture is thought to be due to stimulation of specific parts of the body, promoting circulation. Acupuncture is a commonly practiced therapy for a variety of health problems, including CPP.[9,10] The purpose of this treatment is to decrease pelvic dysfunction and reduce CPP. Acupuncture can be utilized as a standalone treatment, but it is often a part of a multimodal therapy plan including physical therapy and pelvic floor rehabilitation.[10]

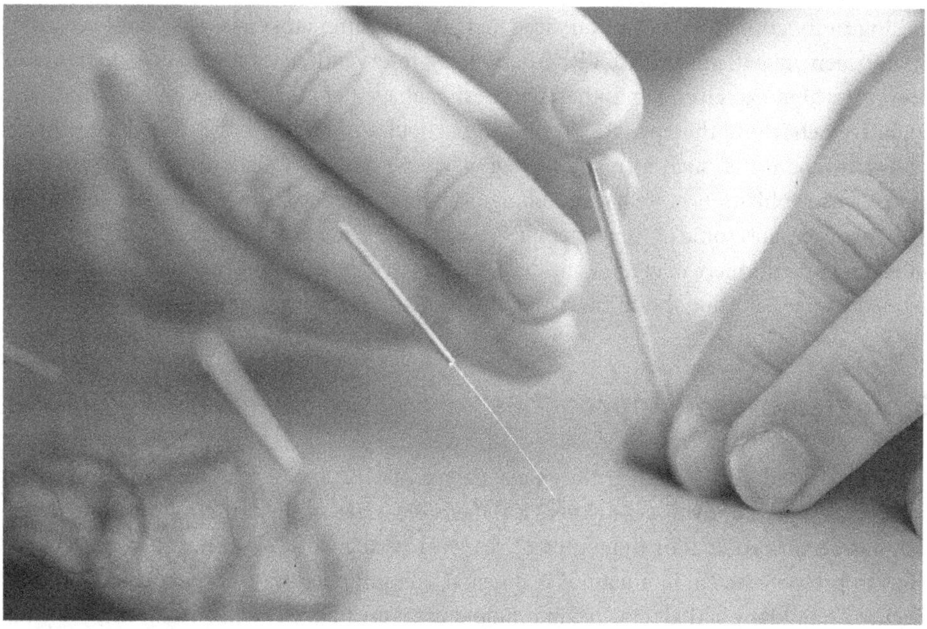

Figure 27.2 Acupuncture technique with placement of needles at skin.
Photo by Katherine Hanlon on Unsplash.

Muscle-Joint Manipulation

Muscle and joint manipulation is a treatment modality that focuses on physical interventions to improve physical functioning and pain. Such interventions include biofeedback; electrical stimulation; and manual therapies, such as myofascial release, trigger point injections, massage therapy, and pelvic floor muscle therapy (PFMT).[1,9,11] PFMT is a modality that seeks to improve pelvic floor muscle strength and function through the repeated contractions of these muscles. This technique was initially described by Kegel et al. as a means of assisting women in managing stress urinary incontinence. Recently, these exercises have become increasingly popular in managing an array of pelvic floor disorders, including CPP.[3]. Massage therapy relies on manual manipulation of soft tissues of skin, muscle, ligament, and fascia. This is meant to improve circulation, reduce stress, and relax contracted musculature.[11–13] One such intervention is the *Thiele technique*, which involves transvaginal digital pressure along the direction of pelvic musculature. This technique is meant to relax the pelvic muscles, improve tone, and increase muscle coordination.[3,14] Improvement in pelvic muscle tone can assist in treating vaginal pain, sexual dysfunction, and urinary incontinence.[3,9]

Mind–Body Interventions

Mind–body interventions focus on interaction between the brain and the body, utilizing the mind to improve physical functioning, reduce stress, and treat the symptoms of CPP.[2,9] Such interventions reduce pain via remodeling of the hypothalamic-pituitary axis, which plays a role in central pain syndromes through dysregulation of cortisol and immune responses, leading to inflammatory activation. This increased inflammatory response has been commonly seen in patients with CPP.[1] Mind–body interventions include such therapies as deep-breathing exercises, hypnotherapy, stress-management techniques, mindfulness, and cognitive behavioral therapy (CBT). CBT in particular has been shown to reduce pain via coping mechanisms, such as restructuring alarming and unrealistic thoughts about pain (pain catastrophizing), as well as mood management.[9] Due to its increasing use in chronic pain management, some of these therapies, such as CBT, are now considered "mainstream," and some practitioners may not consider them CAM modalities.[5] Even so, they are closely aligned with other mind–body interventions.

Biological-Based Approaches

Biological-based approaches to the management of CPP include herbal and supplement therapy, as well as individualized biological therapies.[5] Herbal therapy is a form of medicine that has been practiced for thousands of years across the world. It utilizes herbal formulations to promote health in a natural manner, as compounded by an expert practitioner.[2,15] (Figure 27.3). Many herbal remedies and supplements are utilized in the management of pain. These include pollen extract, green tea extract, cayenne, and numerous traditional Chinese herbs.[1,2,15] (Figure 27.4). These treatments are thought to treat pain via reduction in inflammation and promotion of healing.[6] Another biological-based approach is the use of aromatherapy. Aromatherapy involves the use of essential oils, such as lavender oil, to produce a pleasant aroma that reduces stress and decreases inflammation, thus producing analgesia.[16]

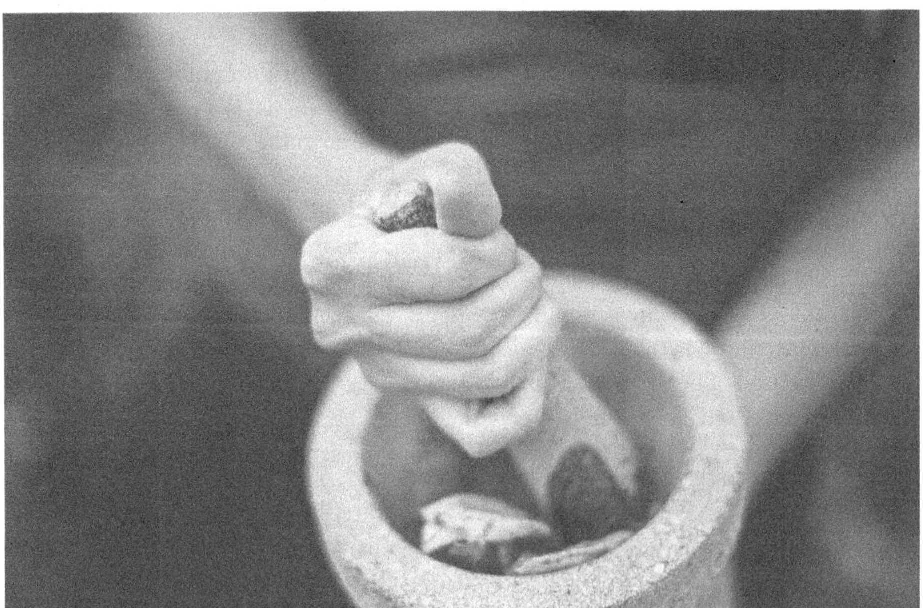

Figure 27.3 Herbal remedy compounding with a mortar and pestle.
Source: Photo by Katherine Hanlon on Unsplash.

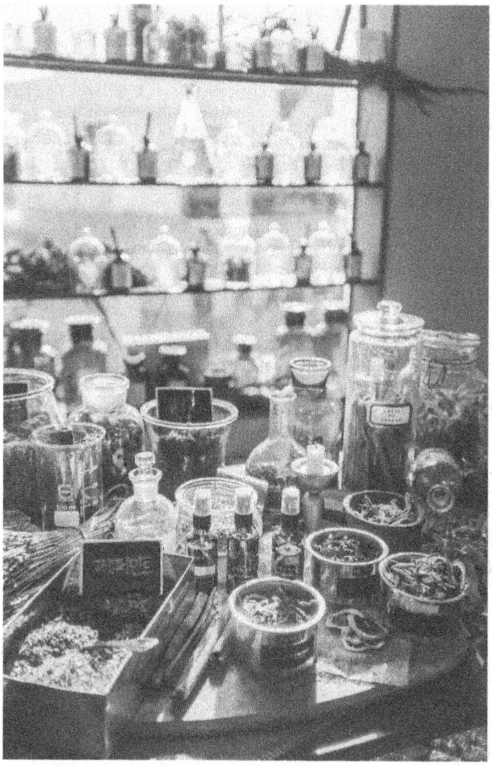

Figure 27.4 Herbs used for compounding for remedies.
Source: Photo by Bundo Kim on Unsplash.

Energy Therapy

Energy therapies involve manipulation of energy fields. These fields may originate within the body (biofields) or from other sources, such as electromagnetic fields. Biofield manipulation relies on manipulation of the body to alter the flow of energy. These therapies include Qi gong, Reiki, and therapeutic touch. Electromagnetic manipulation utilizes pulse fields, magnetic fields, or electric current fields to treat a variety of pain syndromes.[5]

Gender-Specific Considerations

Many of the techniques in this chapter are not specific to any one gender. Because CPP may be caused by disorders of organ systems other than the female reproductive system, many of these techniques, such as acupuncture, chiropractic care, mind–body interventions, biological-based approaches, and energy therapies, are applicable to male and female patients. Other techniques, such as Thiele massage, are specific only to patients with female reproductive anatomy.

Current Research

There are varying degrees of evidence for the therapies described in this chapter. Additionally, there is a paucity of research regarding many of these treatments as they specifically relate to pelvic pain. There is little evidence to suggest a significant benefit in chiropractic care for management of pelvic pain.[8] There is some limited evidence to support the use of acupuncture, particularly in conjunction with pelvic floor rehabilitation techniques, in the management of CPP.[2,10] Of the CAM methods mentioned here, physiotherapy and psychotherapy have the strongest evidence to support their usage in management of CPP, with several studies to support their use in reduction of pain and improvement of quality of life.[11,17,18] A recent retrospective study showed some evidence favoring the use of Chinese herbal medicine in treatment of pelvic pain due to endometriosis.[14] A literature search failed to discover evidence to support the use of energy therapy for pelvic pain, but there is some evidence for its use in other pain conditions.[19]

Clinical Practice Recommendations

It is not necessary for practitioners who do not offer CAM modalities to be intimately familiar with them, but it is helpful to know something about CAM because many patients have an interest in it and may ask for further information. Practitioners should familiarize themselves with providers of CAM modalities in their areas and would be well advised to know when to make appropriate referrals to such providers.

Conclusion

CAM encompasses a wide variety of treatments not commonly well known to medical practitioners. Several of these treatments have some utility in managing CPP, which is often difficult to treat via more conventional means. While not in any way comprehensive, this chapter has provided an overview of many commonly utilized CAM methods for pelvic pain. Utilization of CAM enables a holistic approach to the management of CPP in combination with more commonly known medical treatments. Such an approach to treatment would benefit many who suffer from CPP.

References

1. Srinivasan M, Torres JE, McGeary D, Nagpal AS. Complementary and alternative (CAM) treatment options for women with pelvic pain. Curr Physical Med Rehabil Rep. 2020;8(3):240–248. doi:10.1007/s40141-020-00264-6
2. Carinci AJ, Pathak R, Young M, Christo PJ. Complementary and alternative treatments for chronic pelvic pain. Curr Pain Headache Rep. 2013;17(2):1–5. doi:10.1007/s11916-012-0316-5

3. Arnouk A, De E, Rehfuss A, Cappadocia C, Dickson S, Lian F. Physical, complementary, and alternative medicine in the treatment of pelvic floor disorders. Curr Urol Rep. 2017;18(6):1–13. doi:10.1007/s11934-017-0694-7
4. National Center for Complementary and Alternative Medicine - National Institutes of Health. American adult use of complementary and alternative medicine. J Pain Palliat Care Pharmacother. 2004;18(4):111–114.
5. National Center for Complementary and Alternative Medicine. Complementary and alternative medicine: Information for practitioners and consumers. J Pain Palliat Care Pharmacother. 2002;16(4):89–100.
6. Sai Kong, Yue-Hui Zhang, Chen-Fang Liu, et al. The complementary and alternative medicine for endometriosis: A review of utilization and mechanism. Evidence-Based Complement Altern Med. 2014;2014. doi:10.1155/2014/146383
7. Conner SN, Trudell AS, Conner CA. Chiropractic care for the pregnant body. Clin Obstet Gynecol. 2021;64(3):602–610. doi:10.1097/GRF.0000000000000621
8. Weis CA, Pohlman K, Draper C, daSilva-Oolup S, Stuber K, Hawk C. Chiropractic care for adults with pregnancy-related low back, pelvic girdle pain, or combination pain: A systematic review. J Manipulative Physiol Therap. 2020;43(7):714–731. doi:10.1016/j.jmpt.2020.05.005
9. Jia X, Crouss T, Rana N, Whitmore KE. Complementary and alternative medicine for the management of interstitial cystitis/bladder pain syndrome: A recent update. Curr Bladder Dysfunction Rep. 2020;15(3):214–218. doi:10.1007/s11884-020-00594-0
10. Jie Zheng, Xinsheng Lai, Weifeng Zhu, Yingjie Huang, Chuyun Chen, Jianqin Chen. Effects of acupuncture combined with rehabilitation on chronic pelvic pain syndrome in females: A meta-analysis running head—acupuncture combined with rehabilitation on chronic pelvic pain. J Healthcare Engineer. 2022;2022. doi:10.1155/2022/8770510
11. Fuentes-Márquez P, Cabrera-Martos I, Valenza MC. Physiotherapy interventions for patients with chronic pelvic pain: A systematic review of the literature. Physiotherapy Theory Pract. 2019;35(12):1131–1138. doi:10.1080/09593985.2018.1472687
12. Mak S, Allen J, Begashaw M, et al. Use of massage therapy for pain, 2018–2023: A systematic review. JAMA Netw Open. 2024;7(7):e2422259. doi:10.1001/jamanetworkopen.2024.22259
13. Azima S, Bakhshayesh HR, Kaviani M, Abbasnia K, Sayadi M. Comparison of the effect of massage therapy and isometric exercises on primary dysmenorrhea: A randomized controlled clinical trial. J Pediatr Adolesc Gynecol. 2015;28(6):486-491. doi:10.1016/j.jpag.2015.02.003
14. De Souza Montenegro MLL, Mateus-Vasconcelos EC, Candido dos Reis FJ, Rosa e Silva JC, Nogueira AA, Poli Neto OB. Thiele massage as a therapeutic option for women with chronic pelvic pain caused by tenderness of pelvic floor muscles. J Evaluation Clin Pract. 2010;16(5):981–982. doi:10.1111/j.1365-2753.2009.01202.x
15. Lin Y, Hou R, Zhang T, Chung JPW, Wang CC, Zhao R. Efficacy and safety of Chinese herbal medicine for endometriosis associated pain. Am J Chinese Med. 2022;50(4):1095–1111. doi:10.1142/S0192415X22500446
16. Özel BZ, Quevedo A, Jung C, Shirazi F, Dancz CE. Lavender aromatherapy for anxiety and pain during multichannel urodynamics: A randomized controlled pilot trial. Female Pelvic Med Reconstruct Surg. 2021;27(11):654–658. doi:10.1097/SPV.0000000000001032

17. Nygaard AS, Haugstad GK, Wilsgaard T, Øian P, Stedenfeldt M. Baseline pain characteristics predict pain reduction after physical therapy in women with chronic pelvic pain: Secondary analysis of data from a randomized controlled trial. Scand J Pain. 2020;20(4):793–800. doi:10.1515/sjpain-2020-0026
18. Johnson S, Bradshaw A, Bresnahan R, Evans E, Herron K, Hapangama DK. Biopsychosocial approaches for the management of female chronic pelvic pain: A systematic review. BJOG. 2025;132(3):266–277. doi:10.1111/1471-0528.17987
19. Unal N, Bektaş Akpinar N, Bek D, Yurtsever S. The effect of reiki on pain, functional status, and holistic well-being in patients with knee osteoarthritis: A randomized controlled trial. Orthoped Nurs. 2024;43(2):109–118. doi:10.1097/NOR.0000000000001017

28
Advanced Evidence-Based Interventional Techniques for Pelvic Pain

Katherine Gohres, Peter Sloane, Raj Patel, Karishma Kondapalli, and Magdalena Anitescu

Pelvic Pain Incidence, and Prevalence

Chronic pelvic pain (CPP) is defined as persistent pain in the lower abdomen or pelvic region lasting at least 6 months, excluding pain that occurs exclusively during menstrual periods or intercourse, and is not due to pregnancy.[1] Historically, only noncyclical pain was considered to meet criteria for CPP. The definition has evolved to include cyclic pain if symptoms start affecting cognition, behavior, and sexual and emotional health.[2]

CPP is a significant health issue for women worldwide, with prevalence estimates ranging from 6% to 26% of women, depending on the population and definitions used.[3] Of these women, approximately one-third will have no obvious gynecologic pathology, and one-third will have persistent pain even after hysterectomy.[4] Previous literature estimates that CPP incurs direct healthcare costs of US$208 million, with additional indirect costs as high as $US31 million each year.[4]

History of Pelvic Pain and Common Sources

Historically, women's pelvic pain was poorly understood and often misattributed to purely gynecologic or even psychological causes. In past centuries, many women's pain complaints were dismissed under the diagnosis of "hysteria," a term derived from the Greek word for uterus (*hystera*) and premised on the notion of a wandering or troubled womb.[5] These misconceptions contributed to the widespread dismissal of women's pain complaints and delayed the development of evidence-based approaches.

Modern understanding has reframed CPP as a legitimate, multifactorial condition with overlapping physical and psychosocial dimensions. Pain may originate from one or more systems and can involve somatic or visceral structures. Some theories suggest infection, neurogenic inflammation, hypoxia, and pelvic floor muscle weakness as possible causes of CPP. However, because other chronic pain syndromes are commonly concurrent with CPP in patients, central pain dysfunction remains the more likely source.[6] In addition, transgender men and gender-diverse individuals assigned female at birth may also experience CPP—often related to hormonal therapy, pelvic floor tension, or underlying gynecologic conditions—highlighting the need for gender-affirming, inclusive evaluation practices.[7]

Pelvic pain can severely disrupt daily life activities, pushing emotional boundaries, straining relationships, and hindering advancement toward personal goals.[8] Moreover, a history of sexual abuse has been known to have an association with CPP, and some studies have revealed that those affected tend to have more severe pain.[9]

Differential Diagnoses

CPP has a broad differential diagnosis, although the process should be approached as a syndrome with multifactorial etiology. Other systems, including gastrointestinal, gynecologic, musculoskeletal, neurologic, psychosocial, urologic, and vascular, may all contribute to symptoms. Most commonly associated conditions include irritable bowel syndrome (IBS), endometriosis, myofascial syndromes (such as levator ani syndrome, muscular dystonia, pelvic floor trigger point), and interstitial cystitis. Characteristics of CPP include allodynia and hyperalgesia. The syndrome can be further broken down into subgroups, such as painful bladder syndrome (PBS) and provoked vestibulodynia (PVD). PBS is associated with increased urgency and frequency of urination that affects quality of life. PVD is associated with pain or soreness with vaginal penetration.[6]

Because the etiology of the condition can vary greatly, the current approach to CPP is to start with a thorough history and physical before pursuing more invasive diagnostic tests or interventions. Along with assessing the character, frequency, and triggers of the pain, understanding a patient's other medical history, social history, or other stressors may help elicit a more focal origin that permits targeted treatment. A thorough physical examination may include an abdominal exam along with an external and internal genitourinary exam. At that point, if comprehensive information-gathering still cannot help narrow the etiology, it may indicate that multiple generators of pain are present. Further diagnostics such as pregnancy tests, urine analysis, sexually transmitted disease screening, endometrial biopsy, colonoscopy, cystoscopy, or radiographic imaging may provide more answers based on the concurrent symptoms upon presentation. A clinician should be willing to tailor their investigation of the pain to each patient's unique experience.

Advanced Interventional Treatments

Visceral Pain from the Pelvis and Genital System

Visceral pelvic pain is present in up to 24% of women,[10] and, when chronic, it is associated with anxiety, depression, and recurrent hospitalization.[11] Visceral pain is classically characterized as diffuse, deep, colicky, or achy and can often lead to diagnoses of "functional" pain due to the cryptic nature of visceral sensory mechanisms. Current understanding describes CPP as the result of sensitization of primary afferent fibers directly innervating pelvic viscera, central sensitization,[12] and dysregulation of the descending tracts that regulate spinal nociceptive pathways.[13,14] When evaluating visceral pain originating from the genitals or pelvis, it is important to consider ischemia, luminal distention, inflammation, and malignancy as potential causes before prioritizing a functional etiology. Chronic visceral pelvic pain treatment includes physical therapy, cognitive behavioral therapy, narcotics, interventional techniques.[15]

Superior Hypogastric Nerve Block or Radiofrequency Ablation

Superior hypogastric nerve block or radiofrequency ablation (RFA) neurolysis is a form of sympathetic nerve blockade that has been shown to provide long-lasting relief in 50–70% of patients with chronic pelvis pain.[15] The superior hypogastric plexus typically sits anteriorly to the L5 and S1 vertebral bodies in the retroperitoneum, medial to the psoas. It is posterior to the aorta's bifurcation into the common iliacs. As the plexus descends, it becomes the inferior hypogastric plexus, which provides innervation to the pelvic floor, bladder, urethra, ovaries, genitals, descending colon, and rectum. The superior hypogastric plexus's favorable accessibility relative to the inferior plexus has made it a popular target in treating chronic cases of pain (e.g., malignancy) and in acute settings[16] (e.g., immediately following hysterectomies).

There are currently two main fluoroscopic approaches to super hypogastric nerve block or RFA ablation: classic two-needle and transdiscal single-needle. Ultrasound- and CT-guided approaches are have also been found to be safe and effective techniques.[17,18]

In the classic two-needle approach, the patient is prone with a 22G needle inserted 5–7 cm lateral from the L4–L5 disc space.[19] Under fluoroscopy the anterior aspect of the L5 vertebral body is targeted until loss of resistance[20] with traversal of the psoas fascia is felt. It is common for the transverse process of the L5 and the iliac crest to obstruct the needle's path. Correct placement of the needle is confirmed with contrast before either injecting the provider's choice of neurolysis/anesthetic or performing radiofrequency lesioning. The process is then repeated on the contralateral side. Complications are rare and include unintentional perforation of the bladder or other pelvic viscera and intravascular injection of the iliac vessels. Genito-femoral nerves can also be blocked by this approach, especially if needles are slightly misplaced higher in relation to the L5 vertebral body; this side effect or complication can manifest by consequent motor dysfunction (foot drop) that can be temporary in steroid-based blocks or permanent when neurolytic agents (98% alcohol or 6% phenol) are used for pelvic malignancy pain.

In the transdiscal single-needle approach,[21] the patient is lateral or prone and a needle is advanced 7–8 cm from the midline at the level of L4–L5 toward the L5–S1 disc, navigating inferiorly to the facet joints and intentionally traversing the L5–S1 disc until it is advanced just past the anterior annulus fibrosus.[22] Placement is confirmed with fluoroscopy and then followed by administration of injectate, heat nerve ablation (RFA), or neurolytic agent. This technique avoids the iliac crest as a barrier that may make the classic approach more challenging. Some studies have found the transdiscal approach to be safer and faster than the classic approach,[15] although discitis is a potential complication.

The ultrasound-guided approach has also been described as a safe and effective technique.[17] As the patient lies supine, a curvilinear probe is placed between the umbilicus and pubic symphysis until the L5 vertebra is identified just below the aortic bifurcation. A 22G needle is then carefully advanced, being sure to avoid any bowel, organs, or vessels, until the lower third of the L5 vertebra is reached.[23] After confirmation of placement, injectate or neurolytic agent (98% alcohol or 6% phenol) is administered.

The CT-guided approach utilizes CT scanning to identify the L5–S1 disc, determine the appropriate trajectory, and then confirm appropriate needle placement.[15]

Ganglion Impar Block

The ganglion impar (also referred to as Walther ganglion) sits in the retroperitoneum just anterior to the sacrococcygeal junction (SCJ), and is the final sympathetic ganglion. It contains the visceral afferents to the perineum, distal rectum, anus, distal urethra, vulva, and distal third of the vagina.[24] Indications for blockade of the ganglion impar include management or diagnosis of visceral pain in the perineal or coccygeal regions, with RFA or neurolysis usually reserved for malignant etiologies of pain.[25]

There are two approaches for the ganglion impar block: the classic trans-anococcygeal approach and the trans-sacrococcygeal approach. Generally, the trans-sacrococcygeal approach is more popular due to superior patient comfort and lower risk of anal and rectal injuries.[24]

In the classic trans-anococcygeal approach, the patient is placed in lateral decubitus with the hips flexed. To protect the rectum from puncture, a finger is placed in the rectum. A standard 22-gauge needle is then bent 1 inch from its hub to form a 30-degree angle before being advanced through the anococcygeal ligament up toward the SCJ. Placement is confirmed with fluoroscopy before administration of injectate.

The trans-sacrococcygeal technique involves a 20G needle being placed at the sacral hiatus and then advanced under ultrasound guidance or fluoroscopy through the sacrococcygeal ligament until the tip is just anterior to the sacrum, which is usually associated with loss of resistance.[24] Fluoroscopy can be hindered by impacted stool or rectal gas, while the trans-sacrococcygeal approach may be limited if there is significant calcification of the sacrococcygeal ligament or joint.[25]

Visceral/Neuropathic Pain from General Sources

Advanced neuromodulatory therapies such as dorsal root ganglion stimulation (DRGS) and spinal cord stimulation (SCS) are further avenues for relief. Each addresses the visceral and neuropathic pathophysiology underlying CPP. Additionally, complex pelvic anatomy and unpredictable dermatomes challenge targeting of peripheral nerves. CPP is a mechanistically related entity to complex regional pain syndrome (CPRS) and is thus amenable to similar therapies. Regulatory support for interventional neuromodulation of CPP rests on US Food and Drug Administration (FDA) approval in 2016 of CPRS types I and II lower limb therapies. More central targeting of the DRG or spinal cord itself may better address the central sensitization and autonomic dysregulation featured in visceral and neuropathic etiology of CPP.[26]

Spinal Cord Stimulation

Though SCS is historically reserved for diverse neuropathic pain such as CPRS and ischemic pain, it is now emerging as salvage therapy for chronic visceral pelvic pain refractory to time-limited effects of nerve plexus blocks. Indications for SCS in CPP have broadly included endometriosis, pudendal neuralgia, coccydynia, vulvodynia, and painful bladder syndrome. Large, broadly inclusive trials remain elusive due to the complexity of CPP.[27] Small case series and studies were recently examined in narrative review for SCS in chronic pelvic and abdominal pain, emphasizing methodological, patient selection, size, and procedural heterogeneity offering low-quality evidence. This review, however, offers encouraging insight and opportunity for improved patient selection, larger robust trials, and device development.[28]

Visceral CPP challenges effective management due to complex innervation, peripheral distribution, and central modulation. Typical indications for SCS are CPP due to gynecologic and urologic etiologies. Neuromodulation treatment is not the first-line treatment for CPP. Technological development from the first monopolar spinal cord electrode placed by Shealy in 1967 to current complex, multimodal, closed-loop arrays accounts for SCS adoption and success as much as refined patient selection.[29–32]

SCS uses electrical leads placed in the epidural space of the spinal cord at the vertebral level supplying pelvic dermatomes, roughly corresponding T12–S3. Lead placement targets midline epidural areas over bilateral dorsal columns. An electrical field is applied over the dorsal columns to modulate neuronal transmission; however, clear mechanisms of electrical neuromodulation remain elusive.[33] Mechanistic assumptions rely on Melzack and Wall's gate control theory of pain, which proposes that continuous stimulation of afferent Aβ nerve fibers in the dorsal column causes release of inhibitory neurotransmitter on C fibers to attenuate nociceptive transmission in the dorsal horn, thereby closing the "gate" to central transmission of nociception.[34] SCS efficacy in neuropathic pain suggests more nuanced mechanisms possibly related to electrical neuromodulation of dorsal roots and/or even islet cell dendrites in the dorsal horns of the spinal cord.

SCS placement is an outpatient surgical procedure. A catheter-threaded electrode with spaced leads is placed in the epidural space under fluoroscopy and sedation and local anesthesia or general anesthesia over a desired spinal level. Skin entry is usually two vertebral levels below desired lead target. Ideal electrode placement is several spinal levels above the target dermatomes due to dorsal column anatomy. A second lead is often placed at one vertebral level above the first catheter to anticipate lead migration. The leads are attached to an external programmable pulse generator and trialed over several days. Electrode geometry and pulse qualities are optimized during the trial period. Once successful, the generator is surgically internalized under sedation with local anesthesia or general anesthesia.

Regarding outcomes, SCS intervention for refractory endometriosis produced more satisfactory results and fewer complications compared to nondifferentiated pelvic pain in women.[35] Success of SCS in chronic pain due to urologic disorders, especially voiding pain, relies on careful patient selection based on age and pathology. Despite complications, reported patient satisfaction with SCS has been high.[36–38] However, among indications for SCS, CPP has the highest rate of explantation at 33%, most commonly due to loss of effect.[39]

Complications include lead migration, broken lead, abundant granulation tissue, diminishing effect, and, rarely, infection at site. Newer devices and improved technique limit these.

Dorsal Root Ganglion Stimulation

DRGS for treatment of pelvic pain grows in popularity as an intervention that more selectively stimulates pain-generating centers compared to SCS. DRGS already enjoys some effectiveness for conditions like postsurgical pain, neuropathic pain, and CPRS. Encouraging evidence is yet limited by sample size, limited follow-up, and a relatively high rate of surgical explantation or revision. These limitations are shared with SCS.[40]

Anatomically, the DRG is located on both sides of the spinal cord in the epidural space posterolateral to the spinal foramen. The DRG is a defining anatomic and functional structure of each spinal nerve root. These ganglia, as the name implies, contain neuron cell bodies (soma) of sensory neurons spanning wide areas. The DRG integrates with the sympathetic chain via rami communicantes nerves. Sensory and autonomic integration contributes to neuromodulation of chronic pain sensitization, thus offering a target for intervention.[41,42] Notably, DRGS requires finer target discrimination than does SCS.

Mechanistically, DRGS purportedly inhibits nociceptive and autonomic afferent transmission at the neuronal T junction, an intersection of the neuron's stem axon and central and peripheral processes, and it also activates endogenous opioid release in the dorsal horn of the spinal cord. DRGS inhibits ectopic excitability in nociceptive cell bodies in the DRG. This pattern of central stimulation attenuates peripheral and central sensitization, a hallmark and therapeutic target of chronic pain in general. Additionally, DRGS may modulate nearby glial neuroinflammatory pathways contributing to pain. Thus, DRGS exploits somatic sensory transmission and sympathetic modulation through the DRG.[43] Both upstream and downstream modulation and favorable access to the epidural space make this intervention mechanistically more attractive for specific targeting of neuron groups rather than the broad target areas of the spinal cord dorsal column inherent in SCS. Smaller targets herein permit smaller lead catheters, less energy delivery, resistance to postural variation and lead displacement, greater targeting flexibility, and enhanced diagnostic and therapeutic feedback. Once a salvage therapy for SCS failure, DRGS grows as a primary neuromodulatory intervention for CPP.[44,45]

Historical indications for DRGS have been CPRS, though pathophysiologic overlap with CPP extends its use to CPP. The pivotal ACCURATE trial suggests the superiority of DRGS over traditional column SCS for CPRS types I and II in lower extremities.[30] More recent studies tout its efficacy in improving overall pain and quality of life in diabetic neuropathy, restless leg syndrome, postsurgical pain syndromes, and painful scars,[46] in addition to CPP in small series. To treat CPP, DRGS leads typically are placed at T12/L1 and S2/S3 bilaterally.[47,48]

Close and regular outpatient follow-up is essential. Periprocedural complications have become less frequent; however, patient-centered outcomes of pain relief, functionality, and unwanted stimulation remain variable. Most studies of DRGS report that pain, functional status, and quality of life is improved in a majority of patients.[48] DRGS and SCS complications share a similar profile. Device-related complications like lead fracture and migration were most common at 27%. Procedure-related complications like dural puncture and bleeding were <1%.[49] Catheter site infection pooled rates during the trial period and after implantation are 1% and 4.8%, respectively.[50]

Somatic Pain Within the Pelvis and Genital System

Finding the source of somatic pelvic pain can be difficult because the differential is often broad. If cyclic symptoms are present, gynecological causes such as endometriosis, adenomyosis, or uterine fibroids should be considered. Gastrointestinal and colorectal pathologies should also be considered; IBS has a prevalence of up to 41% in women with CPP,[51] and colorectal malignancies or indirect inguinal hernias are relatively common pathologies that could present as pelvic pain. Providers should also consider endocrine, musculoskeletal, neuropathic, and urologic pathologies. Pudendal neuralgia is a common but often unrecognized and underdiagnosed cause of pelvic pain. Current estimates report up to a 1%

incidence in the general population,[52] though given the underreported nature of the condition, the true incidence is likely much higher. Pudendal neuralgia will often present with perineal pain worse with sitting and is thought to be secondary to nerve entrapment by pelvic ligaments or muscles. It is thought to also be triggered by events such as childbirth, chronic constipation, and radiation therapy, and in those with direct pelvic trauma and patients who experience prolonged sitting or repetitive hip flexion.[53]

Pudendal Nerve Block and Radiofrequency Ablation

Pudendal nerve block and/or ablation can diagnose and treat pudendal neuralgia, with 25% of patients reporting pain relief lasting >1 month.[54] While some studies show decreased efficacy in pain relief after 2 years,[55] these procedures have been shown to improve pain for up to 6 months[56] and are associated with reduced opioid requirements and fewer patient-reported episodes of unacceptable pain.[57] Pudendal blocks can also be used to provide regional anesthesia for obstetric or even urological procedures. The pudendal nerve is both a sensory and motor nerve that rises from the S2–S4 spinal nerve roots in the sacral plexus and then passes through the greater sciatic foramen. It then traverses the sacrospinous and sacrotuberous ligaments before reentering the perineum through the lesser sciatic foramen to reach the pudendal canal (also called Alcock's canal). The pudendal canal houses the pudendal artery, vein, and nerve. After exiting the canal, the pudendal nerve divides into various branches.[58,59]

A pudendal nerve block targets the pudendal nerve trunk as it enters the lesser sciatic foramen, inferomedial to where the sacrospinous ligament attaches to the ischial spine. Various methods such as landmark-based, ultrasound-guided, fluoroscopically guided, and CT-guided approaches are all used via transvaginal, transperineal, or transgluteal approaches.[60] The primary approach utilized in the outpatient pain clinic by these authors is fluoroscopy-guided. The benefits of the fluoroscopy-guided approach include its relative low cost, availability at many outpatient centers, and ease of landmark recognition.[60,61] Fluoroscopy also has been found to facilitate shorter procedure times while maintaining efficacy comparable to ultrasound-guided approaches.[62]

The current fluoroscopic approach described in literature involves positioning the patient on the procedure table in the prone position. Fluoroscopy is positioned in the anteroposterior view with a 5–20 degree ipsilateral oblique and 0–10 degree caudad tilt to bring the ischial spine out from behind the superior pubic ramus and into view.[60] The skin is infiltrated with local anesthetic, and a spinal needle is then advanced under radiographic guidance to reach the medial ischial spine, where the nerve exits the pelvis.[58] Correct needle position is confirmed under fluoroscopy and then injectate is administered.

Transversus Abdominus Plane Block

The transversus abdominis plane (TAP) block has historically treated acute postoperative pain from nonobstetric abdominal surgery and, to a lesser extent, obstetric surgery like caesarean section. Mechanistically, success relies on wide local anesthetic deposition on anterior abdominal wall sensory nerves T6–L1 in the neurofascial plane dividing internal oblique and transversus abdominis muscle. Ultrasound needle guidance is the gold standard and consistently reported as safe without major complications.[63] Needle guidance can be modified for more specific approaches targeting ilioinguinal and/or ileohypogastric nerves as surgically indicated. Effect reaches the parietal peritoneum, anterior muscles, and overlying skin of the anterior abdominal wall. TAP blocks effectively relieve pain after caesarean section and hysterectomy though they have limited benefit over periprocedural intrathecal morphine. The TAP block's primary benefit has been opioid-sparing in the acute postoperative phase; relief of postoperative nausea and vomiting, pruritis, and bowel hypokinesis have been inconclusively demonstrated in meta-analyses. Naturally, choice of local anesthetic and adjuncts limit effect duration to 24–48 hours.[64–66] There is limited study of TAP block for chronic abdominal pain. Local anesthetic with steroid adjunct appears to reduce pain and gabapentin use for weeks after abdominal surgery in women and men for mostly abdominal surgical disease.[44,67] Though the TAP block is commonly relegated to the realm of upper abdominal wall pain, lower abdominal wall pain originating in the abdominal wall itself, rather than in the peritoneal cavity, features commonly in CPP syndromes.[68]

Ilioinguinal Nerve Block and Iliohypogastric Nerve Block

The ilioinguinal nerve block (IINB) and iliohypogastric nerve block (IHNB) offer additional somatic pain relief, especially in the postoperative realm. They share immediate postoperative effectiveness compared to TAP block and may demonstrate reduced incidence of chronic postoperative pain.[69,70] The ilioinguinal nerve arises from the ventral rami of the L1 spinal nerve and occasionally T12 and emerges at the lateral upper border of the psoas major muscle. It travels anterior to the quadratus lumborum muscle, crosses the iliacus muscle, pierces the transversus abdominis and internal oblique muscles at the level of the anterior iliac crest before entering the inguinal canal to provide sensory innervation to the groin, external genitalia, and inner thigh. The iliohypogastric nerve follows a similar but more cephalad course and provides cutaneous innervation to the hypogastric region, to the pubis and lateral buttock.[27] Both provide motor function to the transversus abdominis and internal oblique muscles. Since their sensory territories border the abdomen and pelvis, their pathologies contribute to "border nerve syndrome." Their neuralgias manifest in the lower abdomen, pelvis, genitalia, and medial thigh.[71] IINB and IHNB are amenable to ultrasound-guided nerve block and share an excellent safety profile. In additional to acute postoperative pain indications, both blocks are safe and effective for some to substantial pain relief in women with nonvisceral pelvic pain localized to the lower abdominal wall, both initially (78.9%) and with subsequent blocks; the minor adverse event rate was 5%, mostly limited to injection site pain.[72]

Trigger Point Injections

Trigger points may develop from repeated chronic muscular overload of abdominal, gluteal, and piriformis muscles in CPP and associated pelvic floor syndromes. Myofascial pain is common in women with CPP.[73,74] Additionally, many women diagnosed with bladder pain syndrome or interstitial cystitis also suffered myofascial pain and pelvic floor hypersensitivity causing hypertonicity. Expectedly, myofascial pelvic floor pain is associated with dyspareunia, vulvodynia, or vaginismus.[75] Trigger points refractory to pelvic floor therapy are targets for trigger point injection (TPI) of local anesthetic, steroid, and botulinum toxin injection, the latter of which causes prolonged chemodenervation of the neuromuscular junction. Local anesthetic and steroid-based TPI disrupt contractile tissue structures and desensitize the nerve terminal to noxious and/or inflammatory stimuli.[76,77] Even dry needling has a placebo effect that approaches the effect of botulinum toxin for CPP. Notably, the associated pelvic floor myalgias in CPP could be independent of neuromuscular controls that cause primary trigger points more amenable to injection. Women with CPP and increased pelvic floor tone did, however, benefit from botulinum toxin TPI.[78,79] A recent study demonstrated that transvaginal TPI using local anesthetic for CPP with pelvic floor hypertonicity had immediate pain relief at initial visits and sustained relief with ongoing visits. Adverse effects are transient, limited to minor vaginal bleeding, leg numbness, and light-headedness.[80]

Anterior Cutaneous Nerve Entrapment Syndrome

Anterior cutaneous nerve entrapment syndrome (ACNES) is an elusive and underrecognized cause of chronic anterior abdominal wall pain. Mentioned above, anterior abdominal wall pain features commonly in CPP syndromes.[68] Time to diagnosis averages several years. Anatomically, neurovascular bundles from intercostal nerves T5–T12 entering the rectus sheath via pairs of foramina in the anterior rectus fascia may become compressed. This compression is pathomechanistic for pain that may start focally and generalize.[71] Risk factors for ACNES include abdominal surgery, pregnancy, obesity, and rectus abdominal overuse; however, many women lack these risk factors. Pelvic pain may accompany abdominal pain as well as visceral abdominal symptoms like nausea, diarrhea, and diaphoresis.[81] A systematic review of treatment options for ACNES supports local anesthetic injections and neurectomy for injection-refractory symptoms. Injection success rates are 75% in this review. Neurectomy offers long-term relief, though a step-wise approach starting with TPI or ultrasound-guided injections is recommended.[81,82] Landmark-guided injections have limited success compared to ultrasound-guided injections. Steroid adjuncts increase effectiveness of injections. Chemical neurolysis, TAP blocks, and rectus sheath plane blocks are less studied and have inconclusive efficacy and safety for lasting relief for ACNES.[83,84] Local anesthetic injection superiority over placebo has been demonstrated in a randomized control trial in ACNES.[85] The most common adverse event is pain at injection.

Conclusion

CPP consists of discomfort in the lower abdominal or pelvic region that is not secondary to menstruation, pregnancy, or sexual intercourse and that lasts at least 6 months. It is found in up to 26% of women globally and is often difficult to diagnose and treat, demanding providers to consider a wide-ranging differential. CPP can be characterized as somatic and/or visceral in nature. Chronic visceral pelvic pain treatment includes multidisciplinary treatments, which can include a superior hypogastric nerve block/ablation and ganglion impar block. SCS and DRGS are often reserved as a salvage therapy for multifactorial, resistant neuropathic pain. Interventions for somatic pelvic pain are centered on the specific sources of a patient's symptoms, such as a pudendal nerve block for pudendal neuralgia, and iliohypogastric block, TAP block, ACNES, or even trigger point injections for hypogastric pain.

References

1. Speer LM, Mushkbar S, Erbele T. Chronic pelvic pain in women. Am Fam Physician. 2016;93(5):380–387. PMID: 26926975.
2. Meisenheimer ES, Carnevale AM. Chronic pelvic pain in women: Evaluation and treatment. Am Fam Physician. 2025;111(3):218–229. PMID: 40106288.

3. Ahangari A. Prevalence of chronic pelvic pain among women: An updated review. Pain Physician. 2014;17(2):E141–E147.
4. Collett B. Visceral pain: The importance of pain management services. Br J Pain. 2013;7(1):6–7. doi:10.1177/2049463713480138.
5. Tasca C, Rapetti M, Carta MG, Fadda B. (2012). Women and hysteria in the history of mental health. Clin Pract Epidemiol Mental Health. 2012;8:110–119. https://doi.org/10.2174/1745017901208010110
6. Grinberg K, Sela Y, Nissanholtz-Gannot R. New insights about chronic pelvic pain syndrome (CPPS). Int J Environ Res Public Health. 2020;17(9):3005. doi:10.3390/ijerph17093005
7. Tordoff DM, Lunn MR, Flentje A, et al. Chronic pelvic pain among transgender men and gender diverse adults assigned female at birth. Andrology. 2025;13(3):600–609. doi:10.1111/andr.13703
8. Mellado BH, Pilger TL, Poli Neto OB, et al. Daily life attitudes of women with moderate or severe chronic pelvic pain: A qualitative study. Eur J Obstet Gynecol Reprod Biol. 2020;254:109–113. doi:10.1016/j.ejogrb.2020.09.001
9. Siqueira-Campos VM, de Deus MSC, Poli-Neto OB, Rosa-E-Silva JC, de Deus JM, Conde DM. Current challenges in the management of chronic pelvic pain in women: From bench to bedside. Int J Womens Health. 2022;14:225–244. doi:10.2147/IJWH.S224891.
10. Collett B. Visceral pain: The importance of pain management services. Br J Pain. 2013;7(1):6–7. doi:10.1177/2049463713480138
11. Wie C, Ghanavatian S, Pew S, et al. Interventional treatment modalities for chronic abdominal and pelvic visceral pain. Curr Pain Headache Rep. 2022;26(9):683–691. doi:10.1007/s11916-022-01072-4
12. Ossipov MH, Lai J, Malan TP Jr, Porreca F. Spinal and supraspinal mechanisms of neuropathic pain. Ann N Y Acad Sci. 2000;909:12–24. doi:10.1111/j.1749-6632.2000.tb06673.x
13. Sengupta JN. Visceral pain: The neurophysiological mechanism. Handb Exp Pharmacol. 2009;194:31–74. doi:10.1007/978-3-540-79090-7_2
14. Zeilhofer HU, Wildner H, Yévenes GE. Fast synaptic inhibition in spinal sensory processing and pain control. Physiol Rev. 2012;92(1):193–235. doi:10.1152/physrev.00043.2010
15. Urits I, Schwartz R, Herman J, et al. A comprehensive update of the superior hypogastric block for the management of chronic pelvic pain. Curr Pain Headache Rep. 2021;25(3):13. doi:10.1007/s11916-020-00933-0
16. Doroshenko M, Turkot O, Dua A, Horn DB. Sympathetic nerve block. StatPearls. February 12, 2024. https://pubmed.ncbi.nlm.nih.gov/32491569/
17. Bhatnagar S, Khanna S, Roshni S, et al. Early ultrasound-guided neurolysis for pain management in gastrointestinal and pelvic malignancies: An observational study in a tertiary care center of urban India. Pain Pract. 2012;12(1):23–32. doi:10.1111/j.1533-2500.2011.00467.x
18. Ghoneim AA, Mansour SM. Comparative study between computed tomography guided superior hypogastric plexus block and the classic posterior approach: A prospective randomized study. Saudi J Anaesth. 2014;8(3):378–383. doi:10.4103/1658-354X.136625
19. Plancarte R, Amescua C, Patt RB, Aldrete JA. Superior hypogastric plexus block for pelvic cancer pain. Anesthesiology. 1990;73(2):236–239. doi:10.1097/00000542-199008000-00008
20. Bharti, Neerja; Singla, Navneet1; Batra, Yatindra K. Radiofrequency ablation of superior hypogastric plexus for the management of pelvic cancer pain. Indian J Pain. 2016;30(1):58–60. doi:10.4103/0970-5333.173481

21. Turker G, Basagan-Mogol E, Gurbet A, Ozturk C, Uckunkaya N, Sahin S. A new technique for superior hypogastric plexus block: The posteromedian transdiscal approach. Tohoku J Exp Med. 2005;206(3):277–281. doi:10.1620/tjem.206.277
22. Liliang PC, Hung CM, Lu K, Chen HJ. Fluoroscopically-guided superior hypogastric plexus neurolysis using a single needle: A modified technique for a posterolateral transdiscal approach. Pain Physician. 2018;21(4):E341–E345.
23. Yan L, Wang X, Zhang Z, Li Z, Chi L, Wang L. Safety and efficacy of ultrasound-guided superior hypogastric plexus block combined with conscious sedation in ambulatory patients undergoing percutaneous microwave ablation of uterine myomas: Study protocol for a single-center, double-blinded, randomized controlled trial. Heliyon. 2024;10(4):e26421. doi:10.1016/j.heliyon.2024.e26421
24. de Leon-Casasola O. Neurolysis of the sympathetic axis for cancer pain management. In: Benzon HT, Rathmell JP, Wu CL, Turk DC, Argoff CE, eds. *Raj's Practical Management of Pain*. 4th ed. Mosby; 2008:917–925. https://doi.org/10.1016/b978-032304184-3.50053-4. https://www.sciencedirect.com/science/article/pii/b9780323041843500534
25. Swain BP, Vidhya S, Kumar S. Ganglion impar block: A magic bullet to fix idiopathic coccygodynia. Cureus. 2023;15(1):e33911. doi:10.7759/cureus.33911
26. Lamvu G, Carrillo J, Ouyang C, Rapkin A. Chronic pelvic pain in women. JAMA. 2021;325(23):2381. doi:10.1001/jama.2021.2631
27. Hunter CW. Anatomy, pathophysiology and interventional therapies for chronic pelvic pain: A review. Pain Physician. 2018;1(21;1):147–167. doi:10.36076/ppj.2018.2.147
28. Bieze M, van Haaps A, Kapural L, et al. Spinal cord stimulation for intractable visceral pain originating from the pelvic and abdominal region: A narrative review on a possible new indication for patients with therapy-resistant pain. J Pain Res. 2024;17:691–736. doi:10.2147/jpr.s445616
29. Mekhail N, Visnjevac O, Azer G, Mehanny DS, Agrawal P, Foorsov V. Spinal cord stimulation 50 years later. Regional Anesth Pain Med. 2018;43(4):391–406. doi:10.1097/aap.0000000000000744
30. Deer TR, Levy RM, Kramer J, et al. Dorsal root ganglion stimulation yielded higher treatment success rate for complex regional pain syndrome and causalgia at 3 and 12 months: A randomized comparative trial. Pain. 2016;158(4):669–681. doi:10.1097/j.pain.0000000000000814
31. Deer TR, Russo MA, Sayed D, et al. The neurostimulation appropriateness consensus committee (NACC)®: Recommendations for the mitigation of complications of neurostimulation. Neuromodulation. 2024;27(6):977–1007. doi:10.1016/j.neurom.2024.04.004
32. Deer TR, Thomson S, Pope JE, Russo M, Luscombe F, Levy R. International neuromodulation society critical assessment: Guideline review of implantable neurostimulation devices. Neuromodulation. 2014;17(7):678–685. doi:10.1111/ner.12186
33. Jensen MP, Brownstone RM. Mechanisms of spinal cord stimulation for the treatment of pain: Still in the dark after 50 years. Eur J Pain. 2018;23(4):652–659. doi:10.1002/ejp.1336
34. Melzack R, Wall PD. Pain mechanisms: A new theory. Science. 1965;150(3699):971–979. doi:10.1126/science.150.3699.971
35. Zegrea A, Kirss J, Pinta T, et al. Outcomes of sacral neuromodulation for chronic pelvic pain: A Finnish national multicenter study. Techn Coloproctol. 2020;24(3):215–220. doi:10.1007/s10151–020-02148–2
36. Kapural L, Jameson J, Johnson C, et al. Treatment of nonsurgical refractory back pain with high-frequency spinal cord stimulation at 10 Khz: 12-month results of a pragmatic, multicenter,

randomized controlled trial. J Neurosurg Spine. 2022;37(2):188–199. doi:10.3171/2021.12.spine211301

37. Tate JL, Stauss T, Li S, Rotte A, Subbaroyan J. A prospective, multi-center, clinical trial of a 10-khz spinal cord stimulation system in the treatment of chronic pelvic pain. Pain Pract. 2020;21(1):45–53. doi:10.1111/papr.12932
38. Hagedorn JM, Romero J, Ha CT, D'Souza RS. Patient satisfaction with spinal cord stimulation and dorsal root ganglion stimulation for chronic intractable pain: A systematic review and meta-analysis. Neuromodulation. 2022;25(7):947–955. doi:10.1016/j.neurom.2022.04.043
39. Hayek SM, Veizi E, Hanes M. Treatment-limiting complications of percutaneous spinal cord stimulator implants: A review of eight years of experience from an academic center database. Neuromodulation. 2015;18(7):603–609. doi:10.1111/ner.12312
40. Burns SL, Majdak P, Adler AR, et al. Dorsal root ganglion stimulation for patients with chronic pelvic pain: A retrospective review of patient experiences and long-term outcomes. Intervent Pain Med. 2024;3(1):100397. doi:10.1016/j.inpm.2024.100397
41. Chung J, Chung K. Importance of hyperexcitability of DRG neurons in neuropathic pain. Pain Pract. 2002;2(2):87–97. doi:10.1046/j.1533-2500.2002.02011.x
42. Berger AA, Liu Y, Possoit H, et al. Dorsal root ganglion (DRG) and chronic pain. Anesthesiol Pain Med. 2021;11(2):e113020. doi:10.5812/aapm.113020
43. Koopmeiners AS, Mueller S, Kramer J, Hogan QH. Effect of electrical field stimulation on dorsal root ganglion neuronal function. Neuromodulation. 2013;16(4):304–311. doi:10.1111/ner.12028
44. Abd-Elsayed A, Vardhan S, Aggarwal A, Vardhan M, Diwan SA. Mechanisms of action of dorsal root ganglion stimulation. Int J Mol Sci. 2024;25(7):3591. doi:10.3390/ijms25073591
45. Krames ES. The dorsal root ganglion in chronic pain and as a target for neuromodulation: A review. Neuromodulation. 2015;18(1):24–32. doi:10.1111/ner.12247
46. Huygen FJPM, Kallewaard JW, Nijhuis H, et al. Effectiveness and safety of dorsal root ganglion stimulation for the treatment of chronic pain: A pooled analysis. Neuromodulation. 2020;23(2):213–221. doi: 10.1111/ner.13074
47. Hunter CW, Yang A. Dorsal root ganglion stimulation for chronic pelvic pain: A case series and technical report on a novel lead configuration. Neuromodulation. 2019;22(1):87–95. doi:10.1111/ner.12801
48. Ghorayeb JH, Chitneni A, Rupp A, Parkash A, Abd-Elsayed A. Dorsal root ganglion stimulation for the treatment of chronic pelvic pain: A systematic review. Pain Pract. 2023;23(7):838–846. doi:10.1111/papr.13255
49. Vanloon M, Van Broeckhoven T, Raymaekers V, et al. Noninfectious complications of dorsal root ganglion stimulation: A systematic review and meta-analysis. Neuromodulation. 2025;28(2):234–248. doi:10.1016/j.neurom.2024.10.010
50. Moman RN, Peterson AA, Maher DP, et al. Infectious complications of dorsal root ganglion stimulation: A systematic review and pooled analysis of incidence. Neuromodulation. 2022;25(7):956–964. doi:10.1111/ner.13473
51. Johnson CM, Makai GEH. Fibromyalgia and irritable bowel syndrome in female pelvic pain. Semin Reprod Med. 2018;36(2):136–142. doi:10.1055/s-0038-1676090
52. Spinosa JP, de Bisschop E, Laurençon J, Kuhn G, Dubuisson JB, Riederer BM. Les réflexes sacrés etagés dans l'etude de la névralgie pudendalte: Validation anatomique [Sacral staged reflexes to localize the pudendal compression: An anatomical validation of the concept]. Rev Med Suisse. 2006;2(84):2416–2421.

53. Leslie SW, Antolak S, Feloney MP, et al. Pudendal neuralgia. [Updated 2024 Feb 12]. StatPearls. 2025 Jan. https://www.ncbi.nlm.nih.gov/books/NBK562246/
54. Kaur J, Leslie SW, Singh P. Pudendal nerve entrapment syndrome. [Updated 2023 Aug 21]. StatPearls. 2025 Jan. https://www.ncbi.nlm.nih.gov/books/NBK544272/
55. Basol G, Kale A, Gurbuz H, Gundogdu EC, Baydilli KN, Usta T. Transvaginal pudendal nerve blocks in patients with pudendal neuralgia: 2-year follow-up results. Arch Gynecol Obstet. 2022;306(4):1107–1116. doi:10.1007/s00404-022-06621-1
56. Kale A, Usta T, Basol G, Cam I, Yavuz M, Aytuluk HG. Comparison of ultrasound-guided transgluteal and finger-guided transvaginal pudendal nerve block techniques: Which one is more effective?. Int Neurourol J. 2019;23(4):310–320. doi:10.5213/inj.1938112.056
57. Knox MC, Thiruthaneeswaran N, Zhong G, et al. Efficacy and safety of the pudendal nerve block as a component of multimodal analgesia for cervical brachytherapy. Clin Transl Radiat Oncol. 2025;54:101001. doi:10.1016/j.ctro.2025.101001
58. Modi DJ, Chazen JL, Singh JR. Modified technique for fluoroscopically guided pudendal nerve block for chronic pelvic pain. Interv Pain Med. 2023;2(2):100262. doi:10.1016/j.inpm.2023.100262
59. Ghanavatian S, Leslie SW, Derian A. Pudendal nerve block. [Updated 2024 Sep 2]. StatPearls. 2025 Jan. https://www.ncbi.nlm.nih.gov/books/NBK551518/
60. Levin D, Van Florcke D, Schmitt M, et al. Fluoroscopy-guided transgluteal pudendal nerve block for pudendal neuralgia: A retrospective case series. J Clin Med. 2024;13(9):2636. doi:10.3390/jcm13092636
61. Choi SS, Lee PB, Kim YC, Kim HJ, Lee SC. C-arm-guided pudendal nerve block: A new technique. Int J Clin Pract. 2006;60(5):553–556. doi:10.1111/j.1742-1241.2006.00836.x
62. Bellingham GA, Bhatia A, Chan CW, Peng PW. Randomized controlled trial comparing pudendal nerve block under ultrasound and fluoroscopic guidance. Reg Anesth Pain Med. 2012;37(3):262–266. doi:10.1097/AAP.0b013e318248c51d
63. McDonnell JG, O'Donnell B, Curley G, Heffernan A, Power C, Laffey JG. The analgesic efficacy of transversus abdominis plane block after abdominal surgery: A prospective randomized controlled trial. Anesth Analg. 2007;104(1):193–197. doi:10.1213/01.ane.0000250223.49963.0f
64. Bacal V, Rana U, McIsaac DI, Chen I. Transversus abdominis plane block for post hysterectomy pain: A systematic review and meta-analysis. J Minimally Invasive Gynecol. 2019;26(1):40–52. doi:10.1016/j.jmig.2018.04.020
65. Champaneria R, Shah L, Wilson MJ, Daniels JP. Clinical effectiveness of transversus abdominis plane (TAP) blocks for pain relief after caesarean section: A meta-analysis. Int J Obstet Anesth. 2016;28:45–60. doi:10.1016/j.ijoa.2016.07.009
66. Jakobsson JG, Wickerts L, Forsberg S, Ledin G. Transversus abdominal plane (TAP) block for postoperative pain management: A review. F1000Research. 2015;4:1359. doi:10.12688/f1000research.7015.1
67. Abd-Elsayed A. Transversus abdominis plane block as a treatment modality for chronic abdominal pain. Pain Physician. 2020;4;23(7;4):405–412. doi:10.36076/ppj.2020/23/405
68. Mui J, Allaire C, Williams C, Yong PJ. Abdominal wall pain in women with chronic pelvic pain. J Obstet Gynaecol Canada. 2016;38(2):154–159. doi:10.1016/j.jogc.2015.11.003
69. Faiz SH, Nader ND, Niknejadi S, Davari-Farid S, Hobika GG, Rahimzadeh P. A clinical trial comparing ultrasound-guided ilioinguinal/iliohypogastric nerve block to transversus abdominis plane block for analgesia following open inguinal hernia repair. J Pain Res. 2019;12:201–207. doi:10.2147/jpr.s179506

70. Elahwal L, Elrahwan S, Elbadry AA. Ilioinguinal and iliohypogastric nerve block for acute and chronic pain relief after caesarean section: A randomized controlled trial. Anesthesiol Pain Med. 2022;12(2):e121837. doi:10.5812/aapm.121837
71. Trescot A. Nerve blocks for pelvic pain. In: Manchikanti, ed. *Essentials of Interventional Techniques in Managing Chronic Pain*. Published online 2024:659–682. doi:10.1007/978-3-031-46217-7_34
72. Cooke CM, Flaxman TE, Chen I, Singh S. Safety and efficacy of ilioinguinal and iliohypogastric nerve blocks for treatment of pelvic pain. J Endometriosis Pelvic Pain Dis. 2019;11(1):37–44. doi:10.1177/2284026518823383
73. Tu F, Fitzgerald C, Senapati S, Pozolo K. Musculoskeletal causes of pelvic pain. Chronic pelvic pain. Published online March 21, 2011:115–124. doi:10.1002/9781444391855.ch11
74. Pastore EA, Katzman WB. Recognizing myofascial pelvic pain in the female patient with chronic pelvic pain. J Obstet Gynecol Neonatal Nurs. 2012;41(5):680–691. doi:10.1111/j.1552-6909.2012.01404.x
75. Butrick CW. Interstitial cystitis and chronic pelvic pain: New insights in neuropathology, diagnosis, and treatment. Clin Obstet Gynecol. 2003;46(4):811–823. doi:10.1097/00003081-200312000-00011
76. Srinivasan M, Lam C, Alm J, Chadwick AL. Trigger point injections. Phys Med Rehabil Clin N Am. 2022;33(2):307–333. doi:10.1016/j.pmr.2022.01.011
77. Langford CF, Udvari Nagy S, Ghoniem GM. Levator ani trigger point injections: An underutilized treatment for chronic pelvic pain. Neurourol Urodynamics. 2007;26(1):59–62. doi:10.1002/nau.20393
78. Moldwin RM, Fariello JY. Myofascial trigger points of the pelvic floor: Associations with urological pain syndromes and treatment strategies including injection therapy. Curr Urol Rep. 2013;14(5):409–417. doi:10.1007/s11934-013-0360-7
79. Abbott JA, Jarvis SK, Lyons SD, Thomson A, Vancaille TG. Botulinum toxin type A for chronic pain and pelvic floor spasm in women. Obstet Gynecol. 2006;108(4):915–923. doi:10.1097/01.aog.0000237100.29870.cc
80. Bartley J, Han E, Gupta P, et al. Transvaginal trigger point injections improve pain scores in women with pelvic floor hypertonicity and pelvic pain conditions. Female Pelvic Med Reconstruct Surg. 2018;25(5):392–396. doi:10.1097/spv.0000000000000581
81. Oor JE, Ünlü Ç, Hazebroek EJ. A systematic review of the treatment for abdominal cutaneous nerve entrapment syndrome. Am J Surg. 2016;212(1):165–174. doi:10.1016/j.amjsurg.2015.12.013
82. Kanakarajan S, Dharmavaram S, Tadros A, Pushparaj H, Rose A. Abdominal cutaneous nerve entrapment syndrome: A cross sectional survey of treatment outcomes. Br J Pain. 2022;16(5):538–545. doi:10.1177/20494637221101719
83. Narouze S. Chronic abdominal wall pain: Diagnosis and interventional treatment. Chronic Abdominal Pain. Published online November 3, 2014:189–194. doi:10.1007/978-1-4939-1992-5_18
84. Shian B, Larson ST. Abdominal wall pain: Clinical evaluation, differential diagnosis, and treatment. Am Fam Physician. 2018;98(7):429–436.
85. Boelens OB, Scheltinga MR, Houterman S, Roumen RM. Randomized clinical trial of trigger point infiltration with lidocaine to diagnose anterior cutaneous nerve entrapment syndrome. J Br Surg. 2013;100(2):217–221. doi:10.1002/bjs.8958.

29

Pudendal Nerve Stimulation in the Treatment of Refractory Urethral Discomfort

Katherine Gohres and Magdalena Anitescu

Introduction

Chronic pelvic pain (CPP) affects up 6–26% of women globally.[1] CPP is characterized as discomfort in the lower abdomen or pelvic region that extends beyond 6 months that cannot be attributed to menstruation, sexual intercourse, or pregnancy.[2] In addition to its significant prevalence, the estimated financial expenses associated with managing and evaluating chronic pelvic pain are impressive, with some health systems incurring more than $150 million a year due to the condition.[3] Navigating the wide array of potential etiologies behind a patient's pelvic symptoms and identifying a treatment that provides long-term relief can be challenging for providers. A common but underdiagnosed contributor to CPP is pudendal neuralgia.[4] This vignette describes a 36-year-old woman presenting with persistent urethral pain after undergoing surgical treatment for retroperitoneal liposarcoma. The patient experienced consistent and significant symptom relief with pudendal nerve blocks, leading to implantation of a pudendal peripheral nerve stimulator. Throughout the duration of the peripheral nerve stimulator, the patient reported a consistent >75% improvement in her pain and was able to eliminate oral morphine from her daily pain regimen.

Clinical Vignette

A 36-year-old woman with a history of retroperitoneal liposarcoma presented to the outpatient pain clinic with low back pain, urethral pain, and left leg pain several years after undergoing surgical resection of her malignancy.

The patient reported a history of a retroperitoneal liposarcoma for which she had a surgical resection, followed by recurrence 3 years later requiring an ex-lap and radiation therapy. Her second procedure had a hospital course complicated by postoperative pain requiring a ketamine drip for 4 days. Two years later, she presented to a pain clinic endorsing persistent lower back pain, left anterior thigh pain, and urethral pain despite multidisciplinary treatment. The thigh pain was sudden, stabbing, and random in onset, while her urethral pain was burning and constant. Her back pain was twisting and sharp in nature, with associated numbness and tingling that extended from her hip down to her knee. She had been seen by urologists with a negative workup. For her pain, she was taking oxycodone 15 mg Q6h, morphine 30 mg BID, amitriptyline 75 mg QHS, which only provided moderate relief. She had also worked with physical therapy, cognitive behavioral therapy, and psychiatrists with marginal improvement in symptoms.

Interventions and Outcome

The patient was originally provided with a caudal block, followed by a lumbar epidural steroid injection. While the block had temporarily alleviated her urinary pain and facilitated the weaning of her morphine from 30 mg to 20 mg BID, the patient's symptoms returned about 10 months later despite evidence of stable disease from her oncologist. Her urinary and thigh discomfort progressed to become 6–7/10 in severity with urination, and she described muscle spasms.

Considering the persistence of her urinary and left thigh discomfort, pelvic floor hypertonicity leading to pudendal neuralgia was hypothesized. The patient received a trial left-sided fluoroscopic pudendal nerve block. For this procedure, the patient was positioned prone on the fluoroscopy table. After a sterile prep and drape, the left ischial spine was identified via fluoroscopy. After anesthetizing the skin with 1% lidocaine, a 22G 3.5-inch Touhy spinal needle was advanced toward the medial ischial spine. Correct placement of the needle was confirmed with contrast under fluoroscopy. After confirmation of negative aspiration to avoid intravascular infiltration, 8 mL of 0.25% bupivacaine and 80 mg of triamcinolone were used.

Two months later, the patient returned to clinic reporting 90% improvement in her leg pain and 100% improvement in her urethral pain. She reported she was now able to be more comfortable, tolerate more activity, need less medication, and sleep better. Eight months after her first pudendal block, the patient received a confirmatory repeat pudendal nerve block (see Figure 29.1) that was successful in providing 100% relief from any persisting discomfort. Given the patient had received two successful diagnostic and therapeutic pudendal nerve blocks, she received a pudendal peripheral nerve stimulator (300-micron MicroLead 2.0 by SPRINT PNS) several months later. This device was placed under fluoroscopy in a similar fashion to a pudendal nerve block; a 20G Tuohy needle was advanced towards the L ischial tuberosity. This time, a peripheral nerve stimulator was used to show appropriate muscle group twitch at 12 mAmp. Next, a MicroLead 2.0 peripheral nerve stimulator device was inserted with a stylet, and its lead deployed perineurally. Stimulation capture was confirmed and then the device and its lead secured.

Throughout the 2-month duration of the peripheral nerve stimulator, the patient reported a consistent >75% improvement in her pain and was able to eliminate oral morphine from her daily pain regimen. The stimulator was then removed, with the patient continuing to experience relief.

Discussion

This case describes the presentation of persistent pelvic and thigh pain that is suspected to be pudendal neuralgia secondary to pelvic floor hypertonicity. After fluoroscopy-guided pudendal nerve block confirmed its likely efficacy, a pudendal peripheral nerve stimulator was

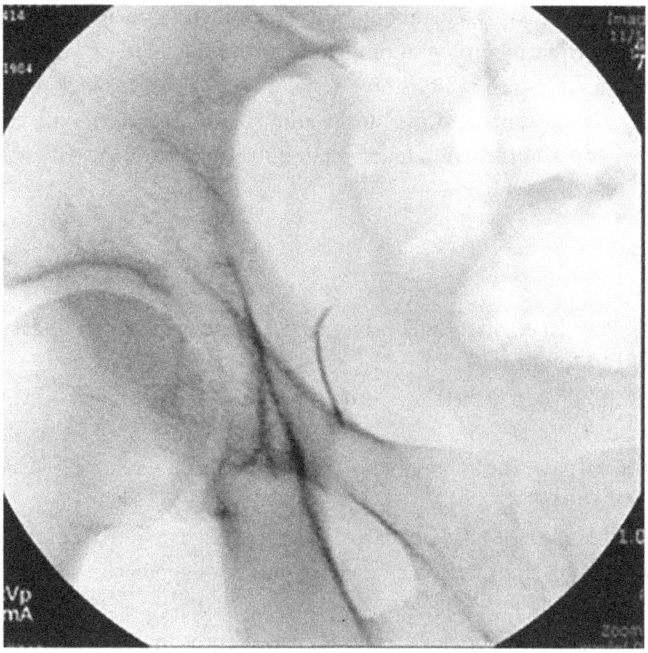

Figure 29.1 X-ray fluoroscopy image exhibiting needle placement for pudendal nerve block.
Source: Courtesy of University of Chicago School of Medicine.

implanted, enabling more than 6 months of comfort that continues to this day. Review of the literature has emphasized the importance of pudendal nerve block in the diagnosis and treatment of pudendal nerve neuralgia[5] and has revealed the pudendal block's association with reduced opioid requirements and fewer patient-reported episodes of unacceptable pain.[6] However, evidence also suggests risk of waning efficacy over time, with only 50% experiencing relief after 3 months and only 25% after 6 months.[7] There is not yet robust literature detailing pudendal peripheral nerve stimulation permanent implantation, nor its efficacy for pelvic pain. Most data on pudendal nerve stimulation are primarily for urologic symptoms, with pelvic pain as a secondary outcome. These small trials show positive implant outcomes with statistically significant improvement in pain and bladder symptoms.[8–10] A limited study of chronic nerve stimulator placement specifically for pudendal neuralgia followed 13 participants who underwent trial stimulator placement, with only 9 opting for permanent placement and only 5 reporting >50% of pain improvement after their postoperative visit (ranging from 6–83 days).[11]

More research will need to be conducted exploring the efficacy of pudendal nerve stimulators for primary treatment of chronic pelvic pain, in addition to investigating the duration of pudendal nerve stimulators' effects.

Conclusion

CPP has a high global prevalence and financial cost to healthcare. Pudendal neuralgia can be implicated in some cases of CPP, meaning interventions targeting the pudendal nerve have potential to provide relief. Most current literature on pudendal peripheral nerve stimulators is on patients with primarily urologic complaints, with little on its efficacy for patients with chronic pelvic pain. This case exhibits how serial pudendal nerve block followed by placement of a 60-day pudendal nerve stimulator resulted in more than 6 months of sustained relief of chronic pelvic pain in addition to facilitation the weaning of the patient's daily opiates.

References

1. Ahangari A. Prevalence of chronic pelvic pain among women: An updated review. Pain Physician. 2014;17(2):E141–E147.
2. Speer LM, Mushkbar S, Erbele T. Chronic pelvic pain in women. Am Fam Physician. 2016;93(5):380–7. PMID: 26926975.
3. Collett B. Visceral pain: The importance of pain management services. Br J Pain. 2013;7(1):6–7. doi:10.1177/2049463713480138
4. Ghoneim AA, Mansour SM. Comparative study between computed tomography guided superior hypogastric plexus block and the classic posterior approach: A prospective randomized study. Saudi J Anaesth. 2014;8(3):378–383. doi:10.4103/1658–354X.136625
5. Li J, Liu H, Qin K, Liu M, Yang H, Li Y. Efficacy and safety of pudendal nerve block for postoperative analgesia of hemorrhoids: A systematic review of 7 randomized controlled trials. Ann Palliat Med. 2021;10(2):2283–2292. doi:10.21037/apm-20–2109
6. Knox MC, Thiruthaneeswaran N, Zhong G, et al. Efficacy and safety of the pudendal nerve block as a component of multimodal analgesia for cervical brachytherapy. Clin Transl Radiat Oncol. 2025;54:101001. doi:10.1016/j.ctro.2025.101001
7. Ran J, Lu F, Xu L, et al. Efficacy of ganglion impar block combined with pudendal nerve pulsed radiofrequency for pudendal neuralgia management-a randomized clinical trial. Trials. 2024;25(1):316. doi:10.1186/s13063–024-08152–3
8. Chen PJ, Lagunas AC, Soriano V, Gupta P, Bruns TM. Perineal and rectal nerve recruitment order varies during pudendal neurostimulator implant surgery. Neurourol Urodyn. 2025;44(4):851–859. doi:10.1002/nau.70010
9. Peters KM, Killinger KA, Boguslawski BM, Boura JA. Chronic pudendal neuromodulation: Expanding available treatment options for refractory urologic symptoms. Neurourol Urodyn. 2010;29(7):1267–1271. doi:10.1002/nau.20823
10. Pinelli M, Malaguti S, Giardiello G, Lazzeri M, Tarantola J, Van Den Hombergh U. A new minimally invasive procedure for pudendal nerve stimulation to treat neurogenic bladder: Description of the method and preliminary data. Neurourol Urodyn. 2005;24(4):305–309. doi:10.1002/nau.20118
11. Hoang Roberts L, Vollstedt A, Volin J, McCartney T, Peters KM. Initial experience using a novel nerve stimulator for the management of pudendal neuralgia. Neurourol Urodyn. 2021;40(6):1670–1677. doi:10.1002/nau.24735

PART VI
MUSCULOSKELETAL PAIN DISORDERS

30

Anatomical Considerations of the Musculoskeletal System in Women

Chitra Ramasubbu, Archana Venkatesan, and Kavya Rajan

Introduction

Musculoskeletal pain conditions are among the most common chronic pain conditions and disproportionately affect women. Specific musculoskeletal problems including neck pain, lower back pain, osteoarthritis, and rheumatoid arthritis occur more frequently and severely affect females.

This chapter aims to provide a comprehensive overview of the female anatomy, hormonal influences in women that contribute to anatomical differences, and regional pain differences in the spine and pelvis. We will also examine the prevalence of musculoskeletal conditions.

Background

The musculoskeletal system comprises a network of bones, muscles, ligaments, tendons, joints, and cartilage. However, the female musculoskeletal system is structurally different from men. Females have a wider pelvis, which has a larger inlet and outlet for childbirth and can contribute to knee, ankle, and foot problems.[1]

Studies indicate the overall prevalence of lower back pain to be 28.8%: 39.0% in men and 60.9% in women.[2] The anatomical differences must be understood to ensure accurate diagnosis and effective treatment of women.

Epidemiology and Risk Factors

Chronic pain has higher prevalence in women across nearly all conditions and age groups. Women also tend to experience an increased intensity and longer duration of pain. Migraine headaches occur at a 3:1 female-to-male ratio. Up to 80–90% of fibromyalgia diagnoses are in women. Osteoarthritis, temporomandibular joint pain, chronic pelvic pain, and autoimmune conditions are more common in women as well. Population-based studies have shown consistent sex differences in pain perception, reporting, and outcomes.[3] Women report greater pain-related disability and lower quality of life even in conditions that are common in both sexes, such as low back pain.[4]

Bone Structure

Women tend to have shorter and lighter bones compared to men of the same age group. With regards to bone density, the thinner cortical bone and less dense trabecular bone contributes to lower bone mineral density.[5] Postmenopausal estrogen decline lowers bone density in the hip, spine, and wrists. Women start losing bone at an earlier age and at a faster rate than men. Women ≥50 years of age have a four times higher rate of osteoporosis and a two times higher rate of osteopenia, and they tend to have fractures 5–10 years earlier compared with men.[5]

Spine Anatomy

Several contributing factors affect the curvature of the spine and posture. Breast size influences thoracic posture and shoulder protraction. Increased anterior load during pregnancy exaggerates lumbar lordosis and pelvic instability.

Overall women have a larger lumbar lordosis than men. They are at an increased risk of spondylolisthesis due to this increased lordosis.[6] They also have slightly more thoracic kyphosis and cervical lordosis, especially after menopause. Women tend to have a narrow lumbar spinal canal, which also contributes to early-onset lumbar stenosis. Lumbar stenosis is more likely to progress and impact quality of life in women. Women are at greater risk of facet joint arthropathy and degenerative spondylolisthesis.[7]

Hormonal Contributors

Estrogen increases central sensitization by increasing the nociceptive neurons in the dorsal horn and brain. Estrogen affects collagen synthesis and soft tissue elasticity, contributing to increased joint laxity. This can lead to repetitive microtrauma, joint instability, hypermobility, and chronic pain.

Chronic pain responses differ between men and women. Estradiol fluctuations can heighten pain, especially around the menstrual cycle. Testosterone does have a protective effect proved by altering central pain pathways in men who have declining testosterone.[8] Elevated relaxin, estrogen, and progesterone during pregnancy increases risk of sacroiliac joint dysfunction, back pain, and pubic symphysis pain.[9] Decline in estrogen during menopause causes loss of muscle mass and reduced collagen content in tendons and ligaments.

Myofascial Differences

Women have a higher prevalence of myofascial pain especially in the neck, shoulder, and pelvic regions. Estrogen does play a role in collagen content as well as viscoelasticity in the fascia by making it more pliable. This does increase flexibility, but it makes the connective tissue and fascia layers more prone to trauma. Men have increased muscle mass, which increases load-bearing capacity.[10]

Imaging studies have also revealed sex-based variations in the orientation and thickness of fascial planes. For example, the thoracolumbar fascia, which is involved in load transfer across the pelvis and trunk, exhibits increased shear mobility and reduced stiffness in women.[11]

Pelvic Anatomy Differences

Women typically exhibit a wider pelvic structure and a greater quadriceps (Q) angle, defined as the angle formed between the quadriceps muscle and the patellar tendon. The larger Q angle in women results in altered knee biomechanics, particularly increased lateral stress on the patella, thereby predisposing females to a higher incidence of patellofemoral pain syndrome and patellar instability. Furthermore, a broader pelvis necessitates compensatory lumbar lordosis, which results in altered spinal load distribution and increased risk of developing low back pain.[12]

Ligament Differences

Evidence suggests that women exhibit greater generalized ligamentous laxity than men, notably in the medial collateral ligament of the knee, hip joint ligaments, ligamentum flavum of the spine, and intrapubic ligaments.[13] This laxity may be further influenced by fluctuations in estrogen and relaxin during the menstrual cycle and pregnancy. These hormones have been shown to reduce type I collagen production and cross-linking, diminishing tensile strength and weakening ligament integrity. Increased ligament compliance may impair joint proprioception and alter neuromuscular control, increasing the risk of joint instability and musculoskeletal injury.

Diagnosis and Assessment

Accurate history-taking and physical exam are required to avoid underrecognition of pain symptoms. Social and cultural influences also play a role in pain behavior. Studies show that women's pain is more likely to be attributed to stress or emotions during diagnosis. The onset, duration, intensity, and fluctuations in pain with menstrual cycle, pregnancy, and menopause should be questioned. Sleep patterns, mood, and caregiving roles play a part in the pain cycle. Clinicians should ask about comorbid conditions including autoimmune conditions, pelvic floor dysfunction, temporomandibular disorder, irritable bowel syndrome, and fibromyalgia. Histories of trauma, abuse, depression, and anxiety are more prevalent in women and should be screened using tools such as PHQ-9, GAD-7, and the McGill Pain Questionnaire.

Imaging modalities may be needed for proper diagnosis. Pelvic structures and soft tissue injury are evaluated better with MRI studies. Overlapping visceral conditions such as endometriosis, irritable bowel syndrome, and interstitial cystitis may mimic musculoskeletal pain and require further testing (Table 30.1).

Table 30.1 Sex-based musculoskeletal differences and clinical implications in women

Domain	Female-specific characteristics	Comparison to men	Clinical implications
Epidemiology of musculoskeletal pain	Higher prevalence, intensity, and duration of chronic musculoskeletal pain; greater pain-related disability and reduced quality of life	Lower prevalence and disability	Increased risk of chronicity; need for early recognition and multimodal management
Bone structure and density	Shorter, lighter bones; thinner cortical bone; less dense trabecular bone; earlier and faster bone loss	Higher peak bone mass; slower age-related loss	Higher rates of osteopenia, osteoporosis, and earlier fractures (5–10 years earlier)
Pelvic anatomy	Wider pelvis with larger inlet/outlet; increased Q angle	Narrower pelvis; smaller Q angle	Altered lower-extremity biomechanics; higher risk of patellofemoral pain, knee instability, low back pain
Spine anatomy	Greater lumbar lordosis; increased thoracic kyphosis and cervical lordosis (especially post-menopause); narrower lumbar spinal canal	Less lumbar lordosis; wider spinal canal	Increased risk of spondylolisthesis, facet arthropathy, lumbar stenosis, and degenerative changes
Pregnancy-related changes	Increased anterior load; pelvic instability; exaggerated lumbar lordosis	Not applicable	Higher incidence of low back pain, sacroiliac joint dysfunction, and pubic symphysis pain
Hormonal influences	Estrogen increases central sensitization and joint laxity; relaxin reduces ligament stiffness; estrogen decline causes muscle and collagen loss	Testosterone provides relative protection via central pain modulation	Heightened pain sensitivity, joint instability, hypermobility, and chronic pain syndromes
Myofascial characteristics	More pliable fascia with increased shear mobility; higher prevalence of myofascial pain (neck, shoulders, pelvis)	Greater muscle mass and load-bearing capacity	Increased susceptibility to myofascial pain, repetitive microtrauma, and soft tissue injury
Ligamentous properties	Greater generalized ligamentous laxity (knee, hip, spine, pelvic ligaments)	Greater ligament stiffness and tensile strength	Increased joint instability, impaired proprioception, higher injury risk
Pain perception and processing	Greater central sensitization; pain fluctuates with menstrual cycle, pregnancy, menopause	More stable pain modulation	Necessitates sex-specific pain assessment and timing-aware management strategies
Diagnosis and assessment considerations	Pain more likely to be underrecognized or attributed to psychosocial causes; higher prevalence of comorbid pain syndromes	Pain more likely to be treated as structural	Importance of comprehensive history, validated screening tools, and avoidance of diagnostic bias
Imaging and differential diagnosis	Pelvic and soft tissue pathology more prevalent; visceral pain often overlaps with musculoskeletal pain	Less overlap with pelvic conditions	MRI often preferred; careful differentiation from visceral pain syndromes

Treatments

Management of musculoskeletal pain in women should be multimodal and individualized. Because of the risk of overlapping pain syndromes, collaborations with multiple specialists may be needed. Nonsteroidal anti-inflammatory drugs; acetaminophen; and topical agents, such as lidocaine patches and diclofenac gel, are used as first-line therapy. Neuropathic agents such as gabapentin, pregabalin, and duloxetine are frequently used. Hormonal replacement therapy and oral contraceptives can help with pain triggered by hormonal fluctuations.

Aggressive physical therapy, aqua therapy, and pelvic floor rehabilitation can help with ligamentous laxity and joint instability and as well as posture correction seen in postpartum and menopausal women. Cognitive behavior therapy, biofeedback, and mindfulness training integrated into treatment will also help with coexisting conditions such as anxiety, depression, and trauma.

Lifestyle modifications including low-impact exercises such as Pilates, yoga, and swimming tend to improve core strength. Nutrition and weight management accelerate healing. Massage, acupuncture, and myofascial release can be used as complementary therapies as well.

When conservative measures fail, interventional pain procedures including epidurals, facet injections, sacroiliac joint injections, trigger point injections, Botox injections, laser therapy, neuromodulation, and regenerative therapies are options. Surgical interventions such as joint surgery, spine surgery, or kyphoplasty may be required in those who fail conservative management.

Conclusion

Clinicians require an in-depth understanding of the female musculoskeletal system to treat specific pain conditions. Recognizing the anatomical and physiological differences helps us diagnose and better manage female patients. A multidisciplinary approach that respects the unique experiences of women and applies scientific knowledge is important to improve outcomes and promote equity in pain medicine.

References

1. Overstreet DS, Strath LJ, Jordan M, Jordan IA, Hobson JM, Owens MA, Williams AC, Edwards RR, Meints SM. A Brief Overview: Sex Differences in Prevalent Chronic Musculoskeletal Conditions. Int J Environ Res Public Health. 2023 Mar 3;20(5):4521. doi: 10.3390/ijerph20054521. PMID: 36901530; PMCID: PMC10001545.
2. Ashton-Miller JA, DeLancey JO. Functional anatomy of the female pelvic floor. Ann N Y Acad Sci. 2007 Apr;1101:266-96. doi: 10.1196/annals.1389.034. Epub 2007 Apr 7. PMID: 17416924.
3. Bartley EJ, Fillingim RB. Sex differences in pain: A brief review of clinical and experimental findings. Br J Anaesth. 2013;111(1):52–58.
4. Mogil JS. Sex differences in pain and pain inhibition: Multiple explanations of a controversial phenomenon. Nat Rev Neurosci. 2012;13(12):859–866.
5. Alswat KA. Gender disparities in osteoporosis. J Clin Med Res. 2017;9(5):382–387.

6. Bonczar M, Koszewski J, Czarnota W, et al. The morphology of the lumbar vertebrae: A systematic review with meta-analysis of 1481 individuals with implications for spine surgery. Surg Radiol Anat. 2024;47(1):22.
7. Mizukoshi R, Yagi M, Yamada Y, et al. Gender differences in spinal mobility during postural changes: A detailed analysis using upright CT. Sci Rep. 2024;14(1):9154.
8. Athnaiel O, Cantillo S, Paredes S, Knezevic NN. The role of sex hormones in pain-related conditions. Int J Mol Sci. 2023;24(3):1866. doi:10.3390/ijms24031866
9. Sandor LF, Ragacs R, Gyori DS. Local effects of steroid hormones within the bone microenvironment. Int J Mol Sci. 2023;24(24):17482.
10. Plotkin LI, Bruzzaniti A, Pianeta R. Sexual dimorphism in the musculoskeletal system: Sex hormones and beyond. J Endocrine Soc. 2024;8(10): bvae153.
11. Langevin HM, Fox JR, Koptiuch C, et al. Reduced thoracolumbar fascia shear strain in human chronic low back pain. BMC Musculoskelet Disord. 2011;12:203.
12. Gant H, Ghimire N, Min K, Musa I, Ashraf M, Lawan A. Impact of the quadriceps angle on health and injury risk in female athletes. Int J Environ Res Public Health. 2024;21(12):1547.
13. Fede C, Pirri C, Fan C, et al. Sensitivity of the fasciae to sex hormone levels: Modulation of collagen-I, collagen-III and fibrillin production. PLoS One. 2019;14(9):e0223195.

31
Musculoskeletal Pain Conditions in Women

Kimberly Templeton and Patrick George

Prevalence of Chronic Musculoskeletal Pain in Women

Chronic musculoskeletal pain is more common among women than men. This may be due, in part, to increased prevalence of pain-generating conditions, such as osteoarthritis, degenerative spondylolisthesis, fibromyalgia, and inflammatory arthropathies (e.g., rheumatoid arthritis) among women. Women represent 60% of patients with osteoarthritis, with sex-based differences increasing after the age of 40.[1] Degenerative spondylolisthesis of the lumbar spine has been reported to be up to 2–4 times more common among women.[2] Rheumatoid arthritis has been reported to be up to 3 times more common among women. In addition, women are more likely to experience low-impact fractures related to low bone mass that can result in chronic pain. While traumatic injuries tend to be more common among men, women are more likely to suffer both short-[3] and long-term pain[4] from these.

Biological Contributors to Increased Pain Prevalence

A variety of explanations have been provided for the increased prevalence of these pain-generating conditions among women. Inflammatory conditions in general are more common among women, and this includes inflammatory arthropathies. In addition, osteoarthritis is more common among women at all ages and at almost every joint. This may be related to inherent sex-based differences in cartilage thickness, estrogen impacts on articular cartilage health, risk for and physiologic responses to injury, lower muscle strength and different firing patterns to protect joints, and differences in inherent (e.g., rheumatoid arthritis) and reactive (e.g., to obesity, after anterior cruciate ligament [ACL] tears) inflammation.

Sex hormones may influence the risk of developing chronic pain because women who have been diagnosed with osteoarthritis and who had lower levels of estradiol, progesterone, and testosterone were more likely to experience increased pain and decreased cartilage mass.[5,6] Ligament hypermobility also differs at various points throughout the menstrual cycle, leading to joint instability and a higher risk of injury.[7]. The presence of obesity impacts the risk of developing musculoskeletal conditions and chronic pain in both women and men, but women experience greater pain at given body mass index (BMI) levels and a stronger association between the level of abdominal fat and widespread chronic musculoskeletal pain.[8] Degenerative spondylolisthesis may be more common in women due to differences in facet joint angles because women tend to have more sagittally oriented joints, or due to increased ligamentous laxity.

Differences in Pain Processing

Almost all studies of chronic musculoskeletal pain indicate that this is more common among women than men. This likely reflects both sex-based differences in how nociceptive signals are processed and gender-based differences in how pain is expressed.

Peripheral Sensitization

Following a fracture, acute pain is modulated, in part, by the release from osteoclasts, osteoblasts, and immune cells of bradykinin, prostaglandin E2, tumor necrosis factor (TNF)-alpha, and nerve growth factor (NGF), further potentiating the slow onset of dull, throbbing pain via C fibers.[9] Alongside C fiber activation, peripheral sensitization can occur due to the surge of pro-inflammatory factors, which lowers the threshold for subsequent nociceptor firing from both Aδ and C fibers.[10]. Peripheral sensitization can also occur due to phosphorylation of various ion channels on both Aδ and C fibers or from an increase in transcription of genes coding for substance P (sP) or calcitonin gene-related peptide (CGRP).[11–13] Release of these inflammatory products is modulated by estrogen,[14] and women can experience fluctuating levels of pain throughout the menstrual cycle.[15]

Central Sensitization

Prolonged exposure to the previously mentioned inflammatory factors released during extensive pathological nociceptive signaling can lead to the development of central sensitization.[16] Prior research suggests increased intracellular calcium promotes intracellular changes that result in enhanced synaptic transmission, diminished inhibitory control, and neuroplastic changes that trigger increased pain perception—occasionally even in the absence of a peripheral stimulus.[16,17] Central sensitization plays a key role in the transition from acute to chronic pain in multiple musculoskeletal conditions such as low back pain, osteoarthritis, and fibromyalgia.[18–20]

Gender-Based Differences in Pain Expression and Behavior

Gender can also impact the expression of pain from musculoskeletal conditions. Views of gendered roles have been found to correlate with musculoskeletal pain-related behaviors.[21] Pain catastrophizing, which is more common among women, has been found to lead to more expressions of pain, lower levels of activity, and significant impact on quality of life among those with osteoarthritis.[22]

After a traumatic musculoskeletal injury, women are more likely than men to develop posttraumatic stress disorder (PTSD), which correlates with higher levels of pain.[23] The experience of depression and anxiety, both more common in women, can also impact expression of musculoskeletal pain, and the relationship between depression and musculoskeletal pain is often bidirectional.[24]

Impact on Function and Quality of Life

Painful musculoskeletal conditions impact quality of life, physical function, the ability to work, and the ability to perform activities of daily living, and they increase the risks for developing other health conditions. Osteoarthritis impacts the ability of women to work and perform tasks of daily living and reduces their quality of life.[25] This tends to worsen with age. Symptomatic osteoarthritis is also associated with an increased risk of developing other health conditions. While both women and men with osteoarthritis are more likely to have comorbidities, this risk is higher among women.

One of the more prevalent conditions among women with osteoarthritis is cardiovascular disease. Women with osteoarthritis of the knee have a higher rate of mortality than those without knee pain; this risk is even higher if degenerative changes are identified on radiographs. While this may be related to interconnected phenomena, such as heightened inflammatory responses or reduced levels of activity, no correlation has been found between painful osteoarthritis of the hand and cardiac disease-related mortality, indicating a more significant role of reduced levels of activity. Similar to women with painful joints, those with painful vertebral compression fractures related to low bone mass demonstrate decreased physical function and quality of life.[26] Chronic musculoskeletal pain, whatever the source, and limited physical function increase the risk of developing depression.

Treatment Access and Differences

While there are no identified sex-based differences in response to most nonsurgical treatments (e.g., nonsteroidal anti-inflammatory drugs [NSAIDs], activity modification, injections) for musculoskeletal conditions, there may be differences in how often and when these treatments are accessed. For example, women are more likely than men to receive opioids, nonopioids, intra-articular injections, and referral to physical therapy in the 12 months prior to joint arthroplasty.[27] This may reflect sex-based differences in the progression of the disease or sex or gender differences in pain. In addition, given the impact of muscle strength and function on the musculoskeletal system, especially for women, exercise may be of benefit to help address chronic musculoskeletal pain.[28]

Surgical Outcomes

Surgery is often the last resort for treatment of painful chronic musculoskeletal conditions. Differences in outcomes after surgery have been described for various musculoskeletal conditions. Men tend to have higher mortality and worse outcomes after treatment of low-impact fractures of the hip. This is likely related to their older age at the time of fracture and related health conditions.

However, women tend to have worse outcomes after surgery for osteoarthritis. Women are more likely than men to have continued pain after joint replacement surgery, especially during the first 6–12 months after surgery. Some of this has been attributed to women being more likely than men to manifest allergies to metals. However, continued pain and worse function after total knee arthroplasty have been found to correlate with worse pain and function and the presence of comorbidities such as depression and anxiety prior to surgery. Worse pain and function prior to surgery may indicate that surgery is delayed longer in women or that their degenerative changes progress more quickly. However, these sex-based differences in response to joint replacement surgery tend to lessen over time.

Women are more likely than men to undergo surgical decompression and fusion for degenerative spondylolisthesis. This has been attributed to differences in anatomy of the spine leading to degenerative changes, which may make the decision for surgery more obvious for women.[29] As seen in women with osteoarthritis, those with spondylolisthesis often come to surgery with more pain and worse function than do men.[30] This can impact the outcomes of surgery. In some studies, however, women tend to report better outcomes than men after spine surgery.[31]

References

1. Segal NA, Nilges JM, Oo WM: Sex differences in osteoarthritis prevalence, pain perception, physical function and therapeutics. Osteoarthr Cartil. 2024;32(9):1045–1053.
2. Devine JG, Schenk-Kisser JM, Skelly AC. Risk factors for degenerative spondylolisthesis: A systematic review. Evid Based Spine Care J. 2012;3(2):25–34.
3. Storesund A, Krukhaug Y, Olsen MV, Rygh LJ, Nilsen RM, Norekvål TM. Females report higher postoperative pain scores than males after ankle surgery. Scand J Pain.2016;12:85–93.
4. Madsen TE, McLean S, Zhai W, et al. Gender differences in pain experience and treatment after motor vehicle collisions: A secondary analysis of the CRASH injury study. Clin Ther. 2018;40(2):204–213.
5. Jin X, Wang BH, Wang X, et al. Associations between endogenous sex hormones and MRI structural changes in patients with symptomatic knee osteoarthritis. Osteoarthr. Cartil. 2017;25:1100–1106.
6. Sniekers YH, Weinans H, Bierma-Zeinstra SM, van Leeuwen JP, van Osch GJ. Animal models for osteoarthritis: The effect of ovariectomy and estrogen treatment – a systematic approach. 2008;Osteoarthr Cartil 16:533–541.
7. Chu SR, Boyer EH, Beynnon B, Segal NA. Pregnancy results in lasting changes in knee joint laxity. PM R. 2019;11:117–124.
8. Kifle ZD, Tian J, Aitken D, Melton PE, Cicuttini F, Jones G, Pan F. MRI-derived abdominal adipose tissue is associated with multisite and widespread chronic pain. Reg Anesth Pain Med. 2025:rapm-2024–105535.
9. Gold MS, Gebhart GF. Nociceptor sensitization in pain pathogenesis. Nature Med. 2010;16(11):1248–1257.
10. Cook AD, Christensen AD, Tewari D, McMahon SB, Hamilton JA. Immune cytokines and their receptors in inflammatory pain. Trends Immunol. 2018;39(3):240–255.
11. Denk F, Bennett DL, McMahon SB. Nerve growth factor and pain mechanisms. Annu Rev Neurosci. 2017;40:307–325.
12. Julius D, Basbaum, A. Molecular mechanisms of nociception. Nature. 2001;413(6852):203–210.
13. Mamet J, Baron A, Lazdunski M, Voilley N. Proinflammatory mediators, stimulators of sensory neuron excitability via the expression of acid-sensing ion channels. J Neurosci. 2002;22(24):10662–10670.

14. Torres HM, Arnold KM, Oviedo M, Westendorf JJ, Weaver SR. Inflammatory processes affecting bone health and repair. Curr Osteoporos Rep. 2023;21(6):842–853.
15. Hellström B, Anderberg UM. Pain perception across the menstrual cycle phases in women with chronic pain. Percept motor Skills. 2003;96(1):201–211.
16. Latremoliere A, Woolf CJ. Central sensitization: A generator of pain hypersensitivity by central neural plasticity. J Pain. 2009;10(9):895–926.
17. Oostinga D, Steverink JG, van Wijck AJM, Verlaan JJ. An understanding of bone pain: A narrative review. Bone. 2020;134:115272.
18. Arendt-Nielsen L, Nie H, Laursen MB, Laursen BS, Madeleine P, Simonsen OH, Graven-Nielsen T. Sensitization in patients with painful knee osteoarthritis. Pain. 2010;149(3):573–581.
19. Arendt-Nielsen L, Graven-Nielsen T. Central sensitization in fibromyalgia and other musculoskeletal disorders. Curr Pain Headache Rep. 2003;7(5):355–361.
20. Desmeules JA, Cedraschi C, Rapiti E, et al. Neurophysiologic evidence for a central sensitization in patients with fibromyalgia. Arthritis Rheum. 2003;48(5):1420–1429.
21. Pedulla R, Glugosh J, Jeyaseelan N, et al. Associations of gender role and pain in musculoskeletal disorders: A mixed-methods systematic review. J Pain. 2024;25(12):104644.
22. Hayashi K, Morishima T, Ikemoto T, Miyagawa H, Okamoto T, Ushida T, Deie M. Pain catastrophizing is independently associated with quality of life in patients with severe hip osteoarthritis. Pain Med. 2019;20(11):2220–2227.
23. Connor JP, Brier ZMF, Price M. The association between pain trajectories with posttraumatic stress disorder, depression, and disability during the acute posttrauma period. Psychosom Med. 2020;82(9):862–868.
24. Hannerz H, Holtermann A, Madsen IEH. Musculoskeletal pain as a predictor for depression in the general working population of Denmark. Scand J Public Health. 2021;49(6):589–597.
25. Mahir L, Belhaj K, Zahi S, Azanmasso H, Lmidmani F, El Fatimi A. Impact of knee osteoarthritis on the quality of life. Ann Phys Rehabil Med. 2016;59(Suppl):e159.
26. Johansson L, Svensson HK, Karlsson J, Olsson LE, Mellström D, Lorentzon M, Sundh D. Decreased physical health-related quality of life: A persisting state for older women with clinical vertebral fracture. Osteoporos Int. 2019;30(10):1961–1971.
27. Bawa HS, Weick JW, Dirschl DR. Gender disparities in osteoarthritis-related health care utilization before total knee arthroplasty. J Arthroplasty. 2016;31(10):2115–2118.
28. Sato, S., Ukimoto, S., Kanamoto, T. et al. Chronic musculoskeletal pain, catastrophizing, and physical function in adult women were improved after 3-month aerobic-resistance circuit training. Sci Rep. 2021;11:14939.
29. Walker TN, Urquhart JC, Rasoulinejad P, et al. Differences in the surgical management of degenerative lumbar spondylolisthesis based on self-reported sex: Analysis of the CSORN prospective DLS study. J Neurosurg Spine. 2024;40(6):723–732.
30. Siccoli A, Staartjes VE, de Wispelaere MP, Schröder ML. Gender differences in degenerative spine surgery: Do female patients really fare worse? Eur Spine J. 2018;27(10):2427–2435.
31. Chan AK, Bisson EF, Bydon M, et al. Women fare best following surgery for degenerative lumbar spondylolisthesis: A comparison of the most and least satisfied patients utilizing data from the Quality Outcomes Database. Neurosurg Focus. 2018;44(1):E3.

32
Back and Neck Pain in Women

Interventional and Comprehensive Approaches

Nyla K. Azam and Farrukh A. Ansari

Introduction

Back and neck pain are two of the most common reasons for patients presenting to their primary care physician. Women are disproportionately affected; they are at higher risk of developing musculoskeletal pain conditions and suffering from a higher severity of disease, with disease burden increasing with age. The prevalence and severity of pain in women can vary based on their phase of life. Optimal management includes a comprehensive approach, combining pharmacologic, physical and lifestyle interventions, and interventional techniques where appropriate.

Background

Musculoskeletal pain affects approximately 1.7 billion people worldwide and is a leading cause of disability. Musculoskeletal pain stems from pathophysiology affecting bones, muscles, ligaments, joints, tendons, and nerves and can often impair movement, affecting functional ability with a downstream economic impact. Women are disproportionately affected, often presenting with more frequent and severe painful episodes. The mechanisms for this disparity are unclear, but it is hypothesized to involve differences in hormone levels and subsequent pain sensitivity, immune system functioning, and anatomic differences with biomechanical changes.[1,2]

Epidemiology and Risk Factors

While there is a vast amount of literature on the prevalence of low back and neck pain, it can be difficult to compare data across studies because of variability in study factors.[3] The Global Burden of Diseases, Injuries, and Risk Factors Study (GBD) systematically quantifies health loss due to disease and injuries by age, sex, year, and location, allowing for comparison of disease burden across the world. The GBD examines the global, regional, and national levels of disease for both back and neck pain. Low back pain is defined as pain along the posterior aspect of the body between the inferior margin of the twelfth ribs and the gluteal folds, with or without leg pain, lasting for 1 day or more. Neck pain is defined as pain ranging from the occiput to the first thoracic vertebra with or without referral into the upper limb(s) for at least 1 day.[4,5]

The GBD revealed low back pain to be the greatest contributor to the world's burden of disability, with a projected increase in prevalence. Back pain had a higher prevalence among females across all groups, with greater differences with increasing age. Neck pain is increasingly common across the world, with similar impacts on quality of life, disability, and healthcare costs. While epidemiological datapoints again show variability, there has similarly been a rise in the prevalence of neck pain. The GBD showed a global prevalence of about 200 million people, an increase of 77.3% from 1990. Similar to low back pain, neck pain had higher prevalence and greater disability among women in all age groups, with a peak in prevalence and disability between the ages of 50 and 74 years.

Data focusing on the US population reveal a similar pattern. The National Health Interview Survey, collected through the National Center for Health, provides estimates of any pain regardless of body region as well as estimates of back and lower and upper limb pain among US adults aged 18 and older. Data collected from respondents (n = 31,997) revealed that 58.9% of adults experienced pain of any kind, with back pain being the most prevalent type (39%), followed by lower limb pain (hips, knees, or feet), then upper limb pain (hands, arms or shoulders). Women were more likely to experience back pain than men (40.6% vs. 37.2%) and more likely to experience pain in all the pain categories examined.[6]

With rising disease burden and costs, it becomes important to understand the reasons contributing to the prevalence of musculoskeletal pain in women. Explanations have included (1) higher likelihood to report pain, (2) greater vulnerability to developing pain due to biological differences, or (3) greater exposure to risk factors for developing pain.[7] The consistency of a higher prevalence, including for other painful conditions, may suggest a sex-related predisposing vulnerability. There is postulation of sex-related differences in central and peripheral pain processing increasing the expression of musculoskeletal pain; the role of hormonal differences on musculoskeletal pain still needs further study.[2] Studies have suggested a greater exposure to risk factors predisposing women to developing painful syndromes, though more research is needed.[7,8]

A longitudinal cohort study of community-based, middle-aged women carried out in Australia over a 9-year period examined the course and contributors of back pain, surveying risk factors for women more likely to report pain. It found that those who had back pain were significantly more likely to have obesity, have a lower educational status, be less likely to engage in vigorous physical activity, and have depressive symptoms. Work- and health-related information were assessed, and additional risk factors included being less likely to participate in paid work and having worse mental and physical health scores.[9]

Pathophysiology

A biopsychosocial model of pain has been well-described, with pain and disability as a dynamic integration between physiological, psychological, and social factors.[10] Biological mechanisms for pain in women can vary based on the phase of their reproductive cycle, with the physiologic responses to pregnancy, the physical and emotional stress related to childrearing, and then perimenopausal abdominal weight gain along with susceptibility to accelerated spinal degeneration all increasing the risk of back pain experienced by women.[1]

Age-related degenerative changes in the spine include a decrease in proteoglycan level, decrease in water content in the nucleus pulposus, and decreased disc height, which in turn can accelerate the development of arthritic changes in the spinal facet joints. Age-related decrease in bone density leads to a decrease in height of the vertebral body, which in turn is correlated with intervertebral arthropathy. An anatomical and MRI study examined sex-related differences in aging in the cervical, thoracic, and lumbar spine. The study found that, for all regions of the spine, vertebral body and adjacent disc height (VBAD) was lower in women compared to men for almost all parts of the cervical spine in almost all age groups, except for C5 and C6 in those aged 80–89 and 30–39, and C4 in those aged 70–79. VBAD was significantly lower in women than in men for thoracic and lumbar vertebrae for all age groups.

Women were noted to have a rapid decrease in the vertebral body height with age in both the cervical and lumbar spine regions. Numerous additional studies have described spinal canal dimensions that are smaller in women compared to men through multiple decades of life, with narrowing proceeding to a greater degree in women and a significant decrease in postmenopausal women.[11]

Low back pain in women is more commonly associated with sacroiliac joint dysfunction relative to men, with unique anatomical and biomechanical differences in the joint. The sacroiliac joint provides stability, facilitating the transmission of force between the body and legs, allowing the ability for bipedal walking. It consists of an articulation between the ilium and sacrum supported by several ligaments and muscles. The joint is relatively fixed, with limited mobility secondary to the tightness of the fibrous ligaments crossing the joint and adjacent vertebrae.

There is well-established sexual dimorphism of the sacroiliac joint with greater degenerative disease in women. The sacroiliac joints of women have more flexible ligaments, a smaller surface area of articulation between the sacrum and the fifth lumbar vertebrae, and more anatomical variants; that and a shorter and more cylindrically oriented pelvic cavity are strongly associated with increased mechanical stress on the joint and subsequent degenerative changes.

The sacroiliac joint is subject to high levels of mechanical strain with walking, standing, and going from sitting to standing positions. Mechanical stress and imbalance on the joint are especially intense during pregnancy and childbirth, when the increased weight and altered center of gravity place additional stress on the joint, exacerbated by the hormone-induced ligament laxity that facilitates widening of the pelvis to allow for childbirth.[12]

Psychological factors are tied to an increase in the pain experience for low back and neck pain and related disability. Depression and anxiety are strong predictors for low back pain, with females being almost twice as likely as males to be diagnosed with both. Early diagnosis and treatment are key to minimize the burden of chronic pain and related disability.[1]

Diagnosis and Assessment

A review of clinical practice guidelines revealed that sex is not typically considered in the assessment, diagnosis, or treatment of back pain. When mentioned, it is typically in the setting of pregnancy or epidemiological factors.[13] Because sex-related factors can impact one's health status, lifespan, disease pathogenesis, and reaction to treatment, future research in diagnosis and assessment should include sex classification for a better understanding of clinical pain outcomes in women.

Back or neck pain can be classified as acute (<6 weeks), subacute (6–2 weeks), or chronic (>12 weeks). Almost 50% of episodes resolve within 1–2 weeks, and 90% resolve within 6–12 weeks.[2] Recurrent or longer-lasting episodes require a thorough evaluation. Back or neck pain can be classified into either specific or nonspecific causes, with nonspecific causes accounting for about 90% of cases. The most common causes for specific low back pain include vertebral fractures, axial spondylarthritis, tumors, infections, and intra-abdominal causes.

Spondyloarthritis is a common cause of low back pain in women, increasing with age and weight. Due to hormone- and pregnancy-induced changes in the pelvis, women are prone to both sacroiliac dysfunction and myofascial pain syndrome of the piriformis muscle, both of which can be mistaken for sciatica. Sacroiliac dysfunction can present with sharp pain radiating down the posterior thigh, while piriformis syndrome can lead to entrapment of the sciatic nerve.[2]

Nonspecific pain often is attributed to musculoskeletal pain, involving muscle strain, ligament sprain, or postural issues. Endometriosis often presents with back pain and should be considered as a differential in women experiencing menstrual cycles.

Treatment Options

Effective treatment targets the specific etiology of pain while keeping a comprehensive overview of a person's health, including considering physical activity, sleep, nutrition, and weight. Physical inactivity can aggravate chronic musculoskeletal pain, and treatment for most conditions will center on starting with rehabilitative modalities including multicomponent exercise (aerobic, strengthening, flexibility, and balance). The greatest benefit occurs with light- to moderate-intensity programs at a frequency of two to three times a week for at least 4 weeks.[14] The relationship between weight, physical activity, and back pain has been studied and has shown the impact of weight on back pain for those with a body mass index >25 kg/m^2 regardless of physical activity, emphasizing the importance of nutrition.[15] Rehabilitative modalities may be limited by pain, though there may be safe ranges for acceptable levels of pain during exercise.[16] Rehabilitative treatment is often supplemented with medications crossing several drug classes, including over-the-counter or prescription strength analgesics, muscle relaxants, and neuropathic agents. Opioids are cautioned against due to their many short- and long-term risks. Interventional therapies are considered when appropriate, with particular attention paid to common sites of arthritis, including the sacroiliac joint and facet joints. Alternative treatments can be an effective adjunctive treatment modality and include acupuncture, tai chi, and osteopathic manipulation.[17]

Complications and Comorbidities

Comorbid factors that can increase the risk of back and neck pain include anxiety, depression, psychiatric illness (including catastrophizing, kinesiophobia, and somatization), rheumatoid arthritis, and diabetes, with the highest-risk comorbidity being anxiety, followed by depression.

Patient-Centered Approaches

A common complaint from patients suffering from chronic pain is that "they don't feel heard." A Kaiser Family Foundation study found that 29% of women report their doctor dismissed a concern they had, and 15% reported that a provider did not believe they were telling the truth about their symptoms.[18] Patient-centered communication is key in strengthening the doctor–patient relationship, helping the physician understand the biopsychosocial context of each patient and empowering patients to facilitate change. A treatment plan is effective only if it is feasible for a patient and needs to be based on a joint discussion taking into consideration the patient's ability and willingness to participate. Medication timing may need to be adjusted to the hours a patient works; physical therapy plans may need to be home-based depending on the patient's ability to travel to a physical location.

Treatment Considerations

For women, treatment must factor in a woman's stage in life and related events, such as whether she is pregnant, breastfeeding, or postmenopausal. Medication therapy may be limited during pregnancy and breastfeeding due to drug safety profiles. Fluoroscopy-based procedures are generally avoided during pregnancy due to the risk of radiation exposure to the developing fetus. Ultrasound-based procedures are safe and can still be offered.

Emerging Trends and Current Research

Healthcare around menopause and the role of hormone replacement therapy is an emerging popular topic of discussion in many forums. The Women's Health Initiative studied hormone replacement therapy and advised that the risks exceeded the benefits, impacting prescribing patterns.[19] The results from a follow-up study show that hormone replacement therapy can play a role in preventing chronic disease when used appropriately.[20] There has been evidence for a slightly higher prevalence of back pain in women on hormone replacement therapy.[21] With the recent increase in attention paid to the topic of hormone replacement therapy, this is an area that will benefit from more study.

Similarly, glucagon-like peptide (GLP-1) receptor agonists have recently received a lot of attention for their ability to facilitate weight loss. Knowing the link between increased weight and back pain, it will be interesting to study whether GLP-1 agonists lead to a decrease in the prevalence of chronic musculoskeletal pain.

Clinical Pearls

- Patient-centered communication is key to understanding the biopsychosocial factors contributing to your patient's pain, with an accurate diagnosis centering on the history and physical.
- To be effective, any treatment plan should be tailored to account for unique considerations that may impact your patient.

References

1. Overstreet DS, Babcock J, Deyo RA, Martin BI, Lee MJ, Jarvik JG. A brief overview: sex differences in prevalent chronic musculoskeletal conditions. Int J Environ Res Public Health 2023;20:4521. https://doi.org/10.3390/ijerph2005452
2. Bizzoca D, Oliva F, Maffulli N, Maffulli G, Longo UG. Gender-related issues in the management of low-back pain: A current concepts review. Clin Pract. 2023;13:1360–1368. https://doi.org/10.3390/clinpract13060122
3. Wang YXJ, Kaplar Z, Deng M, Berven SH, Karppinen J, Cheung KM. Increased low back pain prevalence in females than in males after menopause age: Evidence based on synthetic literature review. Quant Imaging Med Surg. 2016;6(2):199–206.
4. GBD 2021 Low Back Pain Collaborators. Global, regional, and national burden of low back pain, 1990–2020, its attributable risk factors, and projections to 2050: A systematic analysis of the Global Burden of Disease Study 2021. Lancet Rheumatol. 2023;5 e316–329.
5. GBD 2021 Neck Pain Collaborators. Global, regional, and national burden of neck pain, 1990–2020, and projections to 2050: A systematic analysis of the Global Burden of Disease Study 2021. Lancet Rheumatol. 2024;6:e142–155.
6. Lucas JW, Connor EM, Bose J. Back, lower limb, and upper limb pain among U.S. adults, 2019. NCHS Data Brief No. 415. July 2021. Accessed June 17, 2025. https://doi.org/10.15620/cdc:107894
7. Wijnhoven, HAH. Prevalence of musculoskeletal disorders is systematically higher in women than in men. Clin J Pain. 2006;22:717–724.
8. Strazdins L, Bammer G. Women, work and musculoskeletal health. Soc Sci Med. 2004;58(6):997–1005.
9. Brady SRE, Suri P, Jordan KP, Lewis CE, Nguyen U-SDT, Katz JN. Course and contributors to back pain in middle-aged women over 9 years. Spine. 2018;43:1648–1656.
10. Meints SM, Edwards RR. Evaluating psychosocial contributions to chronic pain outcomes. Prog Neuropsychopharmacol Biol Psychiatry. 2018;87(Pt B):168–182.
11. Asai T, Inoue K, Sato K, Takahashi M, Yamamoto H, Nakamura K. Sex- and age-related differences in spinal degeneration: An anatomical and magnetic resonance imaging study of the human spine. Prog Rehabil Med. 2022;7:1–10. doi:10.2490/prm.20220011
12. Ulas ST, Koca TT, Demirag B, Erdem H, Aydın S. Sex disparities of the sacroiliac joint: Focus on joint anatomy and imaging appearance. Diagnostics. 2023;13(642):2–13. https://doi.org/10.3390/diagnostics13040642
13. Rathbone T, Côté P, Wong JJ, Yu H, Sutton D, Yu J. Sex and gender considerations in low back pain clinical practice guidelines: A scoping review. BMJ Open Sport Exercise Med. 2020;6:e000972. doi:10.1136/bmjsem-2020-000972
14. Corte-Rodriguez HDL, Fernández-de-Las-Peñas C, Arias-Buría JL, et al. The role of physical exercise in chronic musculoskeletal pain: best medicine: A narrative review. Healthcare 2024;12(2):242.
15. Brady SRE, Suri P, Jordan KP, et al. Relationships between weight, physical activity, and back pain in young adult women. Medicine. 2016;(95)19:1–7. doi:10.1097/MD.0000000000003368
16. Smith BE, Hendrick P, Smith TO, Rathleff MS, Mills K, Maujean A. Musculoskeletal pain and exercise: Challenging existing paradigms and introducing new. Br J Sports Med. 2019;53(14):907–912.

17. Urits, I., Gress, K., Charipova, K., Habib, K., Lee, D., Lee, C., Kassem, H., Cornett, E. M., Kaye, A. D., & Viswanath, O. (2021). A comprehensive review of alternative therapies for the management of chronic pain patients: Acupuncture, tai chi, osteopathic manipulative medicine, and chiropractic care. *Advances in Therapy, 38*(1), 76–89. https://doi.org/10.1007/s12325-020-01554-0
18. Long M, Freed M, Kub K. Women's experiences with provider communication and interactions in health care settings: Findings from the 2022 KFF Women's Health Survey. February 2023. https://www.kff.org/womens-health-policy/issue-brief/womens-experiences-with-provider-communication-interactions-health-care-settings-findings-from-2022-kff-womens-health-survey/
19. Writing Group for the Women's Health Initiative Investigators. Risk and benefits of estrogen plus progestin in healthy postmenopausal women: Principal results from the Women's Health Initiative randomized control trial. JAMA. 2002;288(3):321–333.
20. Manson JE, Chlebowski RT, Stefanick ML, et al. Menopausal hormone therapy and health outcomes during the intervention and extended poststopping phases of the Women's Health Initiative randomized trials. JAMA. 2013;310(13):1353–1368. doi:10.1001/jama.2013.278040
21. Brynhildsen JO, Ekblad S, Hammar M. Is hormone replacement therapy a risk factor for low back pain among postmenopausal women? Spine. 1998;23(7):809–813.

33

Pelvic Pain and Musculoskeletal Interplay in Women

Patricia Wang, Sharon Marie Mathew, and Leena Mathew

Introduction

The American College of Obstetricians and Gynecologists define chronic pelvic pain (CPP) as noncyclical pain originating from pelvic structures and lasting >6 months. CPP disproportionately affects women, imposing immense suffering and burden on the healthcare system. CPP is a complex condition rising from both gynecological and nongynecological sources.

The diagnostic complexity from overlapping urogenital and colorectal symptoms and viscero-somatic neural convergence in CPP creates a tendency to overlook musculoskeletal contributions. However, a growing understanding of the pelvic anatomy identifies pelvic floor dysfunction (PFD) as a prime driver of CPP.

Epidemiology

CPP affects 15% of women annually in the United States.[1] In 50% cases, CPP has nongynecological etiologies. PFD presents in 50% of reproductive-age women and is often associated with CPP causally or etiologically.[2] The incidence of PFD and CPP increases with age, obesity, smoking, sexual abuse, trauma, sedentarism, diabetes, and chronic constipation.[3]

PFD presents as hypermobility, hypertonicity, laxity, or weakness.[4] Hormonal fluctuations and the shallow female pelvic anatomy with its complex attachments and functional demands increases vulnerability to PFD throughout a woman's lifespan. Pelvic floor damage during childbirth and pregnancy related biomechanical shifts predispose women to PFD and CPP. Additionally pelvic floor laxity stems from collagen degeneration in perimenopause.[4,5]

Musculoskeletal Considerations

The pelvic floor is encased in a ringlike pelvic girdle, fused posteriorly to the sacrococcygeal spine at the sacroiliac (SI) joints. SI ligaments (anterior, posterior, and interosseous) with iliolumbar, sacrospinous, and sacrotuberous ligaments provide stability in the pelvis (Figure 33.1).[6]

The pelvic floor is a dome shaped arrangement of three muscle layers (superficial perineal layer, pelvic diaphragm, and deep urogenital layer).[7] The pelvic diaphragm is the inferior boundary of the abdominopelvic cavity, extending from the symphysis pubis to the coccyx

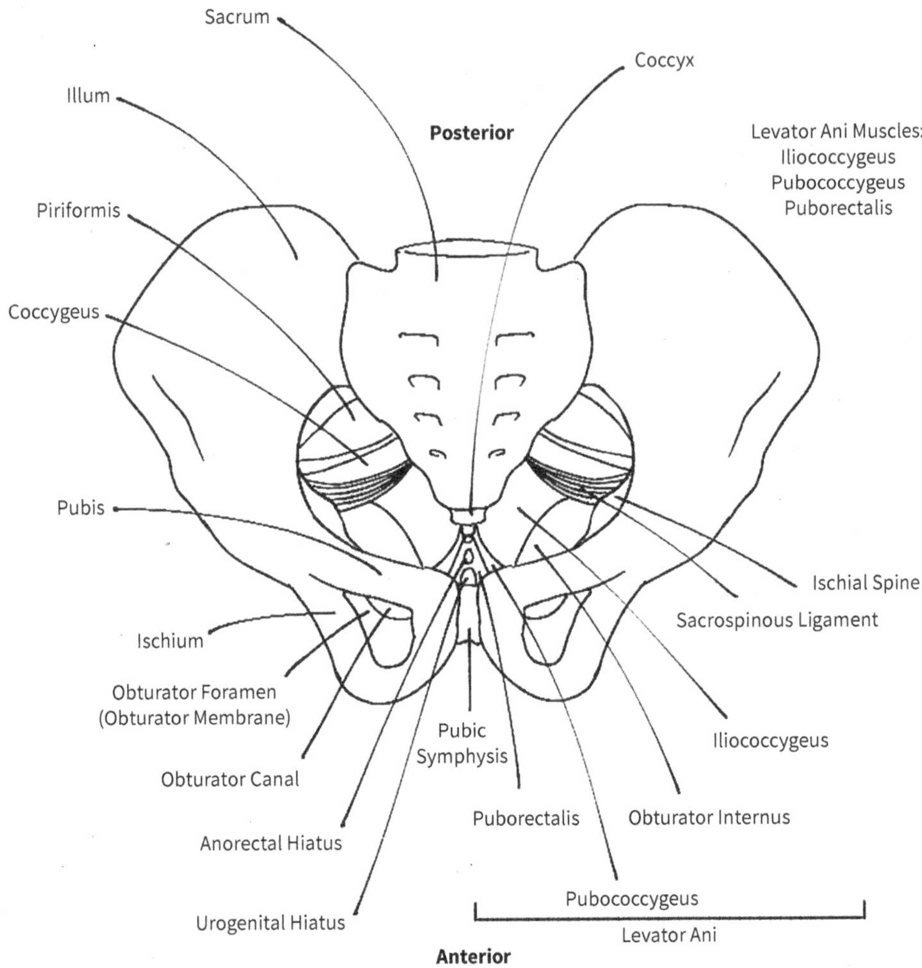

Figure 33.1 Muscles of the pelvic diaphragm and wall.

Source: Lydia Chwang Yuh Wong, Wing Kong Chiu, Matthias Russ, Susan Liew.
Review of techniques for monitoring the healing fracture of bones for implementation in an internally fixated pelvis. Med Engineering Physics. 2012;34(2):140–152.
ISSN 1350-4533, https://doi.org/10.1016/j.medengphy.2011.08.011.

and osseous sidewalls.[8] The obturator internus, an internal rotator of the hip, forms the lateral wall, and the piriformis, an external rotator, forms the posterolateral wall.

The bulk of the pelvic floor is formed by the levator ani, comprised of pubococcygeus, puborectalis, and iliococcygeus muscles.[9] The puborectalis surrounds the rectum in a sling, which is confluent with the urogenital hiatus. Rectal circular and longitudinal smooth muscles extend caudally to form the internal and external anal sphincters, respectively. Thus, contraction of the puborectalis closes the urethra, vagina, and anal sphincters impacting continence and orgasmic mechanisms.[10,11]

The integral theory suggests that four oppositional vectors in the pelvic floor sustain position and shape of pelvic organs. Anterior vectors from the pubococcygeus and puborectalis muscles oppose posterior vectors from the levator plate and rectal longitudinal muscle.

Caudal force from the longitudinal muscle is countered by the uterosacral suspensory ligament.[12]

The suspensory ligaments, formed by the endopelvic fascia, invest the entire pelvic floor and merge with periosteum, sacral ligaments, and urogenital diaphragm. Since nerves and vessels are transmitted through them, strain or damage to the suspensory ligaments causes pain and interrupts integrity of pelvic viscera.[13]

Since it is the floor of the core, the pelvic floor functionally and anatomically synergizes with the core muscles (diaphragm, transversus abdominis, quadratus lumborum, multifidi, and glutei).[7] Core weaknesses, as in diastasis recti, dysregulate intrabdominal pressure, initiating pelvic dyscoordination. Postural or biomechanical imbalance also create compensatory pelvic floor tension.

The connection between the hip rotators and the pelvic floor is critical in PFD, with reciprocal impact. Since pelvic rotation occurs around the bicoxofemoral axis, changes in pelvic tilt alter acetabular anteversion.[13] Hip flexor tightness from chronic sitting causes anterior pelvic tilt, predisposing to PFD.

Diagnosis

A systematic history and examination are necessary to prevent misdiagnosis and to detect PFD associated with CPP.[14] Evaluation of osseous elements includes palpation of the SIJ, anterior superior iliac spines, and pubic symphysis. After informed consent, it is imperative to consider a standardized structured digital palpation of pelvic muscles—performed counterclockwise along the right obturator internus, right levator ani, left levator ani, and left obturator internus.

Myofascial lower abdominal wall pain may masquerade as pelvic pain but usually presents with tenderness over the abdominal muscles and positive Carnett's sign.

The thoraco-lumbar spine and hip complex should always be assessed in CPP. Screening should include hip mobility, posture, gait, single-leg stance, leg length, and deep squat assessment. SI arthropathy and hip and spinal pathology should be considered as primary issues or as contributors to CPP.

In case of diagnostic ambiguity, pelvic ultrasound, electromyography, cystoscopy, defecography, and dynamic pelvic floor MRI may be needed.

Management

Management of CPP focuses on mitigating nociceptive input, central sensitization, and psychological factors. Indicators of successful therapy are analgesia, improved function, and decreased medication use.

Pelvic floor physical therapy (PFPT) is first line in the management of PFD and CPP.[4] PFPT utilizes neural mobilization, scar release, electrical stimulation, internal pelvic massage, and prescriptive exercises. Manual therapy lengthens hypertonic muscles and then strengthens them. Neuromuscular education can repattern posture. Incorporation of myofascial release, strain-counter strain, and breathwork decreases pelvic hypertonicity, and peri-pelvic joint mobilization techniques improve gait mechanics by improving arthro-kinematic limitations.

In a multimodal treatment framework, biofeedback and cognitive behavioral therapy (CBT) are key interventions. Ten to twelve biofeedback sessions for 6–8 weeks improve pelvic hypertonicity by relaxing and retraining the pelvic floor to interrupt the pain–hypertonia cycle.[5] CBT exerts its effects by altering conditioned responses to pain and associated stressors.

Pharmacotherapy depends on comorbidities, access, and economics. Topical agents, heat, and ice are well-tolerated. Vaginal diazepam and baclofen suppositories decrease pelvic hypertonicity and pain. Nonsteroidal anti-inflammatory drugs (NSAIDs), acetaminophen, gabapentanoids, muscle relaxants, alpha-2 agonists, and antidepressants help with analgesia, spasm, mood, and sleep.

Invasive interventions decrease nociceptive input and central sensitization. Hypertonic pelvic muscles may be addressed with trigger point injections (TPI) using dry needling, local anesthetics, or botulinum toxin A.[6] Anesthetic blockade of pudendal nerves and sympathetic plexuses (superior hypogastric, inferior hypogastric, and ganglion impar) have diagnostic and therapeutic utility in CPP. In refractory CPP, carefully considered advanced interventions such as neuromodulation may have a role.

Ergonomic assessments and modifications also provide long-term benefits. Integrating smoking cessation, improving sleep management, enhancing mood, and addressing metabolic health improves pain, mental health, and hormonal health. Additionally, counseling and education are essential for optimal outcomes and treatment adherence.

Clinical Vignette

A 52-year-old software engineer presents with 8 months of worsening, noncyclical pelvic pain and dyspareunia. Her gynecological workup is normal. On examination there is pelvic floor hypertonicity, hip flexor tightness, anterior pelvic tilt, and sacroiliac joint dysfunction.

The patient initiated PFPT, biofeedback, and pharmacotherapy using baclofen and duloxetine. Subsequently TPI and SIJ injections were performed to increase tolerance for PFPT. Ergonomic modifications were incorporated at her workspace.

After 16 weeks she reported 75% improvement, eventually discontinuing medications. She maintained therapeutic gains at her 6-month follow-up while continuing a targeted exercise program and CBT.

References

1. Gyang A, Hartman M, Lamvu G. Musculoskeletal causes of chronic pelvic pain. Obstet Gynecol. 2013;121:645–650.
2. Hagen S, Stark D. Conservative prevention and management of pelvic organ prolapse in women. Cochrane Database Syst Rev. 2011:CD003882.
3. Peinado-Molina RA, Hernández-Martínez A, Martínez-Vázquez S, Rodríguez-Almagro J, Martínez-Galiano JM. Pelvic floor dysfunction: prevalence and associated factors. BMC Public Health. 2023 Oct 14;23(1):2005. doi: 10.1186/s12889-023-16901-3. PMID: 37838661; PMCID: PMC10576367.

4. Tim S, Mazur-Bialy AI. The Most Common Functional Disorders and Factors Affecting Female Pelvic Floor. Life (Basel). 2021 Dec 14;11(12):1397. doi: 10.3390/life11121397. PMID: 34947928; PMCID: PMC8704638.
5. Tinelli A, Malvasi A, Rahimi S, et al. Age-related pelvic floor modifications and prolapse risk factors in postmenopausal women. Menopause. 2010;17:204–212.
6. Hansen JT. *Netter's Clinical Anatomy*. Elsevier; 2014.
7. Prather H, Dugan SA, Fitzgerald CM. Review of anatomy, evaluation, and treatment of musculoskeletal pelvic floor pain in women. PMR. 2009;1:346–358.
8. Raizada V, Mittal RK. Pelvic floor anatomy and applied physiology. Gastroenterol Clin North Am. 2008;37:493–509, vii.
9. Betschart C, Chen L, Ashton-Miller JA, Delancey JOL. Comparison of muscle fiber directions between different levator ani muscle subdivisions. Int Urogynecology J. 2014;25:1263–1268.
10. Rosenbaum TY. Pelvic floor involvement in male and female sexual dysfunction and the role of pelvic floor rehabilitation in treatment. J Sex Med. 2007;4:4–13.
11. Messelink B, Benson T, Berghmans B, et al. Standardization of terminology of pelvic floor muscle function and dysfunction: report from the pelvic floor clinical assessment group of the International Continence Society. Neurourol Urodyn. 2005;24(4):374–380.
12. Quaghebeur J, Petros P, Wyndaele JJ, De Wachter S. The Integral Theory, Pelvic Floor Biomechanics, and Binary Innervation. Int Neurourol J. 2024 Sep;28(3):181–184. doi: 10.5213/inj.2448092.046. Epub 2024 Sep 30. PMID: 39363408; PMCID: PMC11450246.
13. Khalife T, Hagen AM, Alm JEC. Retroperitoneal causes of genitourinary pain syndromes. Sex Med Rev. 2022;10:529–542.
14. Laurenzana L, Fitzgerald C, Bennis S. Pelvic pain and pelvic floor disorders in women. Phys Med Rehabil Clin N Am. 2025;36:311–328.

34
Chronic Musculoskeletal Pain in Women

Diagnosis, Treatment, and Management

Hirsch K. Srivastava, Sharon Marie Mathew, and Leena Mathew

Introduction

Chronic musculoskeletal pain (CMP) affects 47% of the population, and lifetime prevalence approaches 85% in women.[1] CMP conditions, especially myofascial pain syndrome (MPS) and fibromyalgia (FM) disproportionately impact women: 85% of patients at pain clinics have MPS, and 40% of patients at pain clinics have FM.[2–4] Provider biases attribute pain to emotional sources in women, leading to an overestimation of its prevalence in women. Although 80–95% of patients diagnosed with FM in practice are women, unbiased studies indicate that the female-to-male ratio is 3:2.[5] Thirty percent of women with FM feel they are not taken seriously, 46% believe their diagnosis is misunderstood, and 54% perceive physicians are unhelpful.[2]

Pathophysiology

MPS is a regional condition with myofascial trigger points (MTrPs), hyperirritable nodules, and taut bands that provoke pain on palpation.[3,4] Postural malalignment, repetitive strain, and microtrauma depletes adenosine triphosphate (ATP), impairing microcirculation and causing localized ischemia leading to sustained muscle contraction.[3,5–7] Inadequate analgesia with prolonged nociceptive input amplifies pain through central sensitization.[5]

Widespread pain in FM is characterized by hyperalgesia and central sensitization.[6,7] Long considered to be a psychosomatic illness, concrete evidence has established neuroinflammation as the underpinning of FM. The concurrence of migraines, depression, temporomandibular disorder, irritable bowel syndrome, dysmenorrhea, and endometriosis in women with FM suggests shared pathophysiology. Chronic stress, anxiety, and depression perpetuate muscle tension and promote central sensitization through neuroinflammatory induction.[8] Symptom severity correlates with hypothalamic-pituitary axis dysregulation and microglial hyperactivity. Cytokine release from microglia causes neuroinflammation, which further dysregulates microglia. Dysfunctional glial activation in the cingulate cortices disrupts the brain's energy allocation systems, impeding neural networks responsible for attention, motivation, and cognitive control corresponding with fatigue severity. Functional neuroimaging reveals heightened activity in the pain neuromatrix and reduced activity in descending inhibitory pathways. FM patients have hyperactive excitatory neurotransmitters (glutamate, substance P) and hypoactive inhibitory neurotransmitters (gamma aminobutyric acid; GABA). Elevated enkephalins in the cerebrospinal fluid desensitize opioid receptors, possibly explaining the decreased responsiveness to opioids in FM.[6] Systemic factors, including vitamin D and iron deficiency and endocrine and metabolic dysfunction increase pain signaling in the neuromatrix.[7,6] Increasing age, poor ergonomics, smoking, stress, and depression are common risk factors.

Hormonal fluctuations may account for variable pain severity through the menstrual cycle.[7] The hormonal changes in puberty, pregnancy, postpartum, and menopause connect to alterations in pain perception, sleep, mood, and fatigue. Estrogen modulates serotonin and norepinephrine. Progesterone withdrawal and estrogen decline exacerbate central sensitization and lower pain threshold.[9]

Assessment

Nineteen diagnostic criteria have been used across studies, making diagnosis of MPS challenging.[3] Most clinicians adhere to the 2018 International Delphi Consensus, which achieved 80% agreement on three core criteria: palpable taut bands, hypersensitive points, and referred pain.[4]

ACR 2016 uses the Widespread Pain Index (WPI) and Somatic Severity Scale (SSS). The WPI survey includes 19 areas: arms (left/right shoulder girdle, upper arm, lower arm), legs (left/right hip, upper leg, lower leg), and central (jaw, chest, upper back, lower back, neck). SSS measures fatigue, unrefreshed waking, and cognitive and somatic symptoms on a 0–3 severity scale.[10] FM is diagnosed when WPI ≥7 + SSS ≥5 or WPI 4–6 + SSS ≥9 and pain for >3 months.

Management

The Fibromyalgia Impact Questionnaire-Revised (FIQR) is the gold standard for functional assessment in FM and is used to guide therapy. The FIQR looks at 21 items under three subscales: function, impact, and symptoms in the past 7 days. Every item is rated on a 0≥10 Likert scale from lowest to highest severity. Subscales are normalized and added for a global FIQR scale of 0–100, with higher scores indicating higher severity.

Behavioral therapy has first-tier evidence in management of MPS and FM. Cognitive-behavioral therapy (CBT) decreases stress-mediated neuroinflammation and increases functional capacity by modulating cognitive and emotional responses to pain. Biofeedback increases awareness of muscle tension to break the pain–hypertonia cycle. Coping strategies, resiliency building, commitment therapy, and mindfulness-based stress reduction improve pain and increase compliance.[11]

Physical therapy (PT) is a first-line therapy in FM and MPS. Personalized programs improve adherence, function, and fatigue. Aqua therapy, aerobics, and resistance training improve function, improve resilience, and promote neuroplasticity. PT for MPS includes MTrP release using massage and stretching. Joint mobilization improves range of motion.[3,5] During pregnancy, massage and postural optimization is beneficial. Postpartum care includes attention to mental health, sleep, fatigue, and mood. Ergonomics and neuromuscular education are essential to rectify strength and postural imbalances. Topical heat improves spasm and inflammation by decreasing muscle excitability and increasing blood flow and collagen extensibility. Additionally, emerging treatments like near-infrared light therapy and transcranial stimulation may also reduce neuroinflammation and reduce microglial activation.

Pharmacotherapy for FM restores neurotransmitter balance. US Food and Drug (FDA)-approved first-line agents duloxetine (20–60 mg/d), milnacipran (100–200 mg/d), and pregabalin (150–600 mg/d) are comparable for analgesia but differ in adverse effects and specific symptom reduction. Glial activation may be mitigated with low-dose naltrexone. Pharmacotherapy for MPS relies on nonsteroidal anti-inflammatory drugs (NSAIDs), topical analgesics, and muscle relaxants. The challenges of pharmacotherapy in pregnancy and lactation can be countered through the use of acetaminophen, topical agents, and nonpharmacologic modalities.

Deactivation of MPTr with trigger point injections (TPI) may provide relief in MPS. Needle insertion causes local trauma to improve microcirculation and restores length to muscle fibers. Ultrasound guidance increases the efficacy of TPI by accurately identifying myofascial planes. Local anesthetic injections are superior to dry needling and botulinum toxin injection.

Some nutraceuticals are thought to be beneficial in MPS and FM. Tier 1 evidence suggests that 1,000–4,000 IU of vitamin D daily (until serum level is >50 ng/mL) improves pain and function.[12] Acetyl-L-carnitine 1–1.5 g/d may improve cognition through neurotrophic factors.[13] Omega 3 fatty acids 1–3 g and curcumin 500 mg–1 g decrease inflammation. Melatonin 300 mcg–5 mg helps restore circadian rhythm and 300 mg/d of coenzyme Q10 for 90 days improves mitochondrial function to decrease fatigability.[14]

Lifestyle modifications addressing sleep, smoking cessation, and metabolic health improve microglial function and decrease neuroinflammation, pain, and somatic symptoms. Comprehensive care contextualizes comorbidities and patient preferences and uses self-management strategies, counseling, and education to encourage long-term commitment.

Clinical Vignette

A 34-year-old executive presents with fatigue, headache, and pain in all extremities, abdomen, and pelvis for 18 months. She feels stressed at work, and her mood feels "off." She does not feel rested after 7 hours of sleep. Pain intensifies around her menstrual period. She is diffusely tender. Diagnostic studies are normal. FIQR is 59. She is frustrated with her care and being told that she is normal.

Based on ACR 2016 criteria, this patient has FM with moderate severity according to the FIQR score. Treatment was initiated with validation, CBT, duloxetine 30 mg/d, and aqua therapy.

Menstrual tracking was used to guide adjuvant therapy during the luteal phase. Six months later she endorsed improvement in all symptoms with an improved FIQR of 25.

References

1. El-Tallawy SN, Nalamasu R, Salem GI, LeQuang JAK, Pergolizzi JV, Christo PJ. Management of musculoskeletal pain: An update with emphasis on chronic musculoskeletal pain. Pain Ther. 2021;10(1):181–209.
2. Homma M, Ishikawa H, Kiuchi T. Association of physicians' illness perception of fibromyalgia with frustration and resistance to accepting patients: A cross-sectional study. Clin Rheumatol. 2016;35(4):1019–1027.
3. Steen JP, Jaiswal KS, Kumbhare D. Myofascial Pain Syndrome: An Update on Clinical Characteristics, Etiopathogenesis, Diagnosis, and Treatment. Muscle Nerve. 2025 May;71(5):889-910. doi: 10.1002/mus.28377. Epub 2025 Mar 20. PMID: 40110636; PMCID: PMC11998975.
4. Cao QW, Peng BG, Wang L, et al. Expert consensus on the diagnosis and treatment of myofascial pain syndrome. World J Clin Cases. 2021;9(9):2077–2089.
5. Lam C, Francio VT, Gustafson K, Carroll M, York A, Chadwick AL. Myofascial pain: A major player in musculoskeletal pain. Best Pract Res Clin Rheumatol. 2024;38(1):101944.
6. Brummett C, Clauw DJ. Fibromyalgia and centralized pain states. In: Benzon HT, Raja SN, Liu SS, Fishman SM, Cohen SP, eds. *Essentials of Pain Medicine*. Elsevier; 2018:213–222.e2.
7. Sarzi-Puttini P, Giorgi V, Marotto D, Atzeni F. Fibromyalgia: An update on clinical characteristics, aetiopathogenesis and treatment. Nat Rev Rheumatol. 2020;16(11):645–660.
8. Hassamal S. Chronic stress, neuroinflammation, and depression: An overview of pathophysiological mechanisms and emerging anti-inflammatories. Front Psychiatry. 2023;14:1130989.
9. Stieger A, Asadauskas A, Luedi MM, Andereggen L. Women's pain management across the lifespan: A narrative review of hormonal, physiological, and psychosocial perspectives. J Clin Med. 2025;14(10):3427.
10. Wolfe F, Clauw DJ, Fitzcharles MA, et al. 2016 Revisions to the 2010/2011 fibromyalgia diagnostic criteria. Semin Arthritis Rheum. 2016;46(3):319–329.
11. Fischer S, Doerr JM, Strahler J, Mewes R, Thieme K, Nater UM. Stress exacerbates pain in the everyday lives of women with fibromyalgia syndrome: The role of cortisol and alpha-amylase. Psychoneuroendocrinology. 2016;63:68–77.
12. Shipton EE, Shipton EA. Vitamin D deficiency and pain: Clinical evidence of low levels of vitamin d and supplementation in chronic pain states. Pain Ther. 2015;4(1):67–87.
13. Rossini M, Di Munno O, Valentini G, et al. Double-blind, multicenter trial comparing acetyl l-carnitine with placebo in the treatment of fibromyalgia patients. Clin Exp Rheumatol. 2007;25(2):182–188.
14. Campisi L, La Motta C. The use of the coenzyme Q10 as a food supplement in the management of fibromyalgia: A critical review. Antioxid Basel Switz. 2022;11(10):1969.

35
Exercise-Based Interventions for Musculoskeletal Pain

Mohammad Husain Bawany, Sharon Marie Mathew, and Leena Mathew

Introduction

Fibromyalgia (FM) and myofascial pain syndrome (MPS) are the most common chronic musculoskeletal pain (CMP) conditions, with a disproportionate prevalence in women. CMP conditions like FM are associated with maladaptive responses that register increased tissue stress and load as a threat, leading to kinesiophobia and causing functional decline. Challenges to comprehensive treatment include comorbid somatic symptoms, mood disorders, cognitive fog, fatigue, and poor sleep. Pharmacotherapy is also limited by adverse effects, lack of access, and economic factors. Additionally, women have biological barriers to pharmacotherapy during pregnancy and lactation, thus necessitating alternative options.

Exercise is an easy-access, low-risk, nonpharmacologic intervention that should be incorporated early into multimodal therapeutic protocols. The World Health Organization recommends 150–300 minutes of moderate-intensity or 75–150 minutes of moderate to high-intensity physical activity weekly for adults.[1] Muscle contractions produce myokines like irisin, a signaling peptide that enhances myogenesis and osteogenesis and increases brain-derived neurotrophic factor (BDNF) to improve cognition and memory. Myokines promote anti-inflammatory M2 macrophages, stimulate anti-inflammatory cytokines (interleukin [IL]-1ra, IL-10), and decrease pro-inflammatory markers (tumor necrosis factor [TNF]-α, IL-1β). Irisin further facilitates cross-organ communication, stimulating hippocampal neurogenesis, synaptic plasticity, and neurotransmitter release (endocannabinoids, serotonin, dopamine, endorphins) to enhance cognition and memory.

In FM and other CMP conditions, exertional malaise and dysautonomia are barriers to exercise. Supervision, coaching, and graduated exposure strategies can reconceptualize kinesiophobia to introduce movements that are perceived as a threat. For optimal outcomes, exercise therapy is prescribed in the framework of a comprehensive multimodal program individualized to patient preference, comorbidities, baseline fitness, and access.

Aquatic Exercise

Immersion in warm water activates thermoreceptors and mechanoreceptors, which suppresses nociceptors.[2] Submergence in water induces weightlessness: a 50% reduction of body weight occurs with immersion to the waist, 60% at the chest, and 85% at neck level.[3] This weightlessness relaxes the gravity muscles to reduce fatigue perception. The hydrostatic pressure of water also enhances balance equilibrium with compressive forces to improve circulation and lymphatic drainage.[4] The resistance of the water creates work without straining joints, allowing higher-intensity exercise with lower cardiovascular burden. Improved blood and lymphatic flow in muscles improves metabolic waste removal and nutrient delivery. Durable evidence supports the efficacy of aquatic therapy in FM and MPS, showing improved pain, stiffness, and strength.[5] Optimal results are seen with supervised sessions of 45–60 minutes for 12–20 weeks and water temperature at 33–36°C.[6]

Aerobic Exercise

Restoration of movement patterns in CMP are essential with increased age and deconditioning to avoid sarcopenia, fragility, and debility. A therapeutic aerobic exercise program improves pain, mood, fatigue, and sleep by regulating microglial dysfunction, recruiting anti-inflammatory M2 macrophages, and increasing neurogenesis and neuroplasticity through increased BDNF-related dendritic branching. Myokines from aerobic activity improve cognition and memory by increasing hippocampal volume.[7,8] All aerobic exercises engage large muscles in rhythmic movements to increase heart rate. The choice of aerobic activity (walking, running, biking, dancing, swimming) depends on patient preferences, baseline fitness, and access. Supervision and guidance helps with adherence, encouragement, and injury avoidance. The intensity of aerobic exercise is measured by the heart rate (HR) response. HR estimates are obtained using "220 − age" × 76% or a FM-specific formula "209 − 0.85 × age" × 76% based on dysautonomia validation studies. A prescriptive regimen may start 1–3 days per week, for 20–25 minutes/day at 40–50% HR max, progressing over 6–12 weeks to 60–70% HR max for 25–40 minutes for 150 minutes per week.[7,8]

Stretching

Anxiety, mood disorders, and fatigue in patients with CMP and FM causes heightened myofascial tension translating to decreased tissue pliability and mobility. In mobility-averse patients, stretching may work as a first step to counter fear avoidance of movement.[9] Flexibility training helps with global well-being and improves stability and mobility [10] A singular stretch session changes the viscoelasticity of muscle tendon units and increases range of motion of a joint.[11] Whole-body stretching by contraction of antagonist muscles with active stretching of agonist muscles helps with global postural reeducation. Noticeable results are attainable with 40 minutes of a daily stretching program for 8 weeks. Each stretch is held for 15–30 seconds, starting with a 5-minute session and increasing to a 40-minute session.

Resistance Training

Prolonged inactivity leads to deconditioning and diminished strength and endurance.[12] Indirectly, resistance training improves pain and function by interrupting the "pain-inactivity-deconditioning" cycle. Resistance training also improves sarcopenia, bone health, and load absorption and stability of the joint. Therapeutic exercise program may start with a supervised regimen on 2–3 nonconsecutive days per week. Starting at 40–50%, one repetition maximum (RM) intensity for 1–2 sets of 8–12 repetitions, patients may progress over 12 weeks to 2–3 days per week at 60–70% one RM for 2–3 sets. Recovery for 24–48 hours between workouts prevents injury and improves adherence. Significant results are noted at 90 days.

Pilates

Regular engagement with core stabilization exercises activate the internal oblique, rectus abdominis, multifidus, and iliocostalis lumborum, resulting in increased pelvic and trunk stability. Pilates improves pain, kinesiophobia, disability, and quality of life in patients with CMP by enhancing balance, strength, and spinal mobility. An 8-week prescriptive training program of 1–4 weekly sessions for 45 minutes improves range of motion, core muscle thickness, and muscle strength. These therapeutic gains are maintained 3 months after training.[13]

Movement and Meditation Practices

Yoga, tai chi, and qigong incorporate mindfulness, acceptance, regulation of movement, and breathwork to improve self-efficacy. They decrease neuroinflammation, stress, and pain perception through parasympathetic stimulation, lowering inflammatory markers (TNF, IL-II, C reactive protein [CRP]) and regulating the hypothalamic-pituitary-adrenal axis by lowering cortisol. By themselves and in conjunction with other programs they improve balance, flexibility, and strength.

Hatha yoga emphasizes relaxation techniques and gentle postures, while Iyengar yoga incorporates physical postures with props to enhance body awareness and breath control. Qigong uses breathwork with rhythmic movement to develop body awareness, mobility, and balance while inducing relaxation. In tai chi, slow-motion weight-shifting improves muscle strength and joint stability. These movement meditation techniques address the physical and psychological dimensions of chronic pain by modulating sleep, mood, and fatigue. Within the framework of chronic pain, a 3- to 5-day program of yoga, tai-chi, and qigong is best incorporated for at least 6 weeks to see results. Programs of longer duration may achieve better gains.

Although robust evidence supports aerobic exercise, resistance training, and aquatic therapy, combining various exercise modalities is most effective for CMP. The patient's fitness level and access will determine compliance and choice of therapeutic exercise programs. Successful implementation relies on integrating behavioral counseling and empowerment. Collaborative care models that prioritize patient-centered decision-making are associated with reduced attrition and superior outcomes.

References

1. Bull FC, Al-Ansari SS, Biddle S, et al. World Health Organization 2020 guidelines on physical activity and sedentary behaviour. Br J Sports Med. 2020;54(24):1451–1462.
2. Reilly KA, Bird HA. Prophylactic hydrotherapy. Rheumatology (Oxford). 2001 Jan;40(1):4-6. doi: 10.1093/rheumatology/40.1.4. PMID: 11157135.

3. Versey NG, Halson SL, Dawson BT. Water immersion recovery for athletes: Effect on exercise performance and practical recommendations. Sports Med Auckl NZ. 2013;43(11):1101–1130.
4. Zamunér AR, Andrade CP, Arca EA, Avila MA. Impact of water therapy on pain management in patients with fibromyalgia: Current perspectives. J Pain Res. 2019;12:1971–2007.
5. Bidonde J, Busch AJ, Webber SC, et al. Aquatic exercise training for fibromyalgia. Cochrane Database Syst Rev. 2014;2014(10):CD011336.
6. Jentoft ES, Kvalvik AG, Mengshoel AM. Effects of pool-based and land-based aerobic exercise on women with fibromyalgia/chronic widespread muscle pain. Arthritis Rheum. 2001;45(1):42–47.
7. Bidonde J, Busch AJ, Schachter CL, et al. Aerobic exercise training for adults with fibromyalgia. Cochrane Musculoskeletal Group, ed. Cochrane Database Syst Rev. 2017;2017(6): CD012700.
8. Casanova-Rodríguez D, Ranchal-Sánchez A, Rodríguez RB, Jurado-Castro JM. Aerobic Exercise Prescription for Pain Reduction in Fibromyalgia: A Systematic Review and Meta-Analysis. Eur J Pain. 2025 Feb;29(2):e4783. doi: 10.1002/ejp.4783. Erratum in: Eur J Pain. 2025 Oct;29(9):e70105. doi: 10.1002/ejp.70105. PMID: 39805734; PMCID: PMC11730678.
9. Kim SY, Busch AJ, Overend TJ, et al. Flexibility exercise training for adults with fibromyalgia. Cochrane Database Syst Rev. 2019;9(9):CD013419.
10. Costa PB, Graves BS, Whitehurst M, Jacobs PL. The acute effects of different durations of static stretching on dynamic balance performance. J Strength Cond Res. 2009;23(1):141–147.
11. Behm DG, Alizadeh S, Anvar SH, Drury B, Granacher U, Moran J. Non-local acute passive stretching effects on range of motion in healthy adults: A systematic review with meta-analysis. Sports Med. 2021;51(5):945–959.
12. Hawley SE, Bell ZW, Huang Y, Gibbs JC, Churchward-Venne TA. Evaluation of sex-based differences in resistance exercise training-induced changes in muscle mass, strength, and physical performance in healthy older (≥60 y) adults: A systematic review and meta-analysis. Ageing Res Rev. 2023;91:102023.
13. Huang J, Park HY. Effect of Pilates training on pain and disability in patients with chronic low back pain: A systematic review and meta-analysis based on randomized controlled trials. Phys Act Nutr. 2023;27(1):16–29.

36

Interventional Treatments for Musculoskeletal, Fibromyalgia, and Myofascial Pain in Women

Nathaniel Co and Anita Gupta

Introduction

Biological women have a higher prevalence of fibromyalgia, low back pain, and myofascial pain. Studies generally describe women having increased responses to pain and more reported functional impairment. Preclinical studies have described dimorphic patterns in the emotional processing of pain on fMRI and the role of microglia mediating pain hypersensitivity.[1] With that said, more work is warranted in exploring the mechanisms accounting for sex differences in pain perception and therapeutic responsiveness.

Given the significant contribution of musculoskeletal conditions to years lived with disability worldwide, a keen understanding of the wide variety of therapeutic interventions available to patients with musculoskeletal pain syndromes is critical to improving functional and overall health outcomes in women (Table 36.1).

Epidural Steroid Injections

Epidural steroid injections (ESI) are often performed for nonsurgical management of low back pain due to lumbosacral radiculopathy. The injectate often consists of a mixture of corticosteroids and local anesthetics. Recent literature suggests that the strongest predictors of responsiveness to transforaminal ESI treatment within 2–4 weeks include shorter symptom duration and positive sharp wave or fibrillation on electromyography. Despite a robust response to therapy in the short-term, transforaminal ESIs have not demonstrated a reduction in physical disability or incidence of surgery at endpoints beyond 3 months after ESI.[2]

A review on psychosocial factors impacting success of ESI therapy found worse outcomes after ESI for back pain with or without lumbosacral radiculopathy in patients who had substance use disorders, psychiatry conditions, or maladaptive coping strategies. One of the studies in this review found that problem-focused avoidance as a coping strategy was associated with less pain intensity when compared to emotion-focused avoidance.[3] More investigation is needed in refining the role of pretreating psychosocial factors in predicting post-ESI outcomes.

Another important consideration is a decrease in bone mineral density and bone turnover following ESI, particularly in postmenopausal women. A single-center, prospective observational study found reductions in bone formation markers for over 12 weeks, with parameters

Table 36.1 Interventional procedures for musculoskeletal, fibromyalgia, and myofascial pain syndromes in women

Intervention	Target pain syndrome	Key findings	Clinical considerations for women
Dry needling	Myofascial pain (e.g., trigger points)	Reduces localized myofascial pain and improves range of motion; high adherence and safety profile	Generally safe; ideal for abdominal or pelvic trigger points
Trigger point injections (TPI)	Pelvic floor and abdominal myofascial pain	Offers substantial pain relief and improved function; often used when conservative therapies fail	Effective for pelvic pain; tailored techniques may be needed
Botulinum toxin injections	Pelvic floor hypertonicity, dyspareunia	Improves muscle relaxation and sexual function; may reduce spasms in pelvic musculature	Requires EMG guidance; promising for severe levator ani spasm
Transcutaneous electrical nerve stimulation (TENS)/ Neuromodulation devices	Fibromyalgia, chronic musculoskeletal pain	Provides short-term relief, reduces medication use, improves activity tolerance	Safe, low-cost, self-administered adjunct to other therapies
Transcranial stimulation (tDCS/ TMS)	Fibromyalgia, chronic pain	Modest pain and mood improvements; non-invasive brain modulation can improve functional outcomes	May help when other therapies fail; limited long-term data
Radiofrequency ablation (RFA)	Facet joint–related spinal pain	Offers 6–15 months of relief in facet-mediated back or neck pain after diagnostic confirmation	Effective for chronic spinal pain; outcomes not always sex-stratified
Multidisciplinary wellness programs	Fibromyalgia, widespread musculoskeletal pain	Interdisciplinary approaches improve pain, mental health, and quality of life in female populations	Holistic approach crucial in fibromyalgia and widespread pain

returning to normal ranges by around 26 weeks.[4] Consideration of similar perimenopausal physiological changes should be included in the risk–benefit discussion with patients undergoing these interventions.

Facet Joint Interventions

The current American Society of Interventional Pain Physicians (ASIPP) Guidelines on facet joint interventions presents a diagnostic scale for evaluating facet etiologies of lumbar pain, including factors such as axial lumbar pain that improves with rest and patients presenting with more lumbar than leg pain (absence of radicular pattern or present pseudoradicular pattern).[5] Other signs found to correlate with facet joint syndrome include positive Kemp's sign and a recently reported "facet stress sign," which begins with the examiner supporting the distal leg and elevating the patient's leg from a supine position to maximal hip flexion. Next, the patient applies maximal downward resistance, opposing upward force from the provider, followed by the examiner withdrawing their hand and catching the leg near the surface of the examination table. A positive facet stress sign is noted with lumbar pain during the downward motion of the patient's leg (sensitivity 70.3%, specificity 50%, PPV 90.47%, NPV 20%).[5]

ASIPP guidelines support diagnostic and therapeutic facet joint nerve blocks for lumbar, thoracic, and cervical spinal regions (level of evidence I to II) with moderate strength of recommendation. Another treatment modality consists of radiofrequency ablation (RFA), a minimally invasive procedure by which thermal energy destroys nervous tissue responsible for pain modulation/sensation. The ASIPP Guidelines similarly report a level of evidence of II and moderate strength of recommendation for lumbar and cervical RFA, with level of evidence III assigned for thoracic RFA.[5]

Research studies report a higher prevalence of facet joint pain in women compared to men, particularly in women with elevated body mass index (BMI). The higher prevalence of pain alludes to the question of whether these individuals have poorer responses to treatment. One single-center retrospective chart review found reduced improvement in visual analog scale maximum pain scores in patients with elevated BMI undergoing lumbar RFA. They also found a greater proportion of pain relief in women than men (mean = 79.8% vs. 71.6%, $p = 0.046$).[5] With that said, there is otherwise limited evidence comparing treatment outcomes in men and women undergoing facet joint interventions. Given the increased utilization of facet joint interventions as a therapeutic option, it is important for the growing body of literature in support of this treatment modality to determine ideal treatment intervals.

Trigger Point Injections

Trigger point injections (TPIs) have been utilized as a minimally invasive procedure for the management of myofascial pain syndrome. A recent review comparing various injectates for treatment of myofascial pain syndrome, including botulinum toxin A, normal saline, corticosteroids, and local anesthetic agents, found comparable efficacy and minimal risk profiles across all these trigger point injectates. It was hypothesized that diluting pain mediators was sufficient to provide analgesia, and the authors encourage normal saline as a first-line injectate for TPI in consideration of cost and side effects.[6] Variations in technique, local anesthetic type and concentration, and sample size limit the generalizability and validity of these findings. Moreover, many of the included studies had endpoints at 2 weeks, so there is inadequate comparison of the efficacy of these injectates in longer-term follow-up.

While the prevalence of myofascial pain syndrome is increased in women compared to men, there is a lack of research regarding the stratification of outcomes of TPIs by sex. Beyond epidemiologic and historic measures, it is also important to consider etiologies of myofascial pain in women relating to physiologic changes. For example, in the peripartum period, changes to the pelvis during pregnancy may incite sciatic nerve entrapment by the piriformis muscle.[7]

Conclusion

Overall, ESIs, facet joint interventions, and TPIs offer clinical utility as therapeutic options for patients with musculoskeletal pain that is refractory to more conservative treatments. Given the increased prevalence of musculoskeletal pain conditions in women and the relationship between these conditions and functional impairment or disability, it is imperative that physicians educate patients and offer these interventions when clinically indicated. Moreover, maintaining peripartum and perimenopausal considerations in women undergoing these procedures is a necessary step to improve therapeutic outcomes. Psychosocial factors also contribute to the perception of pain and therefore response to treatment. More research is needed regarding the differential perception and mechanisms of pain in women to refine treatments and improve personalized care.

References

1. Queme LF, Jankowski MP. Sex differences and mechanisms of muscle pain. Curr Opin Physiol. 2019;11:1–6.
2. Stensland M, McGeary D, Covell C, et al. The role of psychosocial factors in mediating the treatment response of epidural steroid injections for low back pain with or without lumbosacral radiculopathy: A scoping review. PLoS One. 2025;20(1):e0316366.
3. Park DY, Kang S, Park JH. Factors predicting favorable short-term response to transforaminal epidural steroid injections for lumbosacral radiculopathy. Medicina (Kaunas). 2019;55(5):162.
4. Clare S, Dash A, Liu Y, et al. Epidural steroid injections acutely suppress bone formation markers in postmenopausal women. J Clin Endocrinol Metab. 2022;107(8):e3281–e3287.
5. Manchikanti L, Kaye AD, Soin A, et al. Comprehensive evidence-based guidelines for Facet Joint Interventions in the management of chronic spinal pain: American society of interventional pain physicians (ASIPP) guidelines Facet Joint Interventions 2020 guidelines. Pain Physician. 2020;23(3S):S1–S127.
6. Ting K, Huh A, J. Roldan C. Review of trigger point therapy for the treatment of myofascial pain syndromes. J Anesthesiol Pain Therapy. 2020;1(3):22–29.
7. Bizzoca D, Solarino G, Pulcrano A, et al. Gender-related issues in the management of low-back pain: A current concepts review. Clin Pract. 2023;13(6):1360–1368.

37 Outcomes of Epidural Steroid Injection in Chronic Musculoskeletal Back Pain

Kenzo Lacuarta and Anita Gupta

Introduction

Chronic low back pain (LBP) affects a significant portion of the adult population and impacts patients' daily activities and their overall quality of life. Also referred to as *lumbosacral radicular pain* or *sciatica*, LBP accounts for more than US$100 billion in annual medical costs within the United States, with a global prevalence and incidence as high as 24% and 7%, respectively.[1,2]

The etiology and severity of chronic lumbar pain vary from patient to patient, yielding different approaches to management. A common presentation is herniation of the nucleus pulposus, the shock-absorbing inner core of an intervertebral disc that allows for spinal rotation and flex. The resulting inflammation and stenosis from herniation is the basis of the chronicity of LBP, making it a key target for interventional pain management.

Treatment can be categorized as surgical or nonsurgical, with surgical candidates being those who have already exhausted conservative methods. These nonsurgical treatments include physical therapy, lifestyle changes, analgesic drugs, and epidural steroid injections (ESI).[3] Some studies have looked at gender differences in LBP and its effects on patient outcomes. Bizzoca et al. report that, postoperatively, there is a higher incidence of LBP in women than in men, with female patients showing worse LBP, disability, and quality of life.[4]

The global burden of LBP on women calls for cost-effective treatment, and ESI is a prime candidate given its efficacy. ESI is performed with a Tuohy needle, where the clinician inserts the tip of the needle into the epidural space located between the ligamentum flavum and the dura mater. Corticosteroids and/or anesthetics are then injected into this space, causing immunosuppressive and anti-inflammatory effects.

Several studies have shown the efficacy of ESIs in relieving lumbosacral radicular pain in patients while also preventing or delaying more invasive treatment or surgery.[5] For LBP arising from disk herniation, there is evidence of pain relief and improvements in sleep and daily activities.[6–8] Similar findings were shown in patients with LBP arising from canal stenosis.[9–11] However, while patients report pain relief after ESI, it is unclear whether it is more or less effective than surgical approaches. Some studies have shown surgical treatment for lumbar disc herniation is more effective for long-term pain relief.[12,13]

Despite the lack of consensus within the literature, ESI remains an important tool in the pain management toolbox. More research is needed to help clinicians differentiate which patients would benefit from ESI compared to surgery. Furthermore, pain management clinicians should continue to find ways that ESI can be tailored for women to improve its efficacy in treating chronic LBP in the long-term.

Clinical Vignette

A 54-year-old female presents to the outpatient pain management clinic with an 11-month history of chronic LBP, rated 7/10 on the numeric pain scale, and radiating to the calf and left posterior thigh. The pain was described as a dull ache, with intermittent sharp components, made worse by sitting, walking, and moderate exercise. This has interfered with her work as a secretary at a law firm and her ability to get quality sleep at night. She reports that she makes a conscious effort to avoid sitting for long periods of time at work, but the pain has worsened over the past few weeks. She now asks about other treatments available.

Past medical history was significant for well-controlled hypertension and mild osteoarthritis. The patient never smoked and had no prior history of spinal trauma or surgery. Before referral to physical therapy, she was prescribed medications to help control her pain. The medications included lidocaine patches and meloxicam.

Management

The patient was initially managed conservatively. She began physical therapy 2–3 times per week for 5 weeks focusing on interventions such as extension exercises, upper and lower extremity strength training, and postural control exercises. After 5 weeks, the patient reported only feeling a mild improvement in her symptoms. Due to persistent radicular symptoms and functional limitations affecting her work and daily living, she opted to undergo ESI.

Diagnostic Approach and Treatment

Spinal imaging with MRI, plain CT, or CT myelography is ordered to identify the location and amount of epidural fat at the indicated level. The patient is scheduled for a caudal ESI using a 22G spinal needle. The injectate consists of 2 mL of 0.25% bupivacaine, 3 mL of preservative-free normal saline (PFNS), and 2 mL of 40 mg/mL of triamcinolone.

Outcome

At 2 week postinjection, the patient reports 60% improvement in her LBP. She continues her physical therapy biweekly and is scheduled for a repeat ESI to further relieve her pain. She currently reports decreased pain with her daily activities and work. She will be monitored for further developments given her new regimen and pain levels.

Conclusion

ESIs serve as a noninvasive treatment for LBP that can relieve patient pain and delay or prevent surgery. Our case study highlights the efficacy of ESI in treating LBP not responsive to medications, physical therapy, and lifestyle changes.

Studies have shown that sex-based differences exist in the prevalence and severity of LBP among men and women.[4] Further work must identify how these gender differences can inform which treatment is indicated.

References

1. Crow WT, Willis DR. Estimating cost of care for patients with acute low back pain: A retrospective review of patient records. J Am Osteopath Assoc. 2009;109(4):229–233.
2. Fatoye F, Gebrye T, Odeyemi I. Real-world incidence and prevalence of low back pain using routinely collected data. Rheumatol Int. 2019;39(4):619–626.
3. Chen BL, Guo JB, Zhang HW, Zhang YJ, Zhu Y, Zhang J, Hu HY, Zheng YL, Wang XQ. Surgical versus non-operative treatment for lumbar disc herniation: a systematic review and meta-analysis. Clin Rehabil. 2018 Feb;32(2):146-160. doi: 10.1177/0269215517719952. Epub 2017 Jul 17. PMID: 28715939.
4. Bizzoca D, Solarino G, Pulcrano A, et al. Gender-related issues in the management of low-back pain: A current concepts review. Clin Pract. 2023;13(6):1360–1368. doi:10.3390/clinpract13060122
5. Kreiner DS, Hwang SW, Easa JE, et al. An evidence-based clinical guideline for the diagnosis and treatment of lumbar disc herniation with radiculopathy. Spine J. 2014;14(1):180–191. doi:10.1016/j.spinee.2013.08.003
6. Sariyildiz MA, Batmaz İ, Yazmalar L, Güneş M, Turan Y. The effectiveness of transforaminal epidural steroid injections on radicular pain, functionality, psychological status and sleep quality in patients with lumbar disc herniation. J Back Musculoskeletal Rehabil. 2017;30(2):265–270. doi:10.3233/BMR-150438
7. Guclu B, Deniz L, Yuce Y, et al. Transforaminal epidural steroid injection in the treatment of pain in foraminal and paramedian lumbar disc herniations. Turk Neurosurg. 2020;30:394–399.
8. Sencan S, Çelenlio˘glu AE, Asadov R, Gündüz OH. Predictive factors for treatment success of transforaminal epidural steroid injection in lumbar disc herniation-induced sciatica. Turk J Med Sci. 2020;50:126–131.
9. Sabbaghan S, Mirzamohammadi E, Mahabadi MA, et al. Short-term efficacy of epidural injection of triamcinolone through translaminar approach for the treatment of lumbar canal stenosis. Anesthesiol Pain Med. 2020;10:e99764.
10. Farooque M, Salzman MM, Ye Z. Effectiveness of bilateral transforaminal epidural steroid injections in degenerative lumbar spinal stenosis patients with neurogenic claudication: A case series. PMR. 2017;9:26–31.
11. Hammerich A, Whitman J, Mintken P, et al. Effectiveness of physical therapy combined with epidural steroid injection for individuals with lumbar spinal stenosis: A randomized parallel-group trial. Arch Phys Med Rehabil. 2019;100:797–810.
12. Radcliff K, Hilibrand A, Lurie JD, et al. The impact of epidural steroid injections on the outcomes of patients treated for lumbar disc herniation: A subgroup analysis of the SPORT trial. J Bone Jt Surg Am. 2012;94:1353–1358.
13. Pazhouhande F, Bazmi S, Taheri R, Tabrizi R. Comparing Quality of Life: Discectomy Surgery versus Epidural Corticosteroid Injection for Lumbar Disc Herniation. World Neurosurg. 2024 May;185:e1309-e1320. doi: 10.1016/j.wneu.2024.03.077. Epub 2024 Mar 21. PMID: 38521225.

PART VII
PREGNANCY AND PAIN

38

Comprehensive Pain Treatment Considerations During Pregnancy

Sarafina Kankam, Kelsey Gustafson, and Katherine Adams

Introduction

During pregnancy, a woman's body undergoes a range of physiological and anatomical changes that are essential for supporting fetal development and preparing for childbirth. However, these adaptations can also significantly influence the presentation and perception of pain. Understanding these changes is critical for clinicians managing pain in pregnant patients.

Pathophysiology

This section outlines the anatomical and neurophysiological changes that underlie pain in pregnancy, providing a framework for recognizing and managing common pain conditions in this population.

Anatomical and Physiological Changes in Pregnancy

Hormonal fluctuations—particularly involving relaxin, estrogen, and progesterone—play a key role in tissue remodeling and musculoskeletal flexibility.[1] These hormones support pelvic expansion and prepare the uterus for delivery but also increase joint laxity, alter biomechanics, and contribute to nerve compression, potentially leading to new or worsening pain syndromes.[2]

Pain perception is further influenced by physiological changes during pregnancy. Endogenous opioids, such as beta-endorphins, rise particularly in the third trimester and during labor, while estrogen and progesterone modulate central and peripheral pain thresholds.[3] Psychological factors, including anxiety, past trauma, and social support, also shape the pain experience, reinforcing the need for a holistic approach.

Common Musculoskeletal Pain Conditions

Pain is a highly prevalent complaint during pregnancy, with studies reporting that >60% of women experience some form of discomfort.[4] A substantial portion of this pain arises from musculoskeletal changes related to anatomical, biomechanical, and hormonal adaptations.

Pelvic Girdle Pain and Sacroiliac Joint Pain

Pelvic girdle pain is a common concern, typically presenting as discomfort over the pubic symphysis, lower back, or perineal region, and is often aggravated by walking or leg abduction. Sacroiliac joint pain may also occur, presenting as posterior pelvic pain that worsens with weight-bearing activities and progressive uterine enlargement.

Round Ligament Pain and Piriformis Syndrome

Additional sources of musculoskeletal pain include round ligament pain, characterized by sharp groin discomfort triggered by movement; thoracic pain resulting from intercostal muscle strain; and piriformis syndrome, which manifests as deep gluteal pain with possible radiation into the lower extremities.

Neuropathic and Entrapment Syndromes

Low Back Pain

During pregnancy, certain anatomical and physiological changes can predispose patients to nerve-related pain syndromes. Notably, lumbar disc herniation remains relatively uncommon during pregnancy, with an estimated incidence of approximately 1 in 10,000. This indicates that pregnant individuals are not at increased risk for lumbar disc abnormalities compared to the general population.[5] Instead, radicular symptoms during pregnancy are more often the result of compressive neuropathy caused by the enlarging uterus.

Carpal Tunnel Syndrome

Carpal tunnel syndrome results from compression of the median nerve beneath the carpal ligament, causing pain and paresthesia in the median nerve distribution. It is more common in women, with increased prevalence and more rapid symptom onset during pregnancy.[6] The etiology is multifactorial, largely attributed to hormone-induced edema and fluid retention. As symptoms often resolve postpartum, conservative management—including activity modifications and nocturnal wrist splinting—can be effective without the need for pharmacologic intervention. In more severe or refractory cases, corticosteroid injections or surgical decompression may be warranted.

Meralgia Paresthetica

Meralgia paresthetica is a compressive neuropathy caused by entrapment of the lateral femoral cutaneous nerve beneath the inguinal ligament. It presents with numbness, paresthesia, and pain along the lateral thigh. Diagnosis may involve the lateral compression test and nerve conduction studies, while also ruling out lumbar radiculopathy or disc herniation. Treatment includes stretching, physical therapy, and nerve blocks for more severe cases. Symptoms often improve or resolve postpartum.

Anterior Cutaneous Nerve Entrapment Syndrome

Anterior cutaneous nerve entrapment syndrome (ACNES) results from compression of the cutaneous intercostal nerves from a gravid uterus. As the nerves are compressed within the abdominal wall muscles, patients will have a positive Carnett's sign, which can help differentiate it from visceral abdominal pain. Transverse abdominus plane or rectus sheath blocks can serve as both diagnostic and therapeutic interventions.[7]

Headaches and Migraines

Headaches are a common complaint during pregnancy, often related to estrogen fluctuations and increased vascular sensitivity. It is important to distinguish between primary headaches—such as migraines and tension-type headaches, which account for most cases during pregnancy—and secondary headaches, which may signal more serious conditions such as preeclampsia, subarachnoid hemorrhage, or cerebral venous thrombosis.[8] A thorough evaluation of clinical presentation, medical history, and precipitating factors is essential to differentiate between these entities and guide appropriate management.[9]

Diagnosis and Assessment

In most cases, additional diagnostic workup such as imaging is not routinely indicated during pregnancy as diagnoses can typically be made based on a thorough history and physical examination. Moreover, minimizing fetal exposure to radiation remains a priority. Exceptions include cases presenting with concerning neurological findings such as motor or sensory deficits, or red-flag symptoms suggestive of cauda equina syndrome. In such scenarios, MRI may be warranted to facilitate timely diagnosis and intervention. While MRI is generally considered safe during pregnancy, particularly when performed without gadolinium contrast, there are currently no long-term studies assessing the effects of fetal exposure to strong magnetic fields.[4]

Treatment Options: Pain Management Modalities in Pregnancy

A wide range of pharmacologic and nonpharmacologic strategies are currently available to help manage pain and discomfort during pregnancy and childbirth. The following section explores several of these treatment options in greater detail.

Pharmacologic Strategies

In 1979, the US Food and Drug Administration (FDA) introduced a five-category classification system to assess the teratogenic risk of medications based on available evidence (Table 38.1). Clinicians should use this framework to guide individualized, patient-centered treatment decisions, carefully balancing risks and benefits.

When pharmacologic treatment is necessary for persistent pain during pregnancy, acetaminophen is considered first-line due to its established safety when used appropriately.[10] Nonsteroidal anti-inflammatory drugs (NSAIDs) are contraindicated in the third trimester due to risks including premature closure of the ductus arteriosus, uterine vasoconstriction, oligohydramnios, and hemorrhage.[5] Opioids should be used judiciously, given the risk of neonatal abstinence syndrome (NAS), which may lead to nervous system and gastrointestinal symptoms, poor feeding, and irritability.[11]

For chronic neuropathic pain, selective serotonin and norepinephrine reuptake inhibitors (SNRIs) and gabapentinoids may be effective but require caution in pregnancy due to limited safety data.[12] SNRIs cross the placenta and blood–brain barrier, potentially affecting fetal neurodevelopment by altering monoamine levels. Although some studies suggest possible neurodevelopmental effects, long-term outcomes remain unclear.[13]

Animal studies link gabapentin exposure to fetal growth restriction and congenital anomalies, such as neural tube and craniofacial defects, though these findings have not been confirmed in human populations.[5,14] The use of SNRIs and gabapentinoids during pregnancy should involve shared decision-making and a thorough discussion of risks and benefits.

Tricyclic antidepressants (TCAs) are generally avoided during pregnancy, especially in the first trimester, due to associations with congenital malformations, preterm birth, low birth weight, and persistent pulmonary hypertension in some studies[15] (Table 38.1).

Regional and Local Anesthetic Techniques

Regional and neuraxial anesthesia methods including epidurals and combined spinal epidurals (CSEs) are frequently used for labor and cesarean delivery.[16] Pregnancy-related changes such as increased epidural fat and reduced cerebrospinal fluid (CSF) can alter anesthetic spread and dosing, largely due to epidural venous plexus engorgement from uterine compression. As a result, lower local anesthetic doses are often sufficient.[17]

During pregnancy, interventional modalities such as peripheral nerve blocks and targeted joint injections may be beneficial for managing pain refractory to conservative treatments. When performing interventional procedures, it is important to minimize fetal exposure to radiation by avoiding fluoroscopy when possible and prioritizing landmark-based or

Table 38.1 Fetal risk and medication safety during pregnancy: US Food and Drug Administration (FDA) classification overview

FDA classification	Category definition	Examples
Category A	Human studies show no risk Medications in this class are considered safe to use in pregnancy	
Category B	No risk in animal studies No well-controlled human studies Medications in this class are considered safe to use in pregnancy	Acetaminophen Cyclobenzaprine NSAIDs (in 1st and 2nd trimester) Lidocaine/bupivacaine Oxycodone/Oxycontin Nalbuphine
Category C	Animal studies show an adverse effect There are no satisfactory studies in pregnant women Potential benefits of the drug may outweigh the risks	Morphine Fentanyl Hydromorphone Tramadol Hydrocodone Gabapentin/Pregabalin Dexamethasone/triamcinolone acetonide TCAs/SNRIs Migraine medications: propranolol, nifedipine, verapamil, sumatriptan
Category D	Evidence of fetal risk Drugs in this class may be used in pregnancy if the benefits to the mother outweigh the risk to the fetus	NSAIDs (in 3rd trimester) Carbamazepine
Category X	Drugs in this category are contraindicated in pregnancy	Ergotamine

NSAID, nonsteroidal anti-inflammatory drug; TCA, tricyclic antidepressant; SNRI, serotonin and norepinephrine reuptake inhibitor.

ultrasound-guided approaches. Local anesthetics have been widely used during pregnancy and are considered safe.[18] Additionally, nonsystemic steroid injections have shown no adverse maternal or fetal effects, offering meaningful symptom relief and reduced reliance on systemic medications.[19]

Nonpharmacologic Approaches

Conservative treatment is often preferred for pregnant patients, with multiple nonpharmacologic approaches available for pain management.

Physical therapy focused on posture, ergonomics, and strengthening can significantly reduce low back pain by teaching proper body mechanics and minimizing spinal strain.[5] Techniques such as sacroiliac joint stabilization and prenatal yoga have been shown to improve pain, function, and overall maternal well-being.[20,21]

Transcutaneous electrical nerve stimulation (TENS) is another effective option for low back and pelvic pain, with studies demonstrating improved pain and function.[22] It is considered safe throughout all trimesters when used appropriately, with low current density recommended for comfort and safety.[5]

Cognitive behavioral therapy (CBT) addresses the emotional and cognitive components of pain, enhancing coping strategies and potentially reducing the need for medications.[23] It is safe throughout pregnancy and may be especially beneficial for patients with a history of anxiety, depression, or trauma.[24]

Other modalities such as acupuncture, massage, and aqua therapy may also provide relief, though supporting evidence is variable.[5] Incorporating nonpharmacologic therapies into prenatal care offers a holistic and effective strategy for managing pain during pregnancy.

Clinical Pearls

- Pain during pregnancy is a complex, multifactorial experience influenced by anatomical, hormonal, neurological, and psychosocial changes. While these adaptations support fetal development, they can also contribute to new or worsening pain syndromes affecting maternal quality of life.
- Managing pain requires balancing maternal well-being with fetal safety through an individualized, evidence-based approach grounded in shared decision-making.
- Ethical considerations are especially important when considering pharmacologic treatments.
- Optimal outcomes are achieved through multidisciplinary care involving obstetricians, anesthesiologists, pain specialists, physical therapists, and mental health professionals.
- Despite its prevalence, gaps in research and guidelines persist.
- Clinicians must recognize and validate the unique pain experiences of pregnant patients to ensure they feel supported and empowered.

References

1. Reese ME, Casey E. Hormonal influence on the neuromusculoskeletal system in pregnancy. In: Fitzgerald CM, Segal NA, eds. *Musculoskeletal Health in Pregnancy and Postpartum: An Evidence-Based Guide for Clinicians.* Springer; 2015:19–34. doi:10.1007/978-3-319-14319-4_2
2. Daneau C, Abboud J, Marchand AA, et al. Mechanisms underlying lumbopelvic pain during pregnancy: A proposed model. Front Pain Res (Lausanne). 2021;2:773988. doi:10.3389/fpain.2021.773988
3. Malviya AK, Gupta A, Kumar V, Gupta J, Deepika, Khanna P. Effect of pregnancy hormones on pain perception in the peripartum period: a narrative review. J Anaesthesiol Clin Pharmacol. doi:10.4103/joacp.joacp_174_24
4. Sibai BM. Maternal adaptations to pregnancy: Musculoskeletal changes and pain. Post TW, ed. UpToDate. Accessed March 15, 2025. https://www.uptodate.com/contents/maternal-adaptations-to-pregnancy-musculoskeletal-changes-and-pain
5. Shah S, Banh ET, Koury K, Bhatia G, Nandi R, Gulur P. Pain management in pregnancy: Multimodal approaches. Pain Res Treat. 2015;2015:987483. doi:10.1155/2015/987483

6. Harinesan N, Silsby M, Simon NG. Carpal tunnel syndrome. In: Chalk C, ed. *Handbook of Clinical Neurology*. Vol. 201. Elsevier; 2024:61–88. doi:10.1016/B978-0-323-90108-6.00005-3
7. Kennedy D. Pain in pregnancy. EMRA Pain Management Guide. Emergency Medicine Residents' Association. Accessed April 1, 2025. https://www.emra.org/books/pain-management/pain-in-pregnancy
8. Daneau C, Abboud J, Marchand AA, et al. Mechanisms underlying lumbopelvic pain during pregnancy: A proposed model. Front Pain Res (Lausanne). 2021;2:773988. doi:10.3389/fpain.2021.773988
9. Negro A, Delaruelle Z, Ivanova TA, et al. Headache and pregnancy: a systematic review. J Headache Pain. 2017;18(1):106. doi:10.1186/s10194-017-0816-0
10. Nunge RA, Kendle AM, Alwan S. Pain medication use during pregnancy. Semin Perinatol. 2025;49(4):152074. doi:10.1016/j.semperi.2025.152074
11. American College of Obstetricians and Gynecologists. Opioid use and opioid use disorder in pregnancy: ACOG Committee Opinion No. 711. Obstet Gynecol. 2017;130(2):e81–e94. https://www.acog.org/clinical/clinical-guidance/committee-opinion/articles/2017/08/opioid-use-and-opioid-use-disorder-in-pregnancy
12. Fornasari D. Pharmacotherapy for neuropathic pain: A review. Pain Ther. 2017;6(Suppl 1):25–33. doi:10.1007/s40122-017-0091-4
13. Dubovicky M, Belovicova K, Csatlosova K, Bogi E. Risks of using SSRI/SNRI antidepressants during pregnancy and lactation. Interdiscip Toxicol. 2017;10(1):30–34. doi:10.1515/intox-2017-0004
14. Society for Maternal-Fetal Medicine, Sinkey RG, Ogunsile FJ, et al. Society for Maternal-Fetal Medicine consult series #68: Sickle cell disease in pregnancy. Am J Obstet Gynecol. 2024;230(2):B17–B40. doi:10.1016/j.ajog.2023.10.031
15. Bérard A, Zhao JP, Sheehy O. Antidepressant use during pregnancy and the risk of major congenital malformations in a cohort of depressed pregnant women: An updated analysis of the Quebec Pregnancy Cohort. BMJ Open. 2017;7(1):e013372. doi:10.1136/bmjopen-2016-013372
16. Hill NE, Granlund B. Anesthesia for labor, delivery, and cesarean section in high-risk heart disease. StatPearls. 2025 Jan. Updated February 21, 2023. Accessed March15, 2025. https://www.ncbi.nlm.nih.gov/books/NBK574578/
17. Obstetric Regional Anesthesia. NYSORA. Published July 5, 2018. Accessed May 1, 2025. https://www.nysora.com/topics/sub-specialties/obstetric/obstetric-regional-anesthesia/
18. Lee JM, Shin TJ. Use of local anesthetics for dental treatment during pregnancy: Safety for parturient. J Dent Anesth Pain Med. 2017;17(2):81–90. doi:10.17245/jdapm.2017.17.2.81
19. Filippini C, Saran S, Chari B. Musculoskeletal steroid injections in pregnancy: A review. Skeletal Radiol. 2023;52(8):1465–1473. doi:10.1007/s00256-023-04320-9
20. Teymuri Z, Hosseinifar M, Sirousi M. The effect of stabilization exercises on pain, disability, and pelvic floor muscle function in postpartum lumbopelvic pain: A randomized controlled trial. Am J Phys Med Rehabil. 2018;97(12):885–891. doi:10.1097/PHM.0000000000000993
21. Holden SC, Manor B, Zhou J, Zera C, Davis RB, Yeh GY. Prenatal yoga for back pain, balance, and maternal wellness: A randomized, controlled pilot study. Glob Adv Health Med. 2019;8:2164956119870984. doi:10.1177/2164956119870984
22. Gutke A, Boissonnault J, Brook G, Stuge B. The severity and impact of pelvic girdle pain and low-back pain in pregnancy: A multinational study. J Womens Health (Larchmt). 2018;27(4):510–517. doi:10.1089/jwh.2017.6342

23. Nakao M, Shirotsuki K, Sugaya N. Cognitive-behavioral therapy for management of mental health and stress-related disorders: Recent advances in techniques and technologies. Biopsychosoc Med. 2021;15(1):16. doi:10.1186/s13030–021-00219-w
24. Shapiro M, Sujan AC, Guille C. A clinical trial of a program for pain management and opioid reduction during pregnancy. Reprod Sci. 2022;29(2):606–613. doi:10.1007/s43032–021-00701–4

39

Maternal Pain and Postpartum Recovery

Clinical Implications and Outcomes

Sejal Tamakuwala and Sudheer Potru

Introduction

Pain management during childbirth has evolved substantially over the years, with multimodal therapy being the mainstay of current practice.[1] Societal and cultural norms certainly influence pain management practices.[2] It is important that obstetric practices and cultural attitudes align for birthing persons to have a positive experience.[1] Birthing experience is multifaceted and is affected by variables reported by birthing persons, including but not limited to pain control, duration of labor, support, need for surgical interventions, and education on expectations.[1]

Memories of the birthing experience can affect a person for a lifetime and often have a lasting effect on how they view themselves, their priorities, and their roles and responsibilities.[3] When inadequately managed, perinatal pain contributes to a cascade of adverse maternal outcomes—from chronic pain syndromes and mood disorders all the way to impaired bonding with the infant.[4] We begin with a discussion of etiologies of pain in the pregnancy and postpartum periods.

Common Etiologies of Pain During Pregnancy and Postpartum Recovery

Pain in pregnancy typically stems from musculoskeletal changes, labor, delivery, and post-surgical etiologies. Musculoskeletal pain can affect up to 70% of pregnant individuals and can persist postpartum, which can impair recovery and caregiving. Pain during pregnancy can manifest in numerous regions of the body such as the head/neck, upper and lower back, pelvic girdle, hip, knees, ankle/feet, and wrist/hand.[5] Pain progressively worsens both in severity and number of locations with advancing gestational age and typically improves in the postpartum period.[6] Lumbar and pelvic girdle pain are common in the second and third trimesters due to altered biomechanics, postural shifts, and increased ligamentous laxity driven by relaxin and estrogen. The anterior pelvic tilt, widened gait, and increased lumbar lordosis place continuous strain on spinal and pelvic muscles.[7]

Pregnancy-related pelvic girdle pain (PRPGP) affects 1 in 5 pregnant individuals.[4] While PRPGP is often considered a normal part of pregnancy, it can often significantly affect quality of life, but pregnant individuals often do not receive proper education, and pain complaints may be dismissed.[8] PRPGP can persist postpartum in 33% individuals at 3 months postpartum and 8.5% at 2 years postpartum.[9] In the postpartum period, ergonomic challenges related to infant care—such as breastfeeding posture, prolonged carrying, and interrupted rest—may further aggravate musculoskeletal discomfort. While physical therapy and support devices can be beneficial, underutilization is common, especially in populations with limited postpartum follow-up or financial resources.

Pain following vaginal delivery is driven by continued uterine contractions and perineal lacerations, while breast engorgement and post-cesarean delivery surgical pain account for other etiologies. Given the multifactorial nature, one should use multimodal analgesia such as nonsteroidal anti-inflammatory drugs, acetaminophen, opioids, regional/neuraxial anesthesia (e.g., epidural, fascial plane blockade, etc.), local analgesia, ice packs, heat packs, abdominal binders, etc.[10] Early pain control not only supports mobility and breastfeeding but also reduces the risk of persistent pain and mood complications. Shared decision-making to determine the timing and method of pain control is paramount.[10]

Neurobiological and Hormonal Responses

Pain during and after childbirth is shaped by complex neuroendocrine interactions. During labor, increased oxytocin facilitates uterine contractions but also promotes maternal behaviors and analgesia via central pathways. Endogenous opioids and catecholamines are released in response to pain and stress, modulating both perception and emotional response.[11]

Estrogen and progesterone decrease immediately following delivery, which increases sensitivity to pain and mood changes. Decrease in cortisol in the postpartum setting escalates the inflammatory response, often worsening the pain. These changes in hormones affect pain perception, mood, and maternal–infant bonding. Uncontrolled severe pain in the postpartum setting is an independent risk factor for development of persistent pain, regardless of mode of delivery. Also, individuals with severe acute pain had threefold increased risk of developing postpartum depression.[12]

Psychological and Physical Impact of Pain on Well-Being

Depending on the source cited, chronic pain is often defined as that persisting for >3 months. Per one source, the incidence of development of chronic pain after pain experienced during pregnancy and delivery is approximately 15%.[13] There is a strong association between pain during pregnancy and psychological distress.[14] Catastrophizing, defined as rumination, magnification, or feeling helpless in the presence of pain is of particular concern.[14] Individuals in the moderate pain catastrophizing group are more likely to experience greater pain interference, pain intensity, anxiety, depression, and insomnia at baseline.[13] This group is also more likely to report increased pain intensity pre- and post-delivery and worsened physical recovery in the postpartum setting, which can impact performing activities of daily living. These individuals may benefit from monitoring and managing pain symptoms accordingly throughout pregnancy.[13]

Individuals who experience high pain catastrophizing, pain intensity, anxiety, depression, and insomnia are more likely to have high pain interference in daily social and physical activities. Importantly, early intervention with pain coping strategies and pain management may decrease pain-related disability and improve quality of life.[13]

Uncontrolled pain may also increase the risk of birth trauma, especially among individuals with prior trauma or unmet expectations around delivery.[15] Studies using validated measures have demonstrated that individuals with perineal pain at 4–6 weeks postpartum had an increased risk of depression at 6 months.[16] The relationship between pain and emotional well-being is bidirectional. There is growing evidence that depression influences pain thresholds and that pain can significantly increase risk for depression and anxiety.[17] Postpartum mood disorders such as anxiety, depression, and posttraumatic stress disorder (PTSD) can adversely affect maternal bonding with the infant which, in turn, can have negative impacts on infant health.[15,17,18]

Physical manifestations of pain include trouble performing activities of daily living, social/physical activities, and work obligations. This, in turn, can affect self-esteem, cause loss of identity, and can negatively impact sexual relationships.[19]

Health Disparities in Pain for Women's Health

Equitable pain management continues to be elusive in the current medical system, with deep roots that date back multiple centuries. Certain preconceived notions such as higher pain tolerance and "thicker skin" in minority groups are still pervasive in the lay population and the medical community.[20] Several studies have demonstrated that black and Hispanic patients are less likely to receive neuraxial analgesia during labor and adequate postoperative pain management and more likely to have their pain dismissed or undertreated.[21]

Clinical Practice Recommendations

A team-based approach involving obstetricians, anesthesiologists, physical therapists, mental health professionals, and lactation consultants is essential. Early identification of individuals at risk for chronic pain or mood disorders enables timely intervention prior to or after delivery. Structured follow-up beyond the standard 6-week visit is critical for monitoring pain, especially musculoskeletal and neuropathic pain syndromes that could signal nerve injury during labor.

Enhanced education on pain physiology, trauma-informed care, and equity-focused communication is essential for frontline providers. Institutional protocols should include universal pain assessments that are culturally sensitive and free of bias.

Policy changes are needed to ensure postpartum care includes coverage for physical therapy, mental health support, and lactation services. Medicaid extensions through 12 months postpartum offer an opportunity to embed pain assessment and treatment into routine care.

Conclusion

Pain in the perinatal period is not simply a side effect of childbirth—it is a determinant of physical recovery, emotional well-being, and maternal identity. Addressing pain comprehensively and equitably can improve not only clinical outcomes but also the lived experience of parenthood. By recognizing pain as both a biological and social issue, healthcare systems can support a more equitable and humane postpartum recovery for all.

References

1. DiTomasso D. Bearing the Pain. J Perinatal Neonatal Nurs. 2019;33(4):322–330. doi:10.1097/JPN.0000000000000407
2. Caton D. The influence of social values on obstetric anesthesia. AMA J Ethics. 2015;17(3):253–257. doi:10.1001/journalofethics.2015.17.3.msoc1-1503
3. Hewison A. The language of labour: An examination of the discourses of childbirth. Midwifery. 1993;9(4):225–234. doi:10.1016/0266-6138(93)90006-E
4. National Guideline Alliance (UK). Management of pelvic girdle pain in pregnancy: Antenatal care: Evidence review. National Institute for Health and Care Excellence (NICE). 2021. Accessed June 27, 2025. http://www.ncbi.nlm.nih.gov/books/NBK573945/
5. Munro A, George RB, Chorney J, Snelgrove-Clarke E, Rosen NO. Prevalence and predictors of chronic pain in pregnancy and postpartum. J Obstet Gynaecol Can. 2017;39(9):734–741. doi:10.1016/j.jogc.2017.01.026
6. Dunn G, Egger MJ, Shaw JM, et al. Trajectories of lower back, upper back, and pelvic girdle pain during pregnancy and early postpartum in primiparous women. Womens Health Lond Engl. 2019;15:1745506519842757. doi:10.1177/1745506519842757
7. Sward L, Manning N, Murchison AB, Ghahremani T, McCaulley JA, Magann EF. Pelvic girdle pain in pregnancy: A review. Obstet Gynecol Surv. 2023;78(6):349–357. doi:10.1097/OGX.0000000000001140
8. Mackenzie J, Murray E, Lusher J. Women's experiences of pregnancy related pelvic girdle pain: A systematic review. Midwifery. 2018;56:102–111. doi:10.1016/j.midw.2017.10.011
9. Wuytack F, Daly D, Curtis E, Begley C. Prognostic factors for pregnancy-related pelvic girdle pain: A systematic review. Midwifery. 2018;66:70–78. doi:10.1016/j.midw.2018.07.012
10. American College of Obstetricians and Gynecologists (ACOG). Pharmacologic stepwise multimodal approach for postpartum pain management: ACOG Clinical Consensus No. 1. *Obstetrics & Gynecology*. 2021;138(3):507–517. doi:10.1097/AOG.0000000000004517.
11. Russell JA, Douglas AJ, Ingram CD. Brain preparations for maternity: Adaptive changes in behavioral and neuroendocrine systems during pregnancy and lactation. An overview. Prog Brain Res. 2001;133:1–38. doi:10.1016/s0079-6123(01)33002-9
12. Eisenach JC, Pan PH, Smiley R, Lavand'homme P, Landau R, Houle TT. Severity of acute pain after childbirth, but not type of delivery, predicts persistent pain and postpartum depression. Pain. 2008;140(1):87–94. doi:10.1016/j.pain.2008.07.011
13. Jessa J, Tomfohr-Madsen L, Dhillon A, et al. Trajectories of pain intensity, pain catastrophizing, and pain interference in the perinatal and postpartum period. PAIN Rep. 2024;9(2):e1137. doi:10.1097/PR9.0000000000001137

14. Doğru HY, Özsoy F, Doğru S, et al. Catastrophizing, depression and anxiety during pregnancy: Relation between lumbopelvic pain and physical/social functioning. J Ration-Emotive Cogn-Behav Ther. 2018;36(2):119–136. doi:10.1007/s10942-017-0277-z
15. Dekel S, Stuebe C, Dishy G. Childbirth induced posttraumatic stress syndrome: A systematic review of prevalence and risk factors. Front Psychol. 2017;8. doi:10.3389/fpsyg.2017.00560
16. Chang SR, Chen KH, Lee CN, Shyu MK, Lin MI, Lin WA. Relationships between perineal pain and postpartum depressive symptoms: A prospective cohort study. Int J Nurs Stud. 2016;59:68–78. doi:10.1016/j.ijnurstu.2016.02.012
17. Xiong P, Poehlmann J, Stowe Z, Antony K. Anxiety, depression, and pain in the perinatal period: A review for obstetric care providers. Obstet Gynecol Surv. 2021;76(11):692–713. doi:10.1097/OGX.0000000000000958.
18. Williams C, Patricia Taylor E, Schwannauer M. A web-based survey of mother–infant bond, attachment experiences, and metacognition in posttraumatic stress following childbirth. Infant Ment Health J. 2016;37(3):259–273. doi:10.1002/imhj.21564
19. Dantas THM, Dantas DS, Correia GN, Viana ESR, Pereira ARR, Magalhães AG. Disability and functioning of women with low-risk pregnancy: Assessment using the World Health Organization Disability Assessment Schedule 2.0 (WHODAS 2.0). Int J Gynaecol Obstet Off Organ Int Fed Gynaecol Obstet. 2020;148(1):53–58. doi:10.1002/ijgo.12985
20. Hoffman KM, Trawalter S, Axt JR, Oliver MN. Racial bias in pain assessment and treatment recommendations, and false beliefs about biological differences between blacks and whites. Proc Natl Acad Sci. 2016;113(16):4296–4301. doi:10.1073/pnas.1516047113
21. Johnson JD, Cooper S, Badreldin N, Green C. How can we get to equitable and effective postpartum pain control? *Clin Obstet Gynecol*. Published online June 13, 2022. doi:10.1097/GRF.0000000000000731

40
Managing Pregnancy-Related Pain

Pharmacologic and Nonpharmacologic Approaches

Jarna R. Shah and Aparna Jindal

Introduction

Pain during pregnancy is a very common experience and occurrence. As discussed in the preceding chapters, anatomic and physiologic changes in the pregnancy state can exacerbate and create low back and sacroiliac joint strain. In addition, hormonal changes can worsen and trigger musculoskeletal conditions, pelvic pain, coccydynia, migraines, sciatic pain, and restless legs syndrome.[1,2] Traditionally, pharmacologic treatment options are often limited due to concern for the developing fetus. However, if the pregnant patient is in pain, either during or after the pregnancy, this places them at higher risk for anxiety, depression, disability, and difficulty taking care of their child. Providers must strive to balance treating pregnancy-related pain while weighing the risk of medication exposure on fetal growth.

General Considerations for Pharmacologic Pain Management in Pregnancy

Pharmacologic treatments are typical mainstays of pain management. However, there are limited studies assessing medication use in pregnancy due to this being considered a vulnerable research population.[3] Acetaminophen is generally considered a safe medication for use during pregnancy. This is supported by a large epidemiologic body of evidence.[4] However, if a pregnant patient overdoses on acetaminophen, this has been linked to cases of fetal hepatic toxicity.[5] The Society for Maternal Fetal Medicine recommends avoiding prolonged use of nonsteroidal anti-inflammatory drugs (NSAIDs) during pregnancy. Use in the first trimester is associated with congenital anomalies and spontaneous abortion, while NSAID use in the third trimester may be associated with premature closure of the ductus arteriosus and pulmonary hypertension.[6]

Opioids and Aspirin Use During Pregnancy

Opioids are typically prescribed for acute moderate or severe pain and can be used in pregnancy.[4] There is limited evidence to support long-term use of opioids for chronic pain during pregnancy. Risks include potential associations with congenital malformations, neonatal opioid withdrawal syndrome, and opioid use disorder.[4] The decision to start or maintain opioid therapy, as well as the risks and benefits, should be extensively discussed between the provider and the patient.[7] Daily low-dose aspirin is often used to delay or prevent preeclampsia in pregnancy and is recommended for use by the American College of Obstetricians and Gynecology.[8]

Neuropathic Agents and Muscle Relaxants

Gabapentin, used to treat neuropathic pain and restless legs syndrome, has been associated with higher risk for preterm birth and small-for-gestational age infants.[9] Muscle relaxants such as cyclobenzaprine are not recommended for chronic use in pregnancy but can be used for brief periods to treat acute musculoskeletal conditions.[10]

Nonpharmacologic Pain Management Strategies

Nonpharmacologic treatment options for pain during pregnancy are broad in nature and recommended. These can include ergonomic changes such as supported side sleeping, postural adjustments and corrections, back support, use of a sacral belt, antenatal exercises, and moderate aerobic activity.[11] Other treatment options include relaxation techniques, mindfulness, yoga, massage, reflexology, and acupuncture.[12] However, as compared to pharmacologic treatment modalities, complementary and alternative medication do not yet have strong bodies of supporting evidence.

References

1. Salari N, et al. The global prevalence of low back pain in pregnancy: A comprehensive systematic review and meta-analysis. BMC Pregnancy Childbirth. 2023;23(1):830. doi:10.1186/s12884-023-06151-x
2. Ray-Griffith SL, Wendel MP, Stowe ZN, Magann EF. Chronic pain during pregnancy: A review of the literature. Int J Womens Health. 2018;10:153–164.
3. Biggio JR Jr. Research in pregnant subjects: Increasingly important, but challenging. Ochsner J. 2020;20(1):39–43.
4. Nunge, R. A., Kendle, A. M., & Alwan, S. (2025). Pain medication use during pregnancy. *Seminars in Perinatology, 49*(4), 152074. https://doi.org/10.1016/j.semperi.2025.152074
5. Wilkes, J. M., Clark, L. E., & Herrera, J. L. (2005). Acetaminophen overdose in pregnancy. *Southern Medical Journal, 98*(11), 1118–1122. https://doi.org/10.1097/01.SMJ.0000182493.87188.B7
6. Society for Maternal-Fetal Medicine, Sinkey RG, Ogunsile FJ, et al. Society for Maternal-Fetal Medicine consult series #68: Sickle cell disease in pregnancy. Am J Obstet Gynecol. 2024;230(2):B17–B40.
7. Dowell D, Ragan KR, Jones CM, Baldwin GT, Chou R. CDC clinical practice guideline for prescribing opioids for pain—United States, 2022. MMWR Recommend Rep. 2022;71(3):1–95.
8. American College of Obstetricians and Gynecologists. Low-dose aspirin use during pregnancy. ACOG committee opinion no. 743. Obstet Gynecol. 2018;132:e44–e52.

9. Patorno E, Hernandez-Diaz S, Huybrechts KF, et al. Gabapentin in pregnancy and the risk of adverse neonatal and maternal outcomes: A population-based cohort study nested in the US Medicaid Analytic eXtract dataset. PLoS Med. 2020;17(9):e1003322.
10. Fisher SC, Howley MM, Tran EL, et al. Maternal cyclobenzaprine exposure and risk of birth defects in the National Birth Defects Prevention Study (1997–2011) and Birth Defects Study to Evaluate Pregnancy exposureS (2014–2018). Pharmacoepidemiol Drug Saf. 2023;32(8):855–862.
11. Katonis P, Kampouroglou A, Aggelopoulos A, et al. Pregnancy-related low back pain. Hippokratia. 2011;15(3):205–210.
12. Zuarez-Easton S, Erez O, Zafran N, Carmeli J, Garmi G, Salim R. Pharmacologic and non-pharmacologic options for pain relief during labor: An expert review. Am J Obstet Gynecol. 2023;228(5S):S1246–S1259. doi:10.1016/j.ajog.2023.03.003

41

Pain Relief During Labor and Delivery

Epidural Anesthesia and Alternative Methods

Chadwick Barker, Borys Shturman, and Gary Schwartz

Introduction

Pain is an inevitable aspect of childbirth that nearly every delivering mother expects. Its source is complex and involves both visceral and somatic components. During the first stage of labor the pain originates from uterine contractions and cervical dilation. These pain signals get transmitted via visceral afferent fibers that the enter the spinal cord at the T10–L1 levels. As labor progresses into the second stage, vaginal distension and perineal stretching leads to somatic pain conveyed via the pudendal, ilioinguinal, and genitofemoral nerves. Effective analgesia must address both these phases, with neuraxial techniques being the most time-tested and effective. Despite this, systemic medications and nonpharmacologic techniques have also shown to be useful adjuncts in individualized care plans.[1]

Epidural Analgesia

Epidural analgesia is the gold standard of intrapartum pain management. It works by administering medications into the lumbar epidural space via a catheter, which block the transmission of pain signals from the uterus and vaginal canal. The goal is to produce a dense sensory block while preserving motor function, allowing for limited patient mobility and participation in active pushing during the second stage of labor.

Patient-controlled epidural analgesia (PCEA) allows for additional patient autonomy when it comes to pain management. Studies have shown that PCEA can reduce total anesthetic use, improve patient satisfaction, increase successful spontaneous vaginal delivery rates, and decrease the need for clinician-administered boluses.[3] Nevertheless, epidural analgesia is not without complications. These include but are not limited to transient fetal bradycardia (20%), maternal pruritus (15–20%), postdural puncture headache (1–3%), and more rare complications such as meningitis or epidural hematoma (<0.1%).[1]

From a physiologic standpoint, effective epidural analgesia can reduce the maternal catecholamine surge that typically accompanies labor pain. This reduction leads to decreased uterine vasoconstriction, which assists with uterine perfusion and oxygen delivery to the fetus, a significant benefit for high-risk pregnancies such as those involving preeclampsia, cardiac disease, or fetal growth restriction. Additionally, if an emergency cesarean is required, epidurals establish a reliable route for prompt conversion to surgical anesthesia. This makes them a strategic option in labors with high risk of operative intervention.

Spinal and Combined Spinal-Epidural Techniques

With spinal anesthetics a small volume of opioid with or without a local anesthetic is injected directly into the subarachnoid space. This approach provides rapid-onset analgesia, usually within 1–5 minutes, making it highly effective in emergency clinical scenarios (e.g., cesarian sections) or in patients arriving in advanced labor. The primary disadvantage of this method stems from the relatively short duration of action, which varies depending on the specific medications administered. The inability to extend the block duration after injection makes spinals as a sole anesthetic impractical for standard labor analgesia.

To overcome these limitations, many providers opt for the combined spinal-epidural (CSE) technique, which merges the advantages of both. In this approach, after performing a dural puncture to deliver intrathecal medications, an epidural catheter is inserted to facilitate the maintenance of analgesia. While the intrathecal component provides immediate and often dramatic pain relief, the epidural catheter allows for flexible, titratable dosing throughout the remainder of the labor.

CSE is particularly valuable in clinical settings where rapid analgesia is needed, such as induced labors with strong contractions or in patients arriving in pronounced distress from labor pain. Maternal satisfaction with CSE is consistently high, likely due to the fast onset and consistent, effective pain control.[1]

Indications and Contraindications

Maternal request alone is a sufficient indication for neuraxial anesthesia. Clinical indications could include medical comorbidities (e.g., preeclampsia, cardiac/pulmonary disease), prolonged labor, or anticipated cesarean delivery (see Table 41.1).

Systemic Analgesics

When neuraxial options are contraindicated or declined, intravenous opioids (e.g., fentanyl or remifentanil) may offer an alternative for temporary and partial pain relief. Fentanyl has a fast onset and short duration but crosses the placenta, posing risks of neonatal sedation if given near delivery. It can be administered intermittently or via a patient-controlled analgesia (PCA) pump, offering some degree of autonomy and titration.

Remifentanil, due to its ultra-short half-life, has emerged as an alternative to fentanyl by offering rapid titration. However, because of its potent respiratory depressant effects and the

Table 41.1 Contraindications to neuraxial analgesia

Absolute	Relative
Patient refusal	Coagulopathy
Infection at site of injection	Sepsis
Uncorrected hypovolemia	Fixed cardiac output states
Allergy to medications	Aortic stenosis
Elevated intracranial pressure	Indeterminate neurological states

absence of a ceiling dose, its use mandates continuous one-on-one monitoring with pulse oximetry and immediate access to resuscitative equipment. Maternal desaturation, hypoventilation, and even apnea are all possible. Appropriately, its use is generally limited to tertiary care centers with adequate staffing.[1]

Systemic opioids are a useful but limited option in the obstetric analgesia toolkit. They do not provide the same level of pain relief or physiologic benefit as neuraxial techniques and should be best viewed as bridging or adjunctive measures, not substitutes.[1] Early discussion of realistic anesthetic expectations is essential to prevent patients from anticipating greater pain relief than what can be safely provided.

Nitrous Oxide

Self-administered 50:50 mixture of nitrous oxide (NO) and oxygen offers immediate but mild analgesia and anxiolysis. It is popular for early labor or needle-averse patients and has minimal impact on mobility or uterine tone. Nevertheless, its effectiveness is limited, with many patients ultimately transitioning to epidural analgesia as labor progresses. Studies have demonstrated that only 31% of women who utilize NO during labor do not necessitate a transition to more invasive analgesics.[1,4]

Nonpharmacologic Techniques

Nonpharmacologic methods often receive insufficient recognition, but they have the potential to become essential components of multimodal labor analgesia. These methods enhance maternal satisfaction while supporting natural labor processes and potentially decreasing the need for systemic or neuraxial pain management. The pain relief from these methods does not match epidural effectiveness, yet they help patients cope with pain and feel more relaxed while gaining control over their experience.

1. *Hydrotherapy* requires patients to submerge themselves in warm water either through a shower or birthing tub. Research indicates that hydrotherapy leads to decreased epidural use and shorter labor times and better birth satisfaction ratings.[6] The proposed mechanisms are reduced gravitational strain on muscles, promoted mobility, and decreased circulating stress hormones. Water immersion works best during early labor stages until active pushing starts because infection control requires its discontinuation.
2. A *transcutaneous electrical nerve stimulation* (TENS) device sends low-voltage electrical signals to the lower back area, which targets the dermatomes responsible for uterine pain. Multiple randomized trials have produced inconsistent results, but numerous women describe better pain management and comfort through this method. The safety features and noninvasive nature and portability of TENS make it an appropriate addition to pain management when neuraxial methods are unavailable or unacceptable.[2,5]
3. *Breathing and relaxation techniques* involve teaching patients to perform rhythmic breathing patterns that help them focus on something else while improving oxygenation and reducing anxiety. These approaches achieve their best results when expectant

mothers learn them antenatal with the guidance of a trained support person such as a doula. Research indicates that continuous labor support that includes these techniques leads to reduced cesarean rates and improved patient satisfaction.[1]

Personalizing Pain Treatment to the Patient

The administration of labor pain relief needs an individualized approach since no one method suits all patients. Every decision regarding epidural timing and additional therapy administration needs to evaluate patient preferences along with labor progression and medical history. Informed consent together with shared decision-making are critical to tailoring an individualized care plan. The discussion should include a thorough examination of patient goals, including but not limited to the desired level of pain relief; mobility as a crucial aspect; and past experiences along with current fears affecting perception of delivery.

The medical community recognizes maternal request as a sufficient basis to provide analgesia. The old notion that patients need to achieve specific cervical dilation before receiving epidurals is an outdated requirement. Research findings indicate that starting epidural treatment early does not raise the need for cesarean delivery nor does it negatively impact the labor course. In fact, early epidurals are often associated with better pain management, reduced maternal stress, and comparable or improved maternal satisfaction.[7,8]

The primary factor that determines the selection of analgesic technique after patient preferences is clinical context. Patients with rapid labor progression require a spinal anesthetic or remifentanil PCA to establish adequate pain relief swiftly. On the other hand, patients who are undergoing extended induction would benefit more from early placement of an epidural. The administration of a neuraxial block could also benefit high-risk patients (e.g., cardiac disease and severe preeclampsia) by providing improved hemodynamic control with reduced sympathetic tone in addition to the analgesia.[8]

Impact on Labor and Delivery

Neuraxial analgesia does not negatively affect the natural progression of labor. Epidurals can produce minor delays during the initial and second stages of labor but do not increase the need for cesarean delivery. Current evidence indicates that instrumental delivery rates (e.g., vacuum or forceps) rose slightly but did not result in any adverse effects on newborn health.[8] Research-based meta-analyses have also successfully eliminated the widespread myth that epidurals lead to chronic back pain. Proper management of epidurals combined with judicious dosing results in high patient satisfaction along with safe and positive outcomes.[1]

References

1. Bonarska M, Adasik D, Szymczyk S, Łocik G. A systematic review of contemporary and emerging analgesia techniques for natural labor: Patient-centered approaches and technological advances. J Clin Med. 2025;14(11):3977. https://www.mdpi.com/2077-0383/14/11/3977

2. Michalska A, Blazuk-Fortak A. The impact of transcutaneous electrical nerve stimulation (TENS) on the consecutive stages of labour and perinatal outcomes: A retrospective cohort study. J Clin Med. 2025;14(10):3445. https://www.mdpi.com/2077-0383/14/10/3445
3. Beg T, Daoud BE, Angelo TE. Recent updates in obstetric analgesia. Indian J Pain. 2021;35(3):147–153. https://journals.lww.com/ijpn/fulltext/2021/35030/recent_updates_in_obstetric_analgesia.2.aspx
4. Christensen JR. The use of nitrous oxide in the management of labor pain: Safety and efficacy. 2016. Bethel University Digital Library. https://spark.bethel.edu/etd/123/
5. Czech I, Fuchs P, Fuchs A, et al. Pharmacological and non-pharmacological methods of labour pain relief: Establishment of effectiveness and comparison. Int J Environment Res Public Health. 2018;15(12):2792. https://www.mdpi.com/1660-4601/15/12/2792
6. Blaine AY. Supporting physiologic labor: Effects of hydrotherapy on labor outcomes. Bethel University Electronic Theses and Dissertations. 2020. https://spark.bethel.edu/etd/78/
7. Likis FE, Andrews JC, Collins MR, et al. Nitrous oxide for the management of labor pain: A systematic review. Anesth Analg. 2014;118(1):153–167. https://journals.lww.com/anesthesia-analgesia/fulltext/2014/01000/Nitrous_Oxide_for_the_Management_of_Labor_Pain__A.18.aspx
8. Wong CA, Scavone BM, Peaceman AM, et al. The risk of cesarean delivery with neuraxial analgesia given early versus late in labor. N Engl J Med. 2005;352(7):655–665. https://www.nejm.org/doi/full/10.1056/NEJMoa042573

PART VIII

POSTPARTUM PAIN SYNDROMES

42 Patient-Centered Approaches for Postpartum Pain

Ankita Mathur, Danielle Levin, and Meera Kirpekar

Overview of the Postpartum Period

The postpartum period begins immediately after childbirth and lasts 6–8 weeks. During this time, major changes occur in the body due to physical changes, hormonal shifts, and emotional stressors.

Postpartum pain is common and falls into two categories, pelvic pain and nonpelvic pain.

- Postpartum pelvic pain includes pelvic girdle pain, pudendal neuralgia, perineal pain, scar tissue pain, and pelvic floor dysfunction.
- Postpartum nonpelvic pain includes DeQuervain tenosynovitis, carpal tunnel syndrome, breast pain, and headaches.

Clinical Management and Diagnosis

Chronic postpartum pain occurs at varying rates and can last several months to years postpartum depending on the etiology. Thorough patient history, comprehensive physical exam, and appropriate imaging modalities are needed for management. A multidisciplinary approach with an extensive knowledge of physiology, anatomy, and pharmacology due to lactation are essential for successful treatment. Depending on the etiology of pain, medical, interventional, or surgical treatments may be indicated.

The Patient-Centered Care Model

Managing chronic postpartum pain effectively requires more than a standard treatment algorithm—it calls for a patient-centered approach that recognizes the uniqueness of each individual's symptoms, lifestyle, and treatment goals. Given the complex and often misunderstood nature of chronic postpartum pain, patients frequently report long diagnostic journeys and feelings of frustration or dismissal. A patient-centered strategy emphasizes listening closely to the patient's experiences, validating their pain, and involving them actively in decision-making. This collaborative model fosters trust and improves treatment adherence and satisfaction.

Individualized Care Planning

One key aspect of a patient-centered approach is individualized care planning. Since postpartum pain presents differently in each person—with varying patterns of pain, coexisting pelvic dysfunction, and psychological impacts—treatment must be tailored accordingly. Clinicians should integrate patients' values, preferences, and concerns when recommending treatment modalities, whether they involve conservative management, interventional procedures, or surgery.

Multidisciplinary and Psychosocial Support

Multidisciplinary collaboration is another cornerstone of patient-centered care. A team-based approach ensures that care is comprehensive and holistic, addressing not only the physical condition but also the emotional, social, and functional dimensions of the patient's life. Psychosocial support, including cognitive behavioral therapy or counseling, can be particularly helpful in managing the chronic stress, anxiety, or depression that often accompanies postpartum pain.

Shared Decision-Making and Education

Shared decision-making empowers patients by offering them choices and clearly explaining the benefits and risks of each option. For example, discussing the relative merits of different treatment options allows patients to weigh outcomes and participate actively in shaping their care. Education plays a pivotal role here: patients who understand their condition and treatment options are more likely to be engaged and optimistic, which itself has a positive effect on pain management outcomes.

Suggested Reading

American College of Obstetricians and Gynecologists. Optimizing postpartum care (Committee Opinion No. 736). Obstet Gynecol.2018;131(5):e140–e150. https://doi.org/10.1097/AOG.0000000000002633

Dowell D, Ragan KR, Jones CM, Baldwin GT, Chou R. CDC clinical practice guideline for prescribing opioids for pain—United States, 2022. MMWR.2022;71(3):1–95.

Eisenach JC, Pan PH, Smiley R, Lavand'homme P, Landau R, Houle TT. Severity of acute pain after childbirth, but not type of delivery, predicts persistent pain and postpartum depression. American J Obstet Gynecol.2008;199(5):1–5. https://doi.org/10.1016/j.ajog.2008.08.011

International Association for the Study of Pain. IASP terminology and classification of chronic pain (ICD-11). Pain.2020;161(9):1976–1982. https://doi.org/10.1097/j.pain.0000000000001939

World Health Organization. (2022). *WHO recommendations on maternal and newborn care for a positive postnatal experience*. World Health Organization. https://www.who.int/publications/i/item/9789240045989

43
Pudendal Neuralgia

Ankita Mathur, Danielle Levin, and Meera Kirpekar

Epidemiology and Risk Factors

Pudendal neuralgia is a chronic and often incapacitating neuropathic pain condition that manifests as discomfort in the perineal area. It predominantly affects women, with estimates suggesting it occurs at approximately twice the rate seen in men, impacting around 1 in every 100,000 people, according to the International Pudendal Neuropathy Association.[1]

A range of factors can lead to pudendal neuralgia, especially in women. The most frequent causes include surgical procedures, pelvic trauma, and childbirth. Surgeries that commonly contribute to pudendal nerve injury include prolapse repairs—especially via the vaginal route—sling operations, and hysterectomies. Nerve damage in these cases may result from direct entrapment by sutures or mesh, or secondary to a hematoma compressing the nerve. While symptoms often begin immediately after surgery, the pain may be misattributed to typical postoperative discomfort, thus delaying diagnosis.[2,3]

In vaginal childbirth, overstretching of the pelvic floor can also damage the pudendal nerve. Additionally, a variety of medical conditions may contribute to the development of pudendal neuralgia. These include pelvic floor dysfunction and systemic illnesses such as diabetes, multiple sclerosis, inflammatory bowel disease, and certain viral infections like herpes simplex or HIV, as well as autoimmune or inflammatory disorders.[2,3]

Pathophysiology

Pudendal neuralgia arises from damage, compression, or irritation of the pudendal nerve, which originates from the sacral nerve roots (S2–S4) and supplies motor and sensory innervation to the perineum, genitals, and anus. The nerve's anatomical course makes it vulnerable at specific points, particularly as it passes between the sacrospinous and sacrotuberous ligaments and through Alcock's canal. Compression in these areas—whether due to prolonged sitting, scarring from surgery, pelvic trauma, or childbirth—can result in neuropathic pain.

Mechanistically, nerve compression or trauma leads to demyelination and axonal injury, disrupting normal nerve conduction and leading to spontaneous discharges. Over time, this can trigger peripheral and central sensitization, in which the nervous system becomes hypersensitive, amplifying pain perception even in the absence of ongoing mechanical injury. This process may also involve neuroinflammation and abnormal signaling of pain pathways in the spinal cord and brain.

Ischemia from vascular compression or hematoma can exacerbate nerve dysfunction. Additionally, dysfunction of surrounding pelvic floor muscles often coexists, either contributing to or resulting from altered pudendal nerve signaling, thus creating a cycle of pain and muscular tension.[3,4]

Diagnosis and Assessment

Pudendal neuralgia was initially identified by Amarenco and colleagues in 1987, who referred to it as "cyclist syndrome" due to its early association with competitive cyclists.[2] Today, the condition is diagnosed using the Nantes criteria, which include pain localized to the pudendal nerve region, discomfort that worsens with sitting, absence of nighttime pain, no detectable sensory deficits during a physical exam, and relief following a diagnostic anesthetic nerve block. This nerve block is not only useful for diagnosis but can also provide therapeutic benefits.[3,5]

Treatment Options

Medical Treatment Options

While research on pudendal neuralgia remains relatively limited, there are still several ways to help manage the condition without resorting to invasive procedures. Medical treatments focus on relieving symptoms through a combination of lifestyle changes, physical therapy, cognitive behavioral therapy, medications, and complementary approaches. These options aim to improve quality of life and reduce discomfort while avoiding more aggressive interventions.[2–4,6]

Lifestyle Modifications

Making simple lifestyle adjustments is often the first step in managing pudendal neuralgia as these changes can help reduce irritation to the pudendal nerve. For example, since sitting can worsen the pain, many patients find relief by using specialized cushions, such as a donut-shaped pillow or a customized seat pad, to take pressure off the affected area.

Beyond seating adjustments, broader lifestyle habits play a key role in managing chronic pain. Lifestyle medicine emphasizes six foundational pillars: eating a primarily whole-food, plant-based diet; getting quality sleep; staying physically active; managing stress with healthy coping tools; maintaining strong social connections; and avoiding harmful substances like tobacco, excessive alcohol, and opioids. These habits help lower inflammation in the body, which is crucial since inflammation tends to heighten pain levels.[7,8]

Physical Therapy

Pelvic floor physical therapy offers targeted exercises and treatments designed to either strengthen or relax the pelvic muscles, depending on the patient's specific needs. These muscles support the pelvic organs and can place pressure on nerves, including the pudendal nerve, when dysfunctional. Therapy may help address various issues such as pelvic pain, sexual dysfunction, urinary problems, and constipation.

Rather than applying a one-size-fits-all approach like Kegel exercises, physical therapists begin by assessing the pelvic floor to determine which muscles require strengthening and which need relaxation. Biofeedback tools are often used during this process to track muscle activity and guide treatment. Additional modalities like electrical stimulation or transcutaneous electrical nerve stimulation (TENS) units can also be incorporated to help reduce nerve-related pain by stimulating sacral or perineal nerves.[9,10]

Cognitive Behavioral Therapy

Cognitive behavioral therapy (CBT) is a psychological treatment that has shown promising results in managing chronic pain, including pudendal neuralgia. It focuses on changing negative thought patterns and emotional responses, particularly anxiety, depression, and pain catastrophizing. By addressing these mental health factors, CBT can help reduce pain perception and improve sexual function and quality of life.[11,12]

Pharmacologic Therapy

Medications can also play a helpful role in managing pudendal neuralgia, especially those aimed at calming nerve activity or relaxing muscles. Muscle relaxants such as baclofen, tizanidine, cyclobenzaprine, and methocarbamol can ease tension in the pelvic floor muscles, thereby relieving pressure on the pudendal nerve.

Drugs typically used for nerve pain—such as anticonvulsants (gabapentin, pregabalin, topiramate) and certain antidepressants—can help by working both peripherally on the nerves and centrally on the brain's pain pathways. Tricyclic antidepressants like amitriptyline and nortriptyline, along with serotonin norepinephrine reuptake inhibitors (SNRIs) like duloxetine and venlafaxine, are commonly prescribed for neuropathic pain.

An emerging treatment option is low-dose naltrexone (LDN), which is traditionally used in higher doses to treat opioid and alcohol use disorders. In smaller, off-label doses (0.1–5 mg), LDN has shown potential in managing chronic pain by reducing inflammation, possibly through its effect on Toll-like receptor 4. Studies suggest that LDN is especially helpful for neuropathic pain, making it a promising option for pudendal neuralgia.[13–15]

Interventional Treatment Options

While many noninvasive strategies exist for managing pudendal neuralgia, the condition cannot be formally diagnosed without performing a pudendal nerve block, according to the Nantes criteria.

Nerve Block

A pudendal nerve block serves both diagnostic and therapeutic purposes. The procedure involves injecting a local anesthetic, with or without a corticosteroid. Steroids are often included to potentially extend the duration of relief, though research results vary regarding their effectiveness in doing so. Nonetheless, some studies indicate that adding a steroid can provide symptom relief lasting between 3 and 6 months on average.[5,16]

This block can be administered either without imaging ("blind") or guided by imaging techniques such as ultrasound, fluoroscopy, or CT. The method of delivery often depends on the specialist: obstetricians/gynecologists typically perform the injection through the vaginal canal, targeting Alcock's canal, while pain specialists generally prefer the transgluteal route, targeting the ischial spine. For the latter, using imaging is highly recommended to enhance accuracy and safety.[17]

A randomized, single-blind trial comparing ultrasound-guided and fluoroscopy-guided transgluteal blocks found both techniques equally effective in achieving nerve blockade, with no significant difference in side effects. However, the ultrasound-guided approach took longer to complete. On the downside, fluoroscopy exposes both the patient and medical team to ionizing radiation.[18]

There are limited case reports in the literature detailing the therapeutic use of fluoroscopy-guided pudendal nerve blocks. One such case, documented by Yu et al., involved a patient with severe vulvar pain following bladder cancer surgery and radiation. After undergoing five fluoroscopic nerve blocks, her pain decreased significantly—from a score of 10 down to 3—and she was later able to manage symptoms with oral medications.[19] Another case by Lee et al. described a patient with chronic pelvic pain whose pain level dropped from 9 to 6 after one fluoroscopy-guided injection, with relief lasting about two weeks.[20]

Levin et al.'s retrospective case series of 101 patients with pudendal neuralgia found that fluoroscopy-guided transgluteal pudendal nerve blocks provided effective short-term pain relief (at least 30%) in 49.4% of cases, along with improvements in medication use and daily activities. These findings suggest that this approach may be a valuable option in treating pudendal neuralgia with precision.[17]

If the initial nerve block is only useful in confirming the diagnosis but fails to provide lasting symptom relief, additional options should be considered. One possibility is to repeat the injection because some patients experience increased or prolonged relief after multiple blocks.

Radiofrequency Ablation

Another method for longer-lasting pain control is pulsed radiofrequency ablation. This technique involves delivering pulses of electrical energy to the nerve via a probe; the procedure modulates pain signals without destroying the nerve. It is usually performed under CT guidance, although fluoroscopy or ultrasound may also be used. However, data on its effectiveness for pudendal neuralgia are still limited, and more research is needed.[21,22]

Neuromodulation

Neuromodulation offers yet another route for managing chronic pudendal nerve pain. Three main types of devices currently are available: traditional spinal cord stimulators, dorsal root ganglion (DRG) stimulators, and peripheral nerve stimulators.

Spinal cord stimulators involve implanting electrodes in the epidural space along the spine, connected to a small generator implanted under the skin. Patients can use a remote to send mild electrical pulses, which replace the sensation of pain with a tingling feeling known as *paresthesia*. This method can modulate multiple nerve pathways and potentially change how the brain perceives pain.

DRG stimulation is more targeted, focusing on specific sensory nerve clusters along the spinal cord. These nerves transmit sensory information from particular body areas to the brain. Because each ganglion corresponds to a distinct body region, this technique allows precise targeting—such as the sacral nerves implicated in pudendal neuralgia.

Peripheral nerve stimulators are surgically implanted near nerves outside the brain and spinal cord. The electrode delivers rapid pulses to the targeted nerve, and patients can adjust the intensity as needed. Several case series suggest that stimulation of the sacral nerve roots may benefit patients with pelvic pain. However, studies specifically focused on pudendal nerve stimulation are sparse. Despite this, given the success of neuromodulation for other nerve-related conditions, it remains a promising option—though high costs and insurance barriers may limit access.[23–25]

Surgical Treatment

Surgery may be considered for patients who meet all five Nantes criteria and have not responded to other treatments. Pudendal nerve decompression, or nerve release surgery, is designed to relieve pressure on the nerve by freeing it from surrounding structures. Several surgical routes are available, including transgluteal, transperineal, laparoscopic, and endoscopic gluteal approaches. No single technique proved superior to the others.

However, very few surgeons specialize in this procedure, and insurance coverage can be a significant barrier. When performed on appropriately selected patients, surgical outcomes are promising, with reported success rates between 60% and 80%.[26]

Complications and Comorbidities

Pudendal neuralgia can be a complex and debilitating condition not only because of the chronic pain it causes but also due to its association with several complications and comorbidities. One of the most significant complications is the impact on quality of life. The persistent, sharp, or burning pain in the pelvic region—often worsened by sitting—can severely limit mobility, sexual function, and participation in daily activities. This can lead to emotional distress, anxiety, and depression, which are commonly observed comorbidities. In fact, the chronic nature of the pain and the difficulty in obtaining a timely and accurate diagnosis often exacerbate psychological stress and contribute to a sense of hopelessness in patients.[27]

Other complications can include urinary, bowel, and sexual dysfunction, depending on which branches of the pudendal nerve are affected. Patients may experience urinary urgency, hesitancy, or incontinence, as well as constipation or fecal incontinence. Sexual dysfunction—such as pain during intercourse (dyspareunia), erectile dysfunction, or loss of genital sensation—is also frequently reported and can strain intimate relationships. Additionally, patients may develop muscular imbalances or pelvic floor dysfunction as they unconsciously alter their posture or movement to avoid triggering pain.

Because pudendal neuralgia is often misdiagnosed or underdiagnosed, patients may undergo unnecessary treatments or surgeries, which can lead to further complications. Overall, managing the condition requires a multidisciplinary approach that addresses both the physical and psychological components of the disease.[6,27]

References

1. Hibner M, Desai N, Robertson LJ, Nour M. Pudendal neuralgia. J Minim Invasive Gynecol. 2010;17:148–153. doi:10.1016/j.jmig.2009.11.003
2. Amarenco G, Lanoe Y, Perrigot M, Goudal H. A new canal syndrome: Compression of the pudendal nerve in Alcock's canal or perinal paralysis of cyclists. Presse Med. 1987;16:399.
3. Kaur J, Leslie SW, Singh P. Pudendal nerve entrapment syndrome. StatPearls. February 15, 2026. https://www.ncbi.nlm.nih.gov/books/NBK544272/
4. Khoder W, Hale D. Pudendal neuralgia. Obstet Gynecol Clin North Am. 2014 Sep;41(3):443-52. doi: 10.1016/j.ogc.2014.04.002. Epub 2014 Jul 9. PMID: 25155124.
5. Labat JJ, Riant T, Robert R, Amarenco G, Lefaucheur JP, Rigaud J. Diagnostic criteria for pudendal neuralgia by pudendal nerve entrapment (Nantes criteria). Neurourol Urodyn. 2008;27:306–310. doi:10.1002/nau.20505
6. Leslie SW, Antolak S, Feloney MP, Soon-Sutton TL. Pudendal neuralgia. StatPearls. February 12, 2024. https://pubmed.ncbi.nlm.nih.gov/32965917/
7. Saxena R, Gupta M, Shankar N, Jain S, Saxena A. Effects of yogic intervention on pain scores and quality of life in females with chronic pelvic pain. Int J Yoga. 2017;10:9–15.
8. Levesque A, Bautrant E, Quistrebert V, et al. Recommendations on the management of pudendal nerve entrapment syndrome: A formalised expert consensus. Eur J Pain. 2022;26:7–17.
9. Vallinga MS, Spoelstra SK, Hemel IL, van de Wiel HB, Weijmar Schultz WC. Transcutaneous electrical nerve stimulation as an additional treatment for women suffering from therapy-resistant provoked vestibulodynia: A feasibility study. J Sex Med. 2015;12:228–237.
10. Berghmans B. Physiotherapy for pelvic pain and female sexual dysfunction: An untapped resource. Int Urogynecol J. 2018;29:631–638.
11. Ehde DM, Dillworth TM, Turner JA. Cognitive-behavioral therapy for individuals with chronic pain: Efficacy, innovations, and directions for research. Am Psychol. 2014;69:153–166.
12. Urits I, Callan J, Moore WC, et al. Cognitive behavioral therapy for the treatment of chronic pelvic pain. Best Pract Res Clin Anaesthesiol. 2020;34:409–426.
13. Younger J, Parkitny L, McLain D. The use of low-dose naltrexone (LDN) as a novel anti-inflammatory treatment for chronic pain. Clin Rheumatol. 2014;33:451–459. doi:10.1007/s10067-014-2517-2
14. Nicotra L, Loram LC, Watkins LR, Hutchinson MR. Toll-like receptors in chronic pain. Exp Neurol. 2012;234:316–329.

15. McKenzie-Brown AM, Boorman DW, Ibanez KR, Agwu E, Singh V. Low-dose naltrexone (LDN) for chronic pain at a single institution: A case series. J Pain Res. 2023;16:1993–1998. doi: 10.2147/JPR.S389957
16. Kastler A, Puget J, Tiberghien F, Pellat JM, Krainik A, Kastler B. Dual site pudendal nerve infiltration: More than just a diagnostic test? Pain Physician. 2018;21:83–90.
17. Levin D, Van Florcke D, Schmitt M, Kendall LK, Patel A, Doan LV, Kirpekar M. Fluoroscopy-guided transgluteal pudendal nerve block for pudendal neuralgia: A retrospective case series. J Clin Med. 2024;13(9):2636. doi:10.3390/jcm13092636
18. Bellingham GA, Bhatia A, Chan CW, Peng PW. Randomized controlled trial comparing pudendal nerve block under ultrasound and fluoroscopic guidance. Reg Anesth Pain Med. 2012;37:262–266.
19. Yu JH, Lee YJ, Kim JY, Lee WY, Lim YH. Treatment of radiation-induced vulvar pain via pudendal nerve block under fluoroscopic guidance. Urol Case Rep. 2020;33:101282. doi:10.1016/j.eucr.2020.101282
20. Lee SH, Lee CJ, Lee JY, Kim TH, Sim WS, Lee SY, Hwang HY. Fluoroscopy-guided pudendal nerve block and pulsed radiofrequency treatment: A case report. Korean J Anesthesiol. 2009;56:605–608. doi:10.4097/kjae.2009.56.5.605
21. Collard MD, Xi Y, Patel AA, Scott KM, Jones S, Chhabra A. Initial experience of CT-guided pulsed radiofrequency ablation of the pudendal nerve for chronic recalcitrant pelvic pain. Clin Radiol. 2019;74:897.e17–897.e23.
22. Wang X. Clinical effect and safety of pulsed radiofrequency treatment for pudendal neuralgia: A prospective, randomized controlled clinical trial. J Pain Res. 2018;11:2367–2374.
23. Peters KM, Killinger KA, Jaeger C, Chen C. Pilot study exploring chronic pudendal neuromodulation as a treatment option for pain associated with pudendal neuralgia. Low Urin Tract Symptoms. 2015;7:138–142.
24. Buffenoir K, Rioult B, Hamel O, Labat JJ, Riant T, Robert R. Spinal cord stimulation of the conus medullaris for refractory pudendal neuralgia: A prospective study of 27 consecutive cases. Neurourol Urodyn. 2015;34:177–182.
25. Hunter CW, Yang A. Dorsal root ganglion stimulation for chronic pelvic pain: A case series and technical report on a novel lead configuration. Neuromodulation. 2019;22:87–95.
26. Waxweiler C, Dobos S, Thill V, Bruyninx L. Selection criteria for surgical treatment of pudendal neuralgia. Neurourol Urodyn. 2017;36:663–666.
27. Romão AP, Gorayeb R, Romão GS, Poli-Neto OB, dos Reis FJ, Rosa-e-Silva JC, Nogueira AA. High levels of anxiety and depression have a negative effect on quality of life of women with chronic pelvic pain. Int J Clin Pract. 2009 May;63(5):707–711. doi:10.1111/j.1742-1241.2009.02034.x

44
Pelvic Girdle Pain

Ankita Mathur, Danielle Levin, and Meera Kirpekar

Epidemiology and Risk Factors

Pelvic girdle pain (PGP) is defined as pain felt between the posterior iliac crest and gluteal line, especially near the sacroiliac joint.[1] It is considered among the most common etiologies of musculoskeletal pain in parturients, affecting approximately 50% of pregnant women. The condition is self-limited for the majority of patients, resolving within 3 months after delivery. However, approximately 30% of patients report continued PGP beyond 3 months postpartum.[2]

The main risk factors for postpartum PGP are history of lower back pain or PGP, pelvic trauma, and strenuous physical activity. Interestingly, height, weight, age, smoking, use of oral contraceptives, and time between pregnancies do not contribute to the risk of developing PGP. Neuraxial anesthesia is also not associated with the development of PGP.[3]

Pathophysiology

PGP usually starts in the 18th week of gestation. It often peaks between weeks 24–36. However, it can start as late as 3 weeks postpartum. The exact mechanism underlying the development of PGP is unknown. However, it is hypothesized that it is caused by a combination of hormonal and biomechanical changes.[3]

The pelvis plays an important role in transferring weight from the spine to the lower extremities. The various joints of the pelvis, especially the sacroiliac joint, stabilize the pelvis and allow it to tilt and rotate during ambulation. This helps with shock absorption while walking.[3]

During pregnancy, the corpus luteum and uterine decidua produce the hormone relaxin in increased quantities. This allows for relaxation of connective tissues and thus increased laxity of the joints. Patients with PGP tend to have greater laxity of their pelvic joints. Their pelvic joints tend to have greater motion, which decreases pelvic stabilization. As a result, the shock absorption function of the pelvis is compromised. This increase in shear forces across the joints is thought to be the cause of PGP.[3]

Diagnosis and Assessment

PGP is often described as dull, burning, shooting, or stabbing pain that originates between the posterior iliac crest and gluteal line, often involving the sacroiliac joint. It can radiate to the posterior thigh and is often associated with pubic symphysis pain. The pain is usually

References

1. Burani E, Marruganti S, Giglioni G, Bonetti F, Ceron D, Cozzi Lepri A. Predictive factors for pregnancy-related persistent pelvic girdle pain (PPGP): A systematic review. Medicina (Kaunas). 2023;59(12):2123. doi: 10.3390/medicina59122123
2. Wiezer M, Hage-Fransen MAH, Otto A, et al. Risk factors for pelvic girdle pain postpartum and pregnancy related low back pain postpartum: A systematic review and meta-analysis. Musculoskelet Sci Pract. 2020;48:102154.
3. Vermani E, Mittal R, Weeks A. Pelvic girdle pain and low back pain in pregnancy: A review. Pain Practice. 2010;10(1):60–71.
4. Vleeming A, Albert HB, Ostgaard HC, et al. European guidelines for the diagnosis and treatment of pelvic girdle pain. Eur Spine J. 2008;17(6):794–819.

45

Perineal Pain

Ankita Mathur, Danielle Levin, and Meera Kirpekar

Epidemiology and Risk Factors

Perineal pain following childbirth is a common and significant maternal morbidity, most frequently associated with perineal tears and lacerations sustained during vaginal delivery. Epidemiological studies estimate that approximately 85% of women who undergo vaginal birth experience some form of perineal trauma, with nearly 70% requiring suturing.[1] Among these, a subset—ranging between 3% and 10%—suffer from more severe trauma involving the anal sphincter complex, categorized as third- or fourth-degree obstetric anal sphincter injuries (OASIS).[2]

The incidence and severity of perineal trauma are influenced by several maternal, fetal, and obstetric factors. Primiparous women are at heightened risk due to reduced perineal elasticity. Instrumental deliveries, particularly with forceps, are strongly correlated with higher rates of severe lacerations. Fetal macrosomia, generally defined as a birth weight exceeding 4,000 grams, increases the risk of tissue overstretching and subsequent tearing. Malpresentation, such as occiput posterior positioning, and complications like shoulder dystocia further elevate the likelihood of perineal trauma. A prolonged second stage of labor increases tissue fatigue and pressure, while a precipitous delivery can lead to sudden, unbuffered strain. Midline episiotomy, although less commonly used in contemporary obstetric practice, remains a risk factor for third- and fourth-degree tears, particularly when performed without clear indication. Awareness of these risk factors can inform intrapartum care strategies aimed at minimizing perineal injury.[3–5]

Pathophysiology

Perineal tears result from mechanical overstretching of the perineal tissues during the descent and expulsion of the fetal head and shoulders. The extent of injury is classified by degrees.

- *First degree*: Superficial, involving only the vaginal mucosa and perineal skin.
- *Second degree*: Extends into the underlying perineal muscles without disrupting the anal sphincter.
- *Third degree*: Compromises the external and/or internal anal sphincter.
- *Fourth degree*: Breaches both the anal sphincter and rectal mucosa.

The primary pathological process involves the tearing of connective tissue and muscle fibers, followed by an acute inflammatory response. This cascade includes local edema, leukocyte infiltration, and nociceptor activation, all of which contribute to pain and impaired function. When the injury involves the anal sphincter or surrounding nerve structures—particularly branches of the pudendal nerve—pain may persist beyond the acute phase, resulting in chronic perineal pain or pelvic floor dysfunction. Neuropathic mechanisms, including scar entrapment or nerve damage, may exacerbate the pain and complicate recovery.[6]

Diagnosis and Assessment

Accurate diagnosis of perineal tears is critical to ensure appropriate management and minimize long-term complications. Clinical evaluation should be conducted immediately postpartum, ideally in a well-lit environment with the woman in the lithotomy position to allow complete visualization of the perineal, vaginal, and rectal regions. Digital rectal examination is essential when sphincter involvement is suspected or when lacerations are extensive because superficial inspection alone may fail to identify deeper injuries.

Pain assessment should utilize validated instruments such as the Visual Analog Scale (VAS) or the Numeric Rating Scale (NRS). In cases where anal sphincter integrity is uncertain, further diagnostic tools such as anorectal manometry or endoanal ultrasonography may be warranted. These assessments are particularly useful for detecting occult OASIS, which may otherwise go unrecognized. Postpartum follow-up, typically at 6–12 weeks, should include reassessment of pain, wound healing, continence status, and sexual function.[7]

Medical Management

Initial management involves pharmacologic and supportive strategies. Nonsteroidal anti-inflammatory drugs (NSAIDs), such as ibuprofen, are the cornerstone of therapy. Paracetamol may be added or used as an alternative. Topical anesthetics like lidocaine gel can provide localized relief in the early postpartum period.[8,9]

Stool softeners, such as docusate sodium or polyethylene glycol, are commonly prescribed to prevent constipation and minimize straining.[10] Ice packs or cold compresses applied intermittently during the first 24 hours postpartum can further reduce swelling.[9] Warm sitz baths, beginning after the acute phase, help soothe the region and enhance circulation.

Surgical Management

Surgical intervention is necessary for second- or higher-degree tears. Second-degree lacerations require layered closure using absorbable sutures; continuous suturing techniques are often preferred for reduced postpartum pain.[11]

Repair of third- and fourth-degree tears demands meticulous technique under regional or general anesthesia. The external anal sphincter may be repaired using end-to-end or overlapping methods. Antibiotic prophylaxis and stool softeners are essential adjuncts to reduce the risk of wound infection and dehiscence.[11,12]

Other Interventions

Pelvic floor physiotherapy focuses on strengthening and relaxation of the pelvic floor muscles. Low-level laser therapy has also been shown to significantly reduce pain and improve healing compared to placebo.[13] Furthermore, psychological support, including counseling and music therapy, can be helpful for women experiencing birth-related trauma or anxiety.[14]

Complications and Comorbidities

Failure to adequately manage perineal tears can result in chronic perineal pain, anal and urinary incontinence, and dyspareunia (painful intercourse). Infections, wound dehiscence, and fistula formation are rare but serious sequelae. Moreover, the cumulative effect of pelvic floor injury increases the lifetime risk of pelvic organ prolapse.[15,16]

References

1. Kettle C, Dowswell T, Ismail KM. Continuous and interrupted suturing techniques for repair of episiotomy or second-degree tears. Cochrane Database Syst Rev. 2012;11(11):CD000947.
2. Sultan AH, Thakar R. Lower genital tract and anal sphincter trauma. Best Pract Res Clin Obstet Gynaecol. 2002;16(1):99–115.
3. Marschalek ML, Worda C, Kuessel L, et al. Risk and protective factors for obstetric anal sphincter injuries: A retrospective nationwide study. Birth. 2018;45(4):409–415.
4. Ramm O, Woo VG, Hung YY, Chen HC, Ritterman Weintraub ML. Risk factors for the development of obstetric anal sphincter injuries in modern obstetric practice. Obstet Gynecol. 2018;131(2):290–296.
5. Levin G, Rottenstreich A, Tzur T, Solomayer EF, Meyer R. Risk factors for obstetric anal sphincter injury among parous women. Arch Gynecol Obstet. 2021;303(3):709–714.
6. Macarthur AJ, Macarthur C. Incidence, severity, and determinants of perineal pain after vaginal delivery: A prospective cohort study. Am J Obstet Gynecol. 2004;191(4):1199–1204.
7. East CE, Begg L, Henshall NE, et al. Perineal pain following childbirth: Prevalence, effects on postnatal recovery and analgesia usage. Midwifery. 2012;28(1):93–97.
8. Dekker GA, Chan A, Luke CG, Priest K, McLean M, Forbes JF. Risk of uterine rupture in Australian women attempting vaginal birth after one prior caesarean section: A retrospective population-based cohort study. BJOG. 2010;117(11):1358–1365.
9. Kim HJ, Park HJ, Kim HS, Lee JH, Lee KS, Cho SH. The effects of cryotherapy on perineal pain after childbirth: A systematic review and meta-analysis. Midwifery. 2020;89:102788.
10. Gharehbaghi K, Heidari-Beni M, Rezaie P, Khorasani R, Rahbar N. Treatment of chronic functional constipation during pregnancy and lactation. Z Geburtshilfe Neonatol. 2016;220(1):9–15.
11. Martínez-Galiano JM, Delgado-Rodríguez M, Hernández-Martínez A, Rodríguez-Almagro J. Continuous versus discontinuous suture in perineal injuries produced during delivery in primiparous women: A randomized controlled trial. BMC Pregnancy Childbirth. 2019;19(1):499.

12. Fernando RJ, Sultan AH, Kettle C, Thakar R, Radley S. Repair techniques for obstetric anal sphincter injuries: A randomized controlled trial. Obstet Gynecol. 2006;107(6):1261–1268.
13. Santos Jde O, Pimenta CA, Nobre MR. A randomised clinical trial of the effect of low-level laser therapy for perineal pain and healing after episiotomy: A pilot study. Midwifery. 2012;28(5):e653–659.
14. Maleki A, Youseflu S. The effect of music-based interventions on short-term postpartum episiotomy pain: A systematic review and meta-analysis. Heliyon. 2023;9(4):e14785.
15. Doğan B, Gün İ, Özdamar Ö, Yılmaz A, Muhçu M. Long-term impacts of vaginal birth with mediolateral episiotomy on sexual and pelvic dysfunction and perineal pain. J Matern Fetal Neonatal Med. 2017;30(4):457–460.
16. Saad J, Painter C. Management of postpartum perineal wound complications. Curr Opin Obstet Gynecol. 2023;35(6):505–509.

46
Scar Tissue Pain

Ankita Mathur, Danielle Levin, and Meera Kirpekar

Epidemiology and Risk Factors

Scar tissue pain following cesarean section (C-section) is a relatively underrecognized but clinically significant complication. Studies estimate that between 10% and 30% of women experience some form of persistent pain after cesarean delivery, with a subset attributing symptoms specifically to scar tissue or adhesions.[1,2]

Risk factors are multifactorial. Surgical technique plays a central role; classical vertical incisions and multiple repeat cesarean deliveries increase the likelihood of dense scar formation and intra-abdominal adhesions. Poor wound healing, infection, and hematoma formation can also exacerbate discomfort.[1] Additionally, patients with preexisting conditions such as endometriosis may be predisposed to more extensive fibrosis and nerve entrapment syndromes.[3]

Emerging evidence points to neuropathic components in post-cesarean scar pain, particularly involving iliohypogastric and ilioinguinal nerves, which can become entrapped within scar tissue.[3] Psychosocial factors—such as anxiety and pain catastrophizing—may further modulate the perception and chronicity of pain.[2,4]

Pathophysiology

The pathophysiology of scar pain involves nociceptive, neuropathic, and inflammatory mechanisms. During a C-section, multiple tissue layers are incised. In some individuals, the healing process results in excessive collagen deposition, leading to hypertrophic scarring or keloid formation. Dense fibrous adhesions can tether adjacent structures, causing mechanical traction on the uterus, bladder, and intestines.[3,5]

Nerve involvement is a key driver of persistent pain. Cutaneous sensory nerves can be injured or entrapped, resulting in localized or radiating neuropathic pain described as burning or shooting.[5,6] Persistent nociceptive input can lead to central sensitization, a state where the nervous system becomes hypersensitive, resulting in hyperalgesia and allodynia.[3,7] Furthermore, scar endometriosis—where endometrial tissue implants within the surgical scar—can cause cyclical inflammation and pain.[5,8]

Diagnosis and Assessment

Diagnosis requires a comprehensive clinical evaluation integrating patient history and physical examination.

- *Clinical history*: Clinicians should inquire about pain quality (burning vs. aching) and timing in relation to menstruation or movement.
- *Physical examination*: Inspection for keloids and palpation for point tenderness is essential. Carnett's test—tense abdominal muscles during palpation—can help distinguish superficial from visceral pain.[9]
- *Imaging*: Ultrasound can detect neuromas or scar endometriosis. MRI may be indicated for suspected deep adhesions.[10]
- *Diagnostic blocks*: Temporary pain relief following a local anesthetic injection into the suspected nerve territory supports a neuropathic diagnosis.[11]

Medical Management

First-line treatment involves nonopioid analgesics like acetaminophen and nonsteroidal anti-inflammatory drugs (NSAIDs).[12] For neuropathic components, agents such as gabapentin, pregabalin, or duloxetine are used to modulate pain processing.[13] Topical lidocaine patches can be applied for localized relief.[14]

Physical and Manual Therapies

Manual scar mobilization and myofascial release can improve tissue pliability.[8] Referral to specialized pelvic floor physical therapy is beneficial for patients with deep pelvic pain or dyspareunia.[15]

Interventional and Surgical Treatments

Injection of local anesthetics or corticosteroids into trigger points may provide relief.[16] Diagnostic and therapeutic nerve blocks are often utilized. In refractory cases, radiofrequency ablation (RFA) of peripheral nerves may be considered.

Surgical options include

- *Surgical excision*: For hypertrophic scars or neuromas.
- *Adhesiolysis*: Laparoscopic removal of intra-abdominal adhesions.
- *Neuroma management*: Targeted excision if a specific nerve generator is identified.[8]

Emerging Therapies

Fractional laser therapy and silicone sheets may improve cosmetic and sensory outcomes for hypertrophic scars.[17] Cognitive behavioral therapy (CBT) is recommended for patients where psychosocial factors contribute to pain chronicity.[18]

Complications and Comorbidities

Common complications include intra-abdominal adhesions, which increase surgical risk in future operations.[19] Scar endometriosis remains an underestimated but notable comorbidity, often requiring surgical excision.[20]

Persistent pain can lead to psychological sequelae such as depression or posttraumatic stress disorder (PTSD). It also impacts reproductive health, potentially leading to dyspareunia and increasing the risk of uterine rupture or placenta accreta in future pregnancies.

References

1. Jin J, Peng L, Guo Q, et al. Prevalence and risk factors for chronic pain following cesarean section: A prospective study. BMC Anesthesiol. 2016;16(1):99.
2. Niklasson B, Georgsson Öhman S, Segerdahl M, Blanck A. Risk factors for persistent pain and its influence on maternal wellbeing after cesarean section. Acta Obstet Gynecol Scand. 2015;94(6):622–628.
3. Komatsu R, Carvalho B. Factors associated with persistent pain after childbirth: A narrative review. Br J Anaesth. 2020;124(3):e117–e130.
4. Badreldin N, Grobman WA, Habermann EB,. Maternal psychosocial factors associated with postpartum pain. Am J Obstet Gynecol MFM. 2023;5(5):100908.
5. Nogueira AA, Reis FJ, Poli Neto OB. The potential of cesarean section as a causative factor of chronic pelvic pain. Rev Bras Ginecol Obstet. 2016;38(2):53–55.
6. Møller, M., & Venzo, A. (2014). Entrapped nerve causing severe post-operative pain from scar tissue. *Ugeskrift for Læger, 176*(38), V04140225.
7. Tan HS, Sng BL. Persistent pain after childbirth. BJA Educ. 2022;22(1):33–37.
8. Wasserman JB, Wentz AJ, Koyyalagunta D. Chronic caesarian section scar pain treated with fascial scar release techniques. J Bodyw Mov Ther. 2016;20(4):906–913.
9. Kijima T, Yasui H, Yoshida T, et al. Adhesion-induced chronic abdominal pain: A case report on the diagnostic value of Carnett's test. J Med Case Rep. 2019;13(1):93.
10. Ryu, C., Kim, J., Lee, H., et al. (2022). Postoperative analgesic effectiveness of peripheral nerve blocks in cesarean delivery. *Journal of Personalized Medicine, 12*(4), 634. https://doi.org/10.3390/jpm12040634
11. Mitchell, K. D., Smith, K. J., Yazdi, C. A., et al. (2019). A review of peripheral nerve blocks for cesarean delivery analgesia. *Regional Anesthesia & Pain Medicine, 44*(9), 100752. https://doi.org/10.1136/rapm-2019-100752
12. Altman RD. A rationale for combining acetaminophen and NSAIDs for mild-to-moderate pain. Clin Exp Rheumatol. 2004;22(1):110–117.

13. Finnerup NB, Attal N, Haroutounian S, et al. Pharmacotherapy for neuropathic pain in adults: A systematic review and meta-analysis. Lancet Neurol. 2015;14(2):162–173.
14. Plancarte-Sánchez R, Kuri-Harcuch W, Ortega-López J. Localized neuropathic pain. Gac Med Mex. 2021;157(3):302–308.
15. Wallace SL, Miller LD, Mishra K. Pelvic floor physical therapy in the treatment of pelvic floor dysfunction in women. Curr Opin Obstet Gynecol. 2019;31(6):485–493.
16. Defalque RJ. Painful trigger points in surgical scars. Anesth Analg. 1982;61(6):518–520.
17. Leszczynski R, da Silva CA, Pinto ACPN, Kuczynski U, da Silva EM. Laser therapy for treating hypertrophic and keloid scars. Cochrane Database Syst Rev. 2022;9(9):CD011642.
18. Ehde DM, Dillworth TM, Turner JA. Cognitive-behavioral therapy for individuals with chronic pain. Am Psychol. 2014;69(2):153–166.
19. Pokhrel M, Shrestha R, Shrestha S, et al. Intra-abdominal adhesions among patients undergoing repeat caesarean section. JNMA J Nepal Med Assoc. 2022;60(250):517–520.
20. Wang WY, Chang CY, Lee YC, et al. Abdominal wall endometriosis occurring after cesarean section: An underestimated complication. Clin Exp Obstet Gynecol. 2016;43(5):678–684.

47
Pelvic Floor Dysfunction

Ankita Mathur, Danielle Levin, and Meera Kirpekar

Epidemiology and Risk Factors

The pelvic floor in females is composed of fascia, muscles, ligaments, and nerves that work together to maintain the structural integrity of the pelvis and ensure the designated positioning of pelvic organs. Weakness in any of these structures can compromise the structural integrity of the pelvic floor, leading to malpositioning and dysfunction of the organs. This can have long-term effects and can be significantly debilitating.[1]

Numerous risk factors have been associated with pelvic floor dysfunction (PFD). Individual risk factors, such as age, constipation, obesity, and menopause can weaken the pelvic floor. Lifestyle factors, such as smoking, drinking alcohol or caffeine-containing beverages, and physical activity can also contribute to pelvic floor dysfunction. Among the various risk factors, pregnancy and childbirth are known to majorly increase susceptibility to PFD. During pregnancy and childbirth, there is significant trauma to the pelvic floor, and the prevalence of PFD peaks during the postpartum period. Specific factors during childbirth, such as parity, mode of delivery, prolonged second stage of labor, administration of oxytocin, and increased fetal weight, directly increase the risk of developing PFD.[1]

Pathophysiology

Various structures are involved in maintaining the pelvic floor tone. These include deep muscles, superficial muscles, and their connections and nerve root innervations (2). Physiologic weight gain during pregnancy puts increased pressure on the pelvic floor. This, in conjunction with the increased size of the uterus and the weight of the fetus, causes significant trauma to the pelvic floor and weakens it. Furthermore, prenatal issues and childbirth can damage the pudendal nerve, pelvic floor fascia, external and internal anal sphincters, and levator ani muscles, which can also weaken the pelvic floor.[2,3]

Pregnancy is also associated with changes in collagen, both in quality and quantity. A decrease in the tensile property of collagen decreases the tone of the pelvic floor. A decrease in the collagen content leads to increased laxity of pelvic ligaments and joints. This can also contribute to PFD.[3]

Diagnosis and Assessment

Diagnosis and assessment of pelvic floor pain is clinical. Unfortunately, there is no standardized method of assessing pelvic floor pain. Physical exam plays a key role in assessment.[4] This includes assessment of the pelvic floor tone. This can be done by conducting a digital vaginal exam while asking the patient to contract the pelvic floor muscles.[5]

Meister et al. proposed an organized method of conducting a physical exam for pelvic floor muscles. According to them, the most reproducible way of assessing the pelvic floor is to evaluate both the superficial and deep structures that form the pelvic floor.[6]

The exam involves positioning the patient in a lithotomy position. Then, a unidigital transvaginal exam is performed. The pelvic floor muscles are localized by orienting the pubic symphysis at the 12 o'clock position and the anus at the 6 o'clock position.[6]

The unidigital palpation of the pelvic floor muscles is performed, beginning with the superficial muscles. The bulbospongiosus muscle can be palpated at the 2 o'clock and 10 o'clock positions. The ischiocavernosus muscle can be palpated at the 1 o'clock and 11 o'clock positions. The superficial transverse perineal muscles can be palpated at the 3 o'clock and 9 o'clock positions.[6]

After examination of the superficial muscles, the deep muscles are palpated. The pubococcygeus muscles can be palpated at the 7 o'clock and 11 o'clock positions on the left side, and 1 o'clock and 5 o'clock on the right side. The iliococcygeus muscle can be palpated at the 4 o'clock and 8 o'clock positions. The coccygeus muscle can be palpated at the 5 o'clock and 7 o'clock positions. Following this, the obturator internus muscle can be palpated at the 2 o'clock and 10 o'clock positions.[6]

During the examination, specific pressure at predetermined points on each of the muscles should be applied. A vaginal pressure algometer can be used to ensure the consistency of pressure being applied during examination. A pain assessment scale should be used to record the patient's reported score as each muscle is palpated. Examination of external genitalia, vestibule, urethra, bladder, anus, abdomen, and vaginal wall can also be included.[6]

Physical Therapy

Physical therapy is the mainstay of treating pelvic floor pain. It is also safe for breastfeeding postpartum patients. Techniques such as manual therapy, biofeedback mechanisms, relaxation training, and electrical stimulation have been shown to be helpful with postpartum PFD. Kegel exercises, although useful for strengthening the pelvic floor, can actually exacerbate pelvic floor pain.[4]

Pharmacotherapy

Some patients may not be able to tolerate physical therapy secondary to pain. In such cases, medications can also be incorporated into the treatment plan. A suppository medication containing a combination of baclofen, diazepam, and lidocaine can be helpful.[4] However, it is contraindicated for breastfeeding patients because diazepam can transfer into breast milk and have adverse effects on the breastfeeding infant.[7] Oral pain medications can also be considered while being mindful of safety in breastfeeding patients.

Interventions

Dry needling can be used for pain relief in conjunction with medications and physical therapy. This method involves identifying the most painful point(s) of the pelvic floor muscles via palpation. Then, a very thin needle, such as an acupuncture needle, is inserted into the muscle at the identified point via a transvaginal approach. This is followed by a rapid advancing-and-retracting maneuver with the needle that releases the trigger point of the muscle. Dry needling has only shown to be efficacious as an adjuvant therapy and is not recommended as a first-line treatment or as monotherapy.[8]

For patients with pelvic floor pain refractory to conservative management, off-label onabotulinumtoxinA (onabotA) injection into the pelvic floor muscles can be considered.[8] Total injectate of 100–300 units with a concentration of 100 units/mL can be injected into affected muscles.[4] Consistent with the botulinum toxin A protocol for other pain syndromes, the maximum frequency of injections is every 3 months. Unfortunately, no significant data are available on the safety of onabotA in breastfeeding patients because this population is rarely included in clinical studies. However, due to its large molecular weight, it is unlikely that onabotA is transferred into breast milk, and therefore it can be considered safe for use in breast-feeding patients. Best pain control results are achieved when combined with physical therapy exercises.[8]

Another treatment option for pain refractory to conservative management is injection of local anesthetic into affected pelvic floor muscles. These injections, although effective, provide temporary relief. Long-term relief is only achievable when the underlying physiological cause of the pain is treated.[8]

Complications and Comorbidities

Strain to the various structures of the pelvic floor can compromise pelvic floor tone. This can cause not only pain but also conditions such as, urinary incontinence, fecal incontinence, pelvic organ prolapse, and sexual dysfunction. As a result, in general, women with PFD face a significantly decreased quality of life. Postpartum women face the additional challenge of not being able to embrace motherhood.[1]

References

1. Gao Q, Wang M, Zhang J, et al. Pelvic floor dysfunction in postpartum women: A cross-sectional study. PLoS One. 2024;19(10):e0308563.
2. Wallace SL, Miller LD, Mishra K. Pelvic floor physical therapy in the treatment of pelvic floor dysfunction in women. Curr Opin Obstet Gynecol. 2019;31(6):485–493.
3. Sangsawang B, Sangsawang N. Stress urinary incontinence in pregnant women: A review of prevalence, pathophysiology, and treatment. Int Urogynecol J. 2013;24(6):901–912.
4. Hong MK, Ding DC. Current treatments for female pelvic floor dysfunctions. Gynecol Minim Invasive Ther. 2019;8(4):143–148.
5. Meekins AR, Siddiqui NY. Diagnosis and management of postpartum pelvic floor disorders. Obstet Gynecol Clin North Am. 2020;47(3):477–486.

6. Meister, M. R., Shivakumar, N., Sutcliffe, S., et al. (2018). Physical examination techniques for the assessment of pelvic floor myofascial pain: A systematic review. *American Journal of Obstetrics & Gynecology, 219*(5), 497.e1–497.e13. https://doi.org/10.1016/j.ajog.2018.06.008
7. National Library of Medicine (US). (2024, January 15). *Drugs and Lactation Database (LactMed)*. National Center for Biotechnology Information. https://www.ncbi.nlm.nih.gov/books/NBK501922/
8. Moldwin RM, Fariello JY. Myofascial trigger points of the pelvic floor: Associations with urological pain syndromes and treatment strategies including injection therapy. Curr Urol Rep. 2013;14(5):409–417.

48
DeQuervain Tenosynovitis

Ankita Mathur, Danielle Levin, and Meera Kirpekar

Epidemiology and Risk Factors

DeQuervain tenosynovitis (DQT) is a disease of the hand causing pain along the thumb side of the wrist. DQT occurs at a rate six times higher in females than in males; within the general population, it occurs at a rate of 0.5% in men and 1.3% in women.[1,2] In pregnancy specifically, one large-scale study showed that DQT occurred in 2.1% of pregnant individuals.[3] Onset typically occurs in the third trimester or postpartum with lactation, with a mean onset time of 5.4 months postpartum. The mean duration is approximately 5.15 months.[4]

Multiple risk factors have been noted, including female sex, black race, age >40, and history of thyroid disorders.[5,6] For the postpartum period, specific risk factors include first pregnancy, multiple gestation, cesarean delivery, and underlying rheumatoid arthritis.[3] Primiparity increases risk by more than twofold, often because first-time mothers may be more likely to seek medical attention or have not yet developed ergonomic preventative strategies for holding their child.[4] Interestingly, increased birth weight of the child and diabetic disorders of pregnancy did not significantly increase risk.[3,7] DQT is often self-limited and resolves when lactation ceases.[4]

Pathophysiology

DQT is characterized by stenosing tenosynovitis of the abductor pollicis longus (APL) and extensor pollicis brevis (EPB) tendons. Repetitive motions and increased load are exacerbated in the postpartum period by carrying a baby.[4,7,8] Chronic inflammation leads to neovascularization and thickening of the tendon sheaths.

Hormonal changes, such as increased estrogen and progesterone, cause fluid retention and ligament laxity. DQT can persist due to ongoing hormonal shifts from lactation and typically resolves once pre-pregnancy hormonal levels return.[4,7,8] Anatomical variations, such as accessory tendon slips or a septum within the first dorsal compartment, have also been identified as contributing factors.[8]

Diagnosis and Assessment

Diagnosis requires inquiry regarding the onset, quality, and location of pain (thumb side of the wrist). Pain is often sharp or aching and worsened by twisting or grasping motions. Some patients report numbness, tingling, or weakness in the thumb.

Inspection may show swelling at the base of the thumb. Finkelstein's test—passively deviating the wrist to the ulnar side while flexing the thumb into the palm—is considered the superior diagnostic maneuver.[9] A neurovascular exam should be conducted to rule out other causes.

Diagnostic Imaging

- *Radiographs*: Rule out osteoarthritis or fractures.[9]
- *Ultrasound*: Identifies septa in the dorsal compartment to increase injection success.[10]
- *MRI*: Shows fluid in the tendon sheath, inflammatory changes, and anatomical variants.[11,12]

Treatment Options

First-line treatment includes acetaminophen and nonsteroidal anti-inflammatory drugs (NSAIDs).[13] While NSAIDs require caution in the third trimester, they are generally safe postpartum with minimal transfer into breast milk.

A thumb spica splint offers relief, al though a combination of corticosteroid injection (CSI) and splinting for 3–4 weeks is considered the most effective first-line approach.[13,14] Physical therapy focuses on gliding exercises and strengthening.[15]

Interventional treatments include:

- *CSI*: Ultrasound guidance provides a higher success rate (52–90% relief).[16,17]
- *Regenerative injections*: Platelet-rich plasma (PRP) or prolotherapy may be considered for refractory cases.[18,19]

Surgical release of the compartment is considered if symptoms persist after two CSIs. Complications can include superficial radial nerve injury or hypertrophic scarring.[20]

Laser therapy and therapeutic ultrasound are the most effective emerging modalities.[21] Acupuncture has shown some short-term benefits.[22]

Complications and Comorbidities

Untreated DQT can lead to permanent nerve damage, tendon rupture, or chronic scarring that limits range of motion. The functional impact on a mother's ability to care for her child can also lead to psychological distress.

References

1. Amundsen S, Sørlie T, Bratland S, Helde G, Dietrichs E. Pharmacological treatment of migraine during pregnancy and breastfeeding. Nat Rev Neurol. 2015;11(4):209–219.
2. Shen PC, Hsieh YH, Chen CH, et al. Hand tendinopathy risk factors in Taiwan: A population-based cohort study. Medicine (Baltimore). 2019;98(1):e13795.

3. Bae KJ, Lee HJ, Kim JH, et al. Incidence and risk factors for pregnancy-related de Quervain's tenosynovitis in South Korea. Clin Orthop Surg. 2023;15(1):145–152.
4. Daglan E, Ozkan B, Yildiz C, et al. Risk factors associated with de Quervain tenosynovitis in postpartum women. Hand. 2023;19(4):643–647.
5. Wolf JM, Sturdivant RX, Owens BD. Incidence of de Quervain's tenosynovitis in a young, active population. J Hand Surg Am. 2009;34(1):112–115.
6. Pflibsen LR, Kouloumberis PE, Noland SS. De Quervain's Disease in Postpartum Women. J Womens Health (Larchmt). 2023 Jan;32(1):15-17. doi: 10.1089/jwh.2020.8966. Epub 2021 Feb 23. PMID: 33625265.
7. Schned ES. De Quervain tenosynovitis in pregnant and postpartum women. Obstet Gynecol. 1986;68(3):411–414.
8. Capasso G, Testa V, Maffulli N. Surgical release of de Quervain's stenosing tenosynovitis postpartum. Int Orthop. 2002;26(1):23–25.
9. Wu F, Zhao X, Liu Y, et al. Finkelstein's test is superior to Eichhoff's test. J Hand Microsurg. 2018;10(2):116–118.
10. Allbrook V. "The side of my wrist hurts": De Quervain's tenosynovitis. Aust J Gen Pract. 2019;48(11):753–756.
11. Goyal A, Gupta S, Sharma A, et al. MRI in De Quervain tenosynovitis: Is making the diagnosis sufficient? AJR. 2018;210(3):133–134.
12. Glajchen N, Schweitzer M. MRI features in de Quervain's tenosynovitis of the wrist. Skeletal Radiol. 1996;25(1):63–65.
13. Satteson ES, Tannan SC. De Quervain tenosynovitis. StatPearls. 2025. https://www.ncbi.nlm.nih.gov/books/NBK442005/
14. Challoumas D, Clifford C, Trivedi S, et al. Management of de Quervain tenosynovitis: A systematic review. JAMA Netw Open. 2023;6(10):e2337001.
15. McBain B, Rio E, Cook J, Sanderson J, Docking S. Isometric thumb extension exercise as part of a multimodal intervention for de Quervain's syndrome: A randomised feasibility trial. Hand Ther. 2023 Jun;28(2):72-84. doi: 10.1177/17589983231158499. Epub 2023 Apr 27. PMID: 37904860; PMCID: PMC10584067.
16. Shin, Y. H., Choi, S. W., & Kim, J. K. (2020). Prospective randomized comparison of ultrasonography-guided and blind corticosteroid injection for de Quervain's disease. *Orthopaedics & Traumatology: Surgery & Research, 106*(2), 301–306. https://doi.org/10.1016/j.otsr.2019.11.015
17. Anderson BC, Manthey R, Brouns MC. Treatment of De Quervain's tenosynovitis with corticosteroids. Arthritis Rheum. 1991;34(7):793–8.
18. Asaad SK, Mahmood KA, Arif SO, Abdalla BA, Salih AM, Kakamad FH, Mohammed SH, Salih RQ, Mohammed KK, Salih KM. Efficacy of ultrasound-guided platelet rich plasma injection for the management of de Quervain's tenosynovitis. Med Int (Lond). 2023 Feb 2;3(2):12. doi: 10.3892/mi.2023.72. PMID: 36875820; PMCID: PMC9982492.
19. Zora H, Bayrak G. The impact of prolotherapy and steroid injection on DQT. Acta Med Alanya. 2024;8(1):78–84.
20. Suwannaphisit S, Chuaychoosakoon C. Effectiveness of surgical interventions for treating de Quervain's disease. Ann Med Surg (Lond). 2022;77:103620.
21. Ferrara PE, Codazza S, Galluccio F, et al. Physical modalities for the conservative treatment of wrist and hand's tenosynovitis. Semin Arthritis Rheum. 2020;50(6):1280–1290.
22. Hadianfard M, Sadri L, Saadat S, et al. Efficacy of acupuncture versus local methylprednisolone acetate injection. J Acupunct Meridian Stud. 2014;7(3):115–121.

49
Carpal Tunnel Syndrome

Ankita Mathur, Danielle Levin, and Meera Kirpekar

Epidemiology and Risk Factors

Carpal tunnel syndrome (CTS), a painful condition of the hand caused by pressure on the median nerve, is the most common peripheral nerve entrapment syndrome that affects the upper body. It is particularly frequent in females compared to males and occurs at a ratio of 3:1 to 10:1.[1] CTS occurs bilaterally in up to 87% of patients based on symptoms alone and approximately 50% of patients based on testing.[2] Pregnancy-related carpal tunnel syndrome (PRCTS) occurs at a wide range, from 0.23% to 70% of cases. PRCTS is most commonly seen in the third trimester (63%) followed by the second trimester (26%) and then the first trimester (11%). PRCTS can persist in the postpartum period for up to 3 years post delivery.[3] When comparing PRCTS to CTS in the general population, CTS occurred more often in pregnant women than in nonpregnant women. Furthermore, while the severity of symptoms is most often mild in PRCTS, severe symptoms occurred at a higher rate in PRCTS than in CTS in the general population.[4]

Risk factors for CTS include conditions such as diabetes mellitus, amyloidosis, hypothyroidism, rheumatoid arthritis, tenosynovitis, obesity, and pregnancy.[5–7] With PRCTS, progression and persistence of the disease into the postpartum period has been more frequently noted in two types of instances: initial onset in the first or second trimesters of pregnancy and depression-related disorders.[3]

Pathophysiology

PRCTS results in pain and functional impairment, especially during pregnancy and the postpartum period. The pathophysiology may be multifactorial.

Fluid retention due to the increase in blood volume seen in pregnancy can lead to generalized edema throughout the body or specifically hand edema. Edema leads to a mechanical compression of the median nerve.[2] Starting in the 18th week of pregnancy, the hormone relaxin is released leading to relaxation of the carpal ligament as well as inflammation and flattening of the median nerve. Increased levels of estrogen, aldosterone, cortisol, prolactin, and glucose can also cause decreased venous return and further edema of the carpal tunnel.[3]

Smoking and alcohol consumption have been correlated with development of CTS as well as PRCTS, suggesting an involvement of impairment of microcirculation.[2]

Diagnosis and Assessment

History should include assessment of risk factors such as diabetes, obesity, pregnancy, rheumatoid arthritis, hypothyroidism, amyloidosis, and tenosynovitis. The pain is often in the bilateral hands and wrists but can be unilateral. The pain is typically along the radiocarpal joint and can extend to multiple fingers, with the index finger and thumb most commonly involved. The patient may experience paresthesias of the hand from nerve compression, which could indicate nerve damage. Furthermore, the pain may present at night as well, leading to poor sleep and increased stress, causing possible premature birth.[3]

Physical examination should include inspection and palpation of the area, which may reveal hypotrophy or atrophy of the thenar muscles. The patient may show impaired grip strength and decreased ability to grasp objects. The Tinel and Phalen tests may be performed. The Tinel test, lightly tapping over the wrist where the median nerve crosses, and the Phalen test, pushing the dorsal surfaces of the hands together for 30–60 seconds to increase carpal tunnel pressure, indicate CTS when pain or paresthesias are reproduced.

Classic ultrasound as well as high-frequency ultrasonography (HF-USG) have been used to diagnose PRCTS. Ultrasound has many advantages including low cost, easy availability, no pain, and quick and high yielding information. Ultrasound can show an increase in size of the median nerve, change in the pattern of the nerve due to edema, and compression of the nerve in the carpal tunnel. Doppler examination can also evaluate vascularity.[3]

Electromyographic studies are not typically recommended during pregnancy as nerve stimulation elicits pain, but these can be used in the postpartum period.[3]

Treatment Options

Management of DQT varies by patient, but DQT is often self-limiting and can resolve without intervention. Treatment options range from conservative therapies to interventional and surgical approaches, depending on the severity, duration, and characterization of the pain.

Medical Management

First-line treatment often involves acetaminophen for mild to moderate pain. Aspirin and nonsteroidal anti-inflammatory drugs (NSAIDs) can be used to address nociceptive components including inflammation, but caution must be used during the third trimester of pregnancy, particularly with aspirin as it can cause cryptorchidism and gastroschisis.[8,9] Both can be used safely postpartum.

CTS may be caused by vitamin B_{12} deficiency so its administration may be beneficial for its nerve healing properties.[10] Alpha-lipoic acid, an antioxidant known for decreasing inflammation, may be administered for 3 months to increase nerve conduction and reduce symptoms and may even be started during pregnancy.[10,11] Metabolic syndrome may also occur during pregnancy, leading to the development of CTS due to impact on peripheral nerve metabolism; vitamin D may be used as a treatment though its effect is still under investigation.[12]

Physical and Manual Therapies

Wrist immobilization with a splint can decrease pressure within the carpal tunnel by holding the radiocarpal joint in a neutral position. Correct use of a splint can resolve up to 80% of symptoms in mild to moderate cases of PRCTS. In PRCTS, there is no clear recommendation as to how long a splint should be utilized because symptoms may resolve spontaneously postpartum. However, if symptoms do not resolve, a splint may be recommended for 6 weeks. Wrist splints should be used at night as well as during certain activities during the day that may exacerbate the pain.[10] In the case of postpartum pain, a splint is recommended during activities such as breastfeeding and carrying the baby.

Mechanical traction can also be utilized, which involves traction of the hand using a pneumatic device to increase the space within the carpal tunnel. For CTS, studies have demonstrated improvement in symptoms for at least 7 months. The data for PRCTS are limited.[7,13]

Kinesiotape is useful to increase mobility, reduce edema, activate pain reduction pathways, and decrease muscle tension. In PRCTS, kinesiotape in combination with cupping reduced inflammation.[14]

Physical and occupational therapy for PRCTS is important to increase strength and range of motion as well as to decrease pain; numerous techniques are described in literature. Nerve and tendon gliding exercises and "myofascial release" therapy have both been noted.[15–17]

Interventional Treatments

Corticosteroid injections (CSI) have been found to be effective during pregnancy due to immediate resolution of symptoms and without harmful effects to the fetus.[18] Given the low recurrence rate in the short term, CSI is an indication for acute PRCTS developed in the third trimester. For PRCTS that persists in the postpartum period and becomes a chronic condition, CSI is not generally recommended because its benefits are generally short term and not well established for long-term therapy.[19] CSI is typically done for mild to moderate levels of pain. Potential but rare complications of steroid-based injections into the carpal tunnel include potential axonal and myelin degeneration, thinning of the skin, possible tendon rupture, atrophy of the soft tissue, and crystal-induced synovitis.

Platelet-rich plasma (PRP) therapy and D5W therapy (5% dextrose in water) have been described for CTS. In smaller-scale studies, regenerative medicine for mild to moderate CTS has been effective when conservative measures, including CSI, have failed.[20]

Surgical Interventions

PRCTS remains unpredictable in its need for surgery because symptoms of CTS may resolve spontaneously in the postpartum period. If PRCTS persists beyond the 3-month mark in the postpartum period, surgery may be indicated to prevent worsening symptoms or progression to chronic disease. However, given the unpredictability of spontaneous resolution after childbirth, it is important to decide on surgery for PRCTS on a case-by-case basis, such as worsening pain or functional impairment, particularly in postpartum childcare.[3] Surgical decompression can be performed endoscopically or openly under only local anesthesia.

Emerging and Complementary Therapies

High-frequency laser therapy, ultrasound therapy, iontophoresis, phonophoresis, and hot sand bath therapy have all been described in the literature for PRCTS in very small-scale studies and are generally considered safe therapies.[3] Complementary methods during pregnancy and the postpartum period, such as yoga and acupuncture, have been described to improve grip strength and lower pain.[10]

Complications and Comorbidities

Treatment of PRCTS is important to prevent long-term complications. Complications of untreated CTS include permanent nerve damage with resulting numbness and weakness of the hand and fingers. Muscle atrophy can also occur in the hand. Worsening pain can also occur from untreated CTS, further limiting fine motor skills and reducing overall grip strength. The functional impact of this ultimately affects both physical and mental health and can make caring for a newborn more challenging.

References

1. Randall LB, Braddom RL. *Physical Medicine & Rehabilitation.* 3rd ed. Elsevier Saunders; 2007:1079–1080.
2. Padua L, Padua R, Lo Monaco M, Aprile I, Tonali P. Incidence of bilateral symptoms in carpal tunnel syndrome. Hand Surg. 1998;23B:603–606.
3. Cîmpeanu MC, Popescu A, Ene R, et al. Management of "de novo" carpal tunnel syndrome in pregnancy: A narrative review. J Pers Med. 2024;14:240.
4. Yazdanpanah P, Aramesh S, Mousavizadeh A, et al. Prevalence and severity of carpal tunnel syndrome in women. Iran J Public Health. 2012;41(2):105–110.
5. de Krom MC, Knipschild PG, Kester AD, Thijs CT, Boekkooi PF, Spaans F. Carpal tunnel syndrome: Prevalence in the general population. J Clin Epidemiol. 1992;45:373–376.
6. Becker J, Nora DB, Gomes I, et al. An evaluation of gender, obesity, age, and diabetes mellitus as risk factors for CTS. Clin Neurophysiol. 2002;11(9):1429–1434.
7. Meems M. Carpal tunnel syndrome during pregnancy and the postpartum period and the effect of mechanical traction treatment. 2016. https://research.tilburguniversity.edu/en/publications/carpal-tunnel-syndrome-during-pregnancy-and-the-postpartum-period/
8. Kristensen DM, Hass U, Lesné L, et al. Intrauterine exposure to mild analgesics is a risk factor for development of male reproductive disorders. Hum Reprod. 2011;26:235–244.
9. Baldacci S, Santoro M, Mezzasalma L, Pierini A, Coi A. Medication use during pregnancy and the risk of gastroschisis: A systematic review. Orphanet J Rare Dis. 2024;30:31.
10. Burke FD, Ellis J, McKenna H, Bradley MJ. Primary care management of carpal tunnel syndrome. Postgrad Med J. 2003;79:433–437.
11. Costantino M, Pellicano C, Bottoni G, et al. Peripheral neuropathy in obstetrics: Efficacy and safety of α-lipoic acid supplementation. Eur Rev Med Pharmacol Sci. 2014;18:2766–2771.

12. Stanescu AMA, Simionescu AA, Diaconu CC. Oral Vitamin D Therapy in Patients with Psoriasis. Nutrients. 2021 Jan 6;13(1):163. doi: 10.3390/nu13010163. PMID: 33419149; PMCID: PMC7825555.
13. Tupković E, Redžić A, Šabanović A, et al. Median nerve: Neurophysiological parameters in third trimester of pregnancy. Bosn J Basic Med Sci. 2007;7:84–89.
14. Güner A, Karabay N, Sayın R, et al. The effectiveness of the low-power laser and kinesiotaping in the treatment of CTS. Rheumatol Int. 2018;38:895–904.
15. Keskin Y, Akman MN, Kılıç S, et al. Effectiveness of home exercise in pregnant women with carpal tunnel syndrome. J Pak Med Assoc. 2020;70:202–207.
16. Mezian K, Chang KV, Beekman R, et al. EURO-MUSCULUS/USPRM; Dynamic ultrasound protocols for wrist and hand. Am J Phys Med Rehabil. 2022;101:e132–e138.
17. Hamoda RE, Youssef AR, Alsaeed AM. Effect of myofascial release on electrophysiological and clinical measures of pregnant women with CTS. Physiother Q. 2019;27:18–24.
18. Soad A, Manal Y, Raga E. An epidemiological study of carpal tunnel syndrome among pregnant women at Al-Wahda hospital Derna. Int J Clin Obstet Gynaecol. 2020;4:30–33.
19. Evers S, Overbeek CL, Geelen SJ, et al. Corticosteroid injections for carpal tunnel syndrome: long-term follow-up in a population-based cohort. Plast Reconstr Surg. 2017;140(2):338–347.
20. Wu YT, Chen SR, Chang KV. Ultrasound-guided regenerative injection for carpal tunnel syndrome: A narrative review. Rehabil Pract Sci. 2024;2024(2):Article 5.

50
Breast Pain

Ankita Mathur, Danielle Levin, and Meera Kirpekar

Epidemiology and Risk Factors

Breast pain is among the most common problems faced by lactating mothers in the postpartum period. Young, inexperienced mothers are more likely to be affected.[1] The most common causes are benign conditions, such as mastitis.[2] Approximately 10% of postpartum women suffer from mastitis at some point within the first 3 months of the postpartum period. Approximately 3% of those women have a progression of mastitis into a breast abscess.[3]

Breast pain in the postpartum period can also be associated with masses. Most masses tend to be benign. Of the benign masses, 70% tend to be common nonpregnancy-related masses, such as fibroadenoma, and 30% tend to be pregnancy related, such as hyperplasia.[2] Cancer is a more uncommon etiology of patients presenting with breast pain in the postpartum period. Approximately 2–7% patients with breast pain are diagnosed with breast cancer.[4]

Pathophysiology

The most common etiology of postpartum breast pain is infection. Infection-related breast pain can be classified into three categories: engorgement 2/2 milk stasis, mastitis, and breast abscess. These categories are often the stages of progression as well, with engorgement progressing to mastitis and then breast abscess.[2]

Overall, breast engorgement or poor hygiene can lead to breaks in the breast skin. When the infant breastfeeds, bacteria, commonly *Staphylococcus aureus*, from the infant's mouth can be transferred onto the mother's breast and cause an infection (mastitis) via the break in the breast skin. Mastitis has the potential to progress into an abscess. Most breast abscesses occur within the first month of breastfeeding. They can also occur during the weaning phase as breasts are more likely to be engorged during that time period.[2]

Ductal obstruction can also cause breast pain. Persistent obstruction of a lactiferous duct can lead to the formation of a benign milk retention cyst, known as *galactocele*. Galactoceles can get infected and become painful.[2,5]

Tumors can also present as painful masses during the lactation period. Some tumors, such as fibroadenomas, often respond to pregnancy hormones by increasing in size and becoming painful. They can also get infarcted and cause pain. Although the majority of breast masses are benign, approximately 20% of painful breast masses can be malignant.[2]

Normal physiologic breast enlargement also occurs with pregnancy. Usually there are no issues associated with this. In rare cases, the patient can develop gigantomastia. This exaggerated enlargement of breasts can progress to a point of skin necrosis, ulceration, or hemorrhage.[2]

Diagnosis and Assessment

Assessment and diagnosis of postpartum breast pain involve differentiating between the various benign and malignant etiologies. It is important to decipher between an infection versus a benign tumor versus a malignant tumor. A thorough history and physical exam are key to this process. A baseline physical exam of the breast tissue should be conducted. This should be followed by serial examinations because pregnancy is associated with many physiological changes in the breast tissue that can make evaluation difficult.[2]

If the pain is associated with fever and redness around the affected area, an infectious cause is high on the differential. Further workup can be conducted by obtaining a milk leukocyte count and quantitative breast cultures. If the infection is nonresponsive to antibiotics, then a possible breast abscess should be suspected instead of just mastitis.[2]

If a palpable mass is present on physical exam, malignancy must be ruled out. Benign masses, as compared to malignant masses, tend to be more well-demarcated, smooth, and mobile. Mammography can be helpful. However, pregnancy is associated with increased breast density, vascularity, and water content, which can make it difficult to detect and evaluate smaller lesions via mammography. Ultrasound can be used to differentiate between cystic versus solid masses. Biopsy remains the gold standard to arrive at the most accurate diagnosis.[2]

Treatment Options

Since postpartum breast pain can have multiple etiologies, treatment depends on the diagnosis. In case of mastitis, antibiotics are the standard of care. Breastfeeding can be resumed normally while mastitis is being treated. However, if there is no improvement after a 7- to 10-day antibiotic course, then it is likely that the mastitis may have progressed to an abscess. Treatment for an abscess requires aspiration drainage of the abscess—often multiple drainage procedures—in addition to antibiotics. Milk provides a good culture medium for bacteria, so the breast must be kept empty. Lactation suppressants can be considered. Breastfeeding from the affected breast is contraindicated in the case of breast abscess because it can cause adverse effects in the infant, such as pneumonia, lung abscess, or death. It is safe to continue breastfeeding with the contralateral breast.[2]

For galactoceles, aspiration is diagnostic and curative. Multiple aspirations may be required. Supportive measures include ice packs and breast support. Surgery is rarely required.[2]

Excision and biopsy is the recommended course of treatment for breast masses. Nipple discharge, subareolar masses, and intraductal papillomas require ductal excision. It is recommended to refrain from breastfeeding from the affected breast for at least 1 year after ductal excision. Breastfeeding from the contralateral breast can resume normally.[2]

Complications and Comorbidities

Postpartum breast pain can be significantly distressing for postpartum mothers and can significantly decrease their quality of life.[6] It is the most common cause of premature cessation of breastfeeding.[1] This can be an issue because breastfeeding is proved to be an effective method for improving infant survival and overall health of both infant and the mother. There is a strong association between infant failure to thrive and cessation of breastfeeding at 3 months of age.

Furthermore, breast pain has been associated with greater risk of developing postpartum depression.[7] Early cessation of breastfeeding is associated with feelings of guilt and anxiety, which are thought to contribute to the development of depressive symptoms. Depression can also have a tautological effect on breastfeeding by exacerbating the pain response.[8]

References

1. Leung SSF. Breast pain in lactating mothers. Hong Kong Med J. 2016;22(4):341.
2. Scott-Conner CE, Schorr SJ. The diagnosis and management of breast problems during pregnancy and lactation. Am J Surg. 1995;170(4):401–405.
3. Betzold CM. An update on the recognition and management of lactational breast inflammation. J Midwifery Women Health. 2007;52(6):595–605.
4. Eren T, Aslan A, Ozemir IA, Baysal H, Sagiroglu J, Ekinci O, Alimoglu O. *Factors Effecting Mastalgia*. Breast Care (Basel). 2016;11(3):188–193. doi: 10.1159/000444359
5. Gada PB, Vadakekut ES, Bakhshi G. Galactocele. StatPearls [Internet]. Treasure Island (FL): StatPearls Publishing; updated 2024. https://www.ncbi.nlm.nih.gov/books/NBK539738
6. Douglas P. Re-thinking lactation-related nipple pain and damage. Womens Health (Lond). 2022;18:17455057221087865. doi:10.1177/17455057221087865
7. Gianni ML, Bettinelli ME, Manfra P, et al. Breastfeeding difficulties and risk for early breastfeeding cessation. Nutrients. 2019;11(10):2266.
8. Brown A, Rance J, Bennett P. Understanding the relationship between breastfeeding and postnatal depression: The role of pain and physical difficulties. J Adv Nurs. 2016;72(2):273–282.

51
Postpartum Migraine

Ankita Mathur, Danielle Levin, and Meera Kirpekar

Epidemiology and Risk Factors

Migraine is a neurological disorder characterized by recurring headaches.[1] It is one of the most common neurological disorders with a prevalence of 18.5% worldwide.[2] Women are three times more likely to experience migraines compared to their male counterparts. They are also more likely to experience a higher burden of migraines due to increased severity, longer headaches, increased migraine-related symptoms, and increased migraine-related debilitation. The Global Burden of Disease Study ranked migraine as the leading cause of disability among women of reproductive age.[1–3] Migraine headache pain in women is usually unilateral and often described as pounding, pulsating, or throbbing. Women are also more likely to have associated nausea, photophobia, and phonophobia as compared to men.[1] This is thought to be related to the developmental and activational role played by female sex hormones.[1–3]

Pathophysiology

Recurrence or exacerbation of primary migraine pathology is the most common cause of postpartum migraine. Many physiological and environmental changes in the postpartum period influence this. Drastic fluctuations in estrogen, serotonin, and oxytocin associated with childbirth and breastfeeding can trigger or greatly exacerbate migraine. Environmental factors, such as stress, depression, sleep deprivation, and irregular nutritional intake can also worsen migraine.[4–6]

Diagnosis and Assessment

The most common cause of postpartum headache is exacerbation of the primary headache syndromes, which are usually benign. However, it is important to still start with a broad differential diagnosis and differentiate a benign headache from a life-threatening one. A thorough clinical history must be obtained. This includes the timing and nature of the headache with any associated symptoms; any complications during pregnancy, such as preeclampsia or gestational hypertension; the use of neuraxial anesthesia, etc. A physical exam to rule out any focal neurological deficits must also be performed.[7]

Throbbing, unilateral headaches associated with photosensitivity or nausea are consistent with migraine. Migraine must be differentiated from other types of headaches, both benign and life-threatening. For example, a cluster headache is usually associated with tearing in the ipsilateral eye, congestion, or rhinorrhea. In contrast, if the headache is described as a sudden-onset severe headache, subarachnoid hemorrhage must be ruled out.[7]

Primary headache disorders and postdural puncture headaches usually do not require further workup. Secondary headache disorders, such as those associated with cerebrovascular pathology, infection, etc., may require further workup including imaging and labs.[7]

Treatment Options

The primary consideration for postpartum migraine treatment is breastfeeding. Human breast milk is the ideal source of nutrition for neonates and small infants. Mothers are encouraged to breastfeed as much as possible. When determining a treatment plan for postpartum migraine, it is important to weigh the risks of the infant's exposure via breast milk or not breastfeeding against the benefits of pain and migraine symptom control. The relative infant dose (RID) is a measure of infant drug exposure via breast milk. A RID <10% is generally considered safe.[8]

Lifestyle Modifications

Among the variety of treatment options, good sleep hygiene is most ideal without concern for adverse effects.[9] A placebo-controlled trial of 43 women demonstrated that behavioral sleep modification led to a significant reduction in the frequency and intensity of migraine headaches as compared to placebo.[10]

Migraine Abortive Agents

Most medications used as migraine abortive agents have low risk of transfer through breast milk.

- *Paracetamol (acetaminophen) and nonsteroidal anti-inflammatory drugs (NSAIDs)*: Considered safe. The NSAID of choice is ibuprofen. Diclofenac and naproxen are second-line. Regular use of aspirin is not recommended due to risks of thrombocytopenic purpura and Reye syndrome.[8]
- *Triptans*: Sumatriptan and eletriptan (RID 0.2%) are considered generally safe. Frovatriptan should be avoided due to its long half-life (25–30 hours).[8]
- *Opioids*: Occasional low doses are acceptable for refractory cases, but repeat doses of codeine should be avoided due to CYP2D6 hypermetabolism risks.[8]

Preventative Medications

- *Beta blockers*: Propranolol and metoprolol are first-line for prophylaxis and considered safe.[8]
- *Antiepileptics*: Valproate (RID 1.4–1.7%) and topiramate are generally regarded as safe, although topiramate requires monitoring.[8]

- *Antidepressants*: Amitriptyline and nortriptyline (RID 1.2–2.5%) are safe.[8]
- *Supplements*: Magnesium (RID 0.2%) is safe to use while breastfeeding.[8]

Interventions

OnabotulinumtoxinA-A (onabotA) injections are an option for migraine prevention. Due to its large molecular weight, systemic absorption and transfer into breast milk are negligible, making it likely safe for use in breastfeeding patients.[8,11]

Complications and Comorbidities

Chronic migraine tends to coexist with psychiatric comorbidities like major depressive disorder and anxiety.[12] Women with migraine may also be at increased risk for developing postpartum depression within the first 6 months after delivery.[13]

References

1. Krause, D. N., Warfvinge, K., Haanes, K. A., & Edvinsson, L. (2021). Hormonal influences in migraine — interactions of oestrogen, oxytocin and CGRP. *Nature Reviews Neurology, 17*(10), 621–633. https://doi.org/10.1038/s41582-021-00544-2
2. Broner SW, Lay CL, Seifert TD. Migraine in women. Semin Neurol. 2017;37(6):601–610.
3. Burch R. Epidemiology and treatment of menstrual migraine and migraine during pregnancy and lactation. Headache. 2020;60(1):200–216.
4. Saldanha IJ, Khoshnood B, Roth J, Gill T, Loder E, Buse DC. Management of primary headaches during pregnancy, postpartum, and breastfeeding. Headache. 2021;61(1):11–43.
5. Klein AM, Loder E. Postpartum headache. Int J Obstet Anesth. 2010;19(4):422–430.
6. Lim G. Perinatal depression. Curr Opin Anaesthesiol. 2021;34(3):233–237.
7. Dodick DW. Diagnosing secondary and primary headache disorders. Continuum (Minneap Minn). 2021;27(3):572–585.
8. Amundsen S, Helde G, Bratland S, Dietrichs E. Pharmacological treatment of migraine during pregnancy and breastfeeding. Nat Rev Neurol. 2015;11(4):209–219.
9. Calhoun AH. Migraine treatment in pregnancy and lactation. Curr Pain Headache Rep. 2017;21(11):46.
10. Calhoun AH, Ford S. Behavioral sleep modification may revert transformed migraine to episodic migraine. Headache. 2007;47(8):1178–1183.
11. Russo A, Tessitore A, Silvestro M, Trojsi F, Tedeschi G. Safety of onabotulinumtoxin-A for chronic migraine during pregnancy and breastfeeding. Toxins (Basel). 2025;17(4):192.
12. Halle TM, Thaxter LY, Smitherman TA. Psychiatric comorbidities of migraine. In: *Handbook of Clinical Neurology*. Elsevier: 2024;199:505–516.
13. Gordon-Smith K, Saunders KEA, Ivandic I, et al. Migraine associated with early onset postpartum depression in women with major depressive disorder. Arch Womens Ment Health. 2021;24(6):949–955.

PART IX
AGING AND PAIN

52

Chronic Pain in Aging Women

Challenges and Opportunities

Grace Park

Introduction

The aging process is accompanied by increased susceptibility to chronic pain, particularly in women, due to hormonal shifts, immune system differences, and unique experiences such as childbirth and menopause. Because these chronic, age-related pain conditions cause significant functional limitations, psychological distress, and reduced quality of life, a comprehensive understanding of these conditions is crucial to improve outcomes for older women.

Background

Pain, particularly chronic pain, is a significant issue that negatively impacts a large proportion of the aging population and can lead to functional deficits, cognitive decline, and psychological distress if left unaddressed.[1] As the population in developed countries grows older, the incidence and prevalence of age-related painful conditions are rising and contributing to this pain burden.[2] These conditions encompass a broad spectrum of acute and chronic pain disorders, including osteoarthritis, osteoporosis-related fractures, fibromyalgia, chronic low back pain, and chronic pelvic pain. Interestingly, many of these disorders disproportionately affect women, and the unique interplay of physiological, hormonal, and psychosocial factors in women makes the development and management of these conditions multidimensional.[3]

Epidemiology and Risk Factors

Although estimates on the precise prevalence vary widely, data from the 2019 National Health Interview Survey indicate that 20.5% of adults report chronic pain in the United States.[4] Within this percentage, there is a higher prevalence of chronic pain conditions in women and the elderly.[5] While this prevalence is influenced by socioeconomic disparities in women regarding pain reporting and treatment, factors like postmenopausal hormonal changes lead conditions like osteoarthritis, osteoporosis-related fractures, fibromyalgia, chronic low back pain, and chronic pelvic pain to occur more frequently in older women than in their male counterparts.[6,7] The development of such conditions correspondingly elevates the risk of morbidity and mortality in this population because osteoporotic fractures, particularly hip fractures, are associated with a 1-year mortality rate of 12–17%.[8]

In addition to the risk factors from the natural process of aging, women exhibit significant differences in the mechanisms underlying pain and its transmission that are influenced by sex-specific variations in genes, proteins, hormones, and the immune system.[9] These distinct risk factors contribute to the onset and intensity of age-related painful conditions in women and highlight the critical need for further research to improve pain management strategies for aging women.

Pathophysiology

Estrogen is a powerful hormone that plays a vital role in the human body. Alongside inhibiting bone resorption through antagonization of interleukin (IL)-6 receptors and blockage of IL-6 synthesis to prevent general bone loss,[10] estrogen has been found to have a protective role in pain modulation. By modulating nociceptive sensitization at the level of peripheral, spinal, and supraspinal sites, estrogen alleviates neuropathic pain and hyperalgesia from mechanical and thermal etiologies.[11,12] This effect of estrogen is further supported by the widespread expression of estrogen receptors across neurons within the nociceptive system.[13] Although these findings are primarily from rat studies, sex hormone differences in analgesia and pain have been documented in humans as well, with females experiencing heightened pain sensitivity following a decline in estrogen levels.[14] Therefore, because estrogen plays a protective role in bone turnover and pain modulation, lower estrogen levels in older women contribute to a higher incidence of osteoporosis-related injury and more severe pain associated with age-related conditions.

Often a source of chronic pain, autoimmune diseases are also more prevalent in older women.[15] While immune competence naturally declines with age, women exhibit a stronger immune system and elevated incidence of autoimmune diseases in the setting of hormonal differences. Progesterone and androgens are generally immunosuppressive, whereas estrogen is immune-stimulatory across both innate and adaptive immune systems. Due to this, estrogen has been implicated in the pathogenesis of autoimmune diseases such as systemic lupus erythematosus. However, this hormone has also been shown to exert protective effects in rheumatoid arthritis, so the dual nature of its influence on autoimmune disorders[16] underscores the need for further research to better understand the intricate relationship between sex-specific hormones and the pathogenesis of autoimmune diseases in women as they age.

Unique experiences, such as childbirth, contribute to the pain burden of aging women as well. For example, pelvic floor dysfunction and pudendal neuralgia resulting from the birthing process can lead to prolonged pelvic pain.[17] Chronic pain in older women can also be exacerbated by post hysterectomy pain syndromes and adhesions from prior surgeries.[18]

Diagnosis and Assessment

Given the multifaceted nature of pain in this population, it is crucial for healthcare providers to conduct a detailed assessment of pain patterns, triggers, and associated symptoms while accounting for sex-specific factors like menstrual cycles, childbirth history, or pelvic floor disorders. Common comorbidities that are more prevalent in older females should also be considered while screening for conditions like osteoporosis, autoimmune disorders, metabolic syndromes, and mental health conditions.

Treatment Options

Prevention of age-related painful conditions is key to address the pain burden of the aging population. Healthy aging should be promoted, and targeted strategies focusing on nutrition, exercise, and early interventions are essential to mitigate the risks of developing chronic pain. For example, to prevent age-related deterioration of musculoskeletal health, the European Society for Clinical and Economic Aspects of Osteoporosis and Osteoarthritis (ESCEO) recommend dietary protein intake of 1.0–1.2 g/kg of body weight, vitamin D intake of 800 IU, and calcium intake of 1,000 mg/d alongside regular physical exercise 3–5 times weekly in postmenopausal women.[19]

Alongside lifestyle modifications, clinical interventions targeting hormonal imbalances, such as hormone replacement therapy (HRT), may be considered to address pain conditions in aging women after careful evaluation of risks and benefits. Pain medications, including nonsteroidal anti-inflammatory drugs (NSAIDs), opioids, and adjuvants, should also be used judiciously to avoid polypharmacy risks since women, in comparison to men, are more likely to utilize multiple classes of pain medications.[20] Thus, when formulating individualized approaches to address both physiological and psychological aspects of pain, frequent monitoring and evaluation of pain relief are essential to minimize the side effects associated with polypharmacy.

Incorporating pain management strategies such as physical therapy or cognitive behavioral therapy (CBT) as part of a multidimensional approach to pain management can enhance patient outcomes as well.[21] If these interventions prove insufficient to manage pain from age-related conditions, providers may consider more invasive treatments, such as regional nerve blocks, joint injections, or nerve ablation, when developing a plan of care for these patients.

Complications and Comorbidities

Pain conditions in aging women often coexist with various complications. For example, women experience a higher incidence of obesity that can worsen systemic inflammation and conditions like osteoarthritis.[22] In addition, reduced mobility and increased fall risk, commonly observed in the older population, exacerbate the already heightened risk of osteoporotic fracture development in women. Other coexisting issues like depression and anxiety, which are also more common in females, can amplify pain severity and reduce treatment efficacy in this population.[23] Thus, being mindful of and addressing these comorbidities are integral to effective pain management in older women.

Patient-Centered Approaches

Patient-centered care emphasizes the importance of considering each woman's unique biological, hormonal, and psychosocial profile while recognizing the impacts of the aging process on the human body when facing age-related painful conditions.

Treatment Considerations

The differences in the interplay of hormonal, physiological, and psychosocial factors between males and females necessitate sex-specific approaches to pain management. As hormones themselves impact pain perception and development of painful conditions, addressing hormonal imbalances and being cognizant of distinct cumulative life experiences between men and women are crucial in delivering appropriate care.

Emerging Trends and Current Research

Growing recognition of sex-specific pain mechanisms has led to increased research incorporating both sexes in clinical studies. Advancements in our understanding of sex-specific pain mechanisms have emphasized the importance of targeted therapies and more therapeutic options to address the unmet needs of older women with age-related pain conditions.[24]

Clinical Pearls

- Healthcare providers must prioritize thorough assessments that not only recognize biological and environmental factors, but also the other specific risk factors that women present with.
- To appropriately manage age-related painful conditions, interventions should focus on preventive care, such as lifestyle modifications, and optimization of clinical treatments that address hormonal imbalances and pain management while minimizing polypharmacy and integrating mental health support.

Conclusion

Pain management for aging women is complex. It requires a multifaceted and personalized approach that considers how physiological, hormonal, and psychosocial factors influencing pain perception can alter with age. Thus, addressing these challenges of age-related pain will require continued research and innovation in hopes of the future development of specific targeted therapeutic strategies for the older female population.

References

1. Presto, P., Sehar, U., Kopel, J., & Reddy, P. H. (2024). Mechanisms of pain in aging and age-related conditions: Focus on caregivers. *Ageing Research Reviews, 95,* 102249. https://doi.org/10.1016/j.arr.2024.102249
2. Tinnirello A, Mazzoleni S, Santi C. Chronic pain in the elderly: Mechanisms and distinctive features. Biomolecules. 2021;11(8):1256.
3. Handa R. Low back pain: Myths and facts. J Clin Orthop Trauma. 2019;10(4):828–830.
4. Yong RJ, Mullins PM, Bhattacharyya N. Prevalence of chronic pain among adults in the United States. Pain. 2022;163(2):e328–e32.
5. Tsang A, Von Korff M, Lee S, et al. Common chronic pain conditions in developed and developing countries: Gender and age differences and comorbidity with depression-anxiety disorders. J Pain. 2008;9(10):883–891.
6. Angeli F, Ricci F, Moscucci F, et al. Sex- and gender-related disparities in chest pain syndromes: The feminine mystique of chest pain. Curr Probl Cardiol. 2024;49(4):102457.
7. Hawker GA, King LK. The burden of osteoarthritis in older adults. Clin Geriatr Med. 2022;38(2):181–192.
8. LeBlanc KE, Muncie HL, Jr., LeBlanc LL. Hip fracture: Diagnosis, treatment, and secondary prevention. Am Fam Physician. 2014;89(12):945–951.
9. Osborne NR, Davis KD. Sex and gender differences in pain. Int Rev Neurobiol. 2022;164:277–307.
10. Hadji P, Colli E, Regidor PA. Bone health in estrogen-free contraception. Osteoporos Int. 2019;30(12):2391–2400.
11. Sun LH, Zhang WX, Xu Q, Wu H, Jiao CC, Chen XZ. Estrogen modulation of visceral pain. J Zhejiang Univ Sci B. 2019;20(8):628–636.
12. Chen Q, Zhang W, Sadana N, Chen X. Estrogen receptors in pain modulation: Cellular signaling. Biol Sex Differ. 2021;12(1):22.
13. Shughrue PJ, Lane MV, Merchenthaler I. Comparative distribution of estrogen receptor-alpha and -beta mRNA in the rat central nervous system. J Comp Neurol. 1997;388(4):507–525.
14. Deliu E, Brailoiu GC, Arterburn JB, Oprea TI, Benamar K, Dun NJ, Brailoiu E. Mechanisms of G protein-coupled estrogen receptor-mediated spinal nociception. J Pain. 2012;13(8):742–754.
15. Moulton VR. Sex hormones in acquired immunity and autoimmune disease. Front Immunol. 2018;9:2279.
16. Conrad N, Misra S, Verbakel JY, et al. Incidence, prevalence, and co-occurrence of autoimmune disorders over time and by age, sex, and socioeconomic status: A population-based cohort study of 22 million individuals in the UK. Lancet. 2023;401(10391):1878–1890.
17. Pérez-López FR, Hita-Contreras F. Management of pudendal neuralgia. Climacteric. 2014;17(6):654–656.
18. Brandsborg B, Nikolajsen L. Chronic pain after hysterectomy. Curr Opin Anaesthesiol. 2018;31(3):268–273.

19. Kapoor N, Arora S, Kalra S. Gender disparities in people living with obesity: An unchartered territory. J Midlife Health. 2021;12(2):103–107.
20. Castro-Sánchez AM, Matarán-Peñarrocha GA, López-Rodríguez MM, Lara-Palomo IC, Arendt-Nielsen L, Fernández-de-las-Peñas C. Gender differences in pain severity, disability, depression, and widespread pressure pain sensitivity in patients with fibromyalgia syndrome without comorbid conditions. Pain Med. 2012;13(12):1639–1647.
21. Rizzoli R, Stevenson JC, Bauer JM, et al. The role of dietary protein and vitamin D in maintaining musculoskeletal health in postmenopausal women: A consensus statement from the European Society for Clinical and Economic Aspects of Osteoporosis and Osteoarthritis (ESCEO). Maturitas. 2014;79(1):122–132.
22. Roe CM, McNamara AM, Motheral BR. Gender- and age-related prescription drug use patterns. Ann Pharmacother. 2002;36(1):30–39.
23. Hadley G, Novitch MB. CBT and CFT for chronic pain. Curr Pain Headache Rep. 2021;25(5):35.
24. Ghazisaeidi S, Muley MM, Salter MW. Neuropathic pain: Mechanisms, sex differences, and potential therapies for a global problem. Annu Rev Pharmacol Toxicol. 2023;63:565–583.

53

Pain in Women Across the Lifespan

Considerations in Assessment and Treatment

Vahid Grami and Amna Haider

Introduction

Most literature report that females are more sensitive to pain; however, over a woman's lifespan various underlying changes and factors contribute to pain perception and influence sensitivity. Understanding the prevalence of pain in various age ranges and how biological and psychosocial factors impact pain progression over time, is important in the assessment and treatment of different age groups. Aging introduces challenges to navigating the pain experience and treatment process; this chapter focuses on the underlying changes that occur in each age range to recognize, assess, and optimize care for individuals at different stages of life.

Background

Across the lifespan, from childhood to old age, biological changes, hormonal fluctuations, and psychosocial factors influence the perception and experience of pain. When identifying the source of pain, age has a significant influence on the assessment approach and treatment options. At the biological level, hormonal fluctuations evolve with the stages of life, and each of these stages modulate pain presentation and behavior. Additionally, psychosocial norms and conflicts that arise at varying ages from social acceptance in adolescence to cognitive impairment in older age must equally be considered to treat pain in a multifaceted patient-centric approach. Recognizing and addressing gender-specific variations is essential for providing effective pain management across life stages. A nuanced understanding of how gender influences pain can lead to more accurate assessments, more appropriate interventions, and, ultimately, better health outcomes.

Childhood and Adolescence

Pain conditions in children and adolescence include primary headaches, migraines, abdominal syndromes, juvenile idiopathic arthritis, genetic orthopedic and rheumatologic disorders, cancers, sickle cell disease, and menstrual-related conditions like endometriosis. Approximately 1 in 5 youths experience chronic pain, with girls showing a higher prevalence of chronic headaches and generalized pain compared to boys, although musculoskeletal and back pain show no significant sex difference.[1]

Chronic pain in youth is associated with poorer quality of life, social isolation, missed school, and heightened anxiety and depression risk, with 5–8% being moderately to severely disabled by pain.[1,2] Severe chronic pain prevalence increases up to fourfold after puberty. Studies have shown that sex differences in pain often emerge due to the transition to adolescence at age 12.[3] For girls, menarche brings onset of pain syndromes like dysmenorrhea and endometriosis. Pain symptoms including headache, chronic multisite musculoskeletal pain, chronic upper extremity pain, and increased risk for migraine are more prevalent in girls with early menarche. However, there is no clear association with early menarche and chronic lower back pain.[4] Understanding the hormonal impacts in this age group is important to explain biochemical changes in pain pathways that develop into adulthood.

Adolescents also show differences in pain sensitivity, with younger teens being more sensitive than older ones.[4] Between 20% and 50% of postpubertal adolescents report persistent pain.[5] There is an increase in prevalence of facial pain and back pain in older adolescents. Abdominal pain increases by 8% in girls and decreases by 6% in boys postpuberty. Headache and migraine rates rise in both sexes but more so in females, a trend that persists into adulthood.4

Adulthood

In young adults, chronic disabling pain has a prevalence of 4–14%, and 66.9% experience pain in a 6-month span.[5] Although chronic pain is less common than acute pain, it tends to be more intense and distressing in women. Chronic pain has been found to be 11.1% greater in females than males.[6] Women additionally have higher healthcare expenditures related to chronic pain that increase with age.[6] Longer pain duration is also more common in women: 42.9% of women with chronic pain have symptoms lasting >10 years, compared to only 14.3% of men. Most men report chronic pain durations between 6 months and 1 year.[6]

Older Adults

Pain is common in older adults, with older women consistently demonstrating higher reported prevalence of pain than older men.[7] Seventy percent of older adults have some pain, while 38% have pain that affects their daily living activities.[7] The prevalence of chronic pain is reported to peak at age 60, and chronic widespread pain is associated with a 57% increased risk of early death.[8] Primary causes of pain include neurological and musculoskeletal issues, with common sites being the back, knees, hips, and joints. One out of five adults older than 65 have pain at four or more sites.[7] Institutional living, obesity, lower education, and lower income correlate with higher pain levels. Alarmingly, 80% of institutionalized and 60% of community-dwelling older adults suffer from untreated pain.[8] It is important to identify these older individuals to provide appropriate care for each of their numerous conditions.

Pathophysiology

Age-Related Gender Differences in Pain Pathways

Sex-based differences in pain processing emerge during adolescence. Brain changes include a reduction in gray matter and cortical thickness and increased white matter volume.[4] Testosterone influences these changes more in boys, especially in structures like the amygdala and hippocampus, which are involved in pain regulation. Gray matter plays a role in anti-nociception, and this change may contribute to the differences noted in pain during adolescence between boys and girls.

In adolescents, noxious stimuli cause greater activation in the supramarginal gyrus and prefrontal cortices, and greater deactivation in the orbitofrontal cortex, compared to adults—regions that handle emotional processing and cognitive evaluation of noxious stimuli.[4] The descending pain modulatory system (DPMS)—comprising the prefrontal cortex, anterior cingulate cortex, insula, hypothalamus, amygdala, and periaqueductal gray—which is connected to the release of endogenous opioids, shows gender-specific age responses. With increasing age, males demonstrate increased DPMS response to moderate pain, whereas females show decreased response in areas like the right insula and right anterior cingulate cortex.[9] These brain changes in the perception, processing, and autoregulation of pain are important to understand differences between pain processing across the lifespan. In older adults, there is a decrease in the number of delta nerve fibers that detect sharp localized pain. There is also a proliferation of non-neural glial cells in replacement of pain transmitting neurons.[7] These alterations are progressive but create changes that are important to acknowledge in the evolution of pain.

Hormonal Effects on Pain Tolerance

Age-Related Hormonal Changes

Puberty brings significant hormonal shifts that impact pain tolerance. Many of the sex hormones involved have a concomitant role in pain perception, and changes in the level of these hormones can lead to differences in pain.[4] Early menarche is associated with higher estrogen levels, while in males, testosterone increases in puberty. Testosterone generally has an anti-nociceptive effect, while estrogen can be both pro-nociceptive and anti-nociceptive depending on levels.[4] Hormonal fluctuations have an influence on pain sensitivity. During menarche, estrogen levels are higher, and, considering the pro-nociceptive properties of the hormone, it can potentially contribute to increased pain in girls. However, in girls with high androgen levels, studies found it linked with a potential increased risk of pain in female youth. This is compared to male youth, in whom increased testosterone is protective against pain. The hormonal changes are most drastic in adolescents but are important to be aware of as these patients move into adulthood.

Impact of Hormonal Replacement Therapy

Postmenopausal women on hormonal replacement therapy (HRT) report lower pain thresholds and tolerances compared to non-HRT users and men.[10] In transgender individuals, effects vary by biological sex, endogenous hormone levels, external hormone type, and the nociceptive and anti-nociceptive properties of the external hormone.[11] In the case of oral contraceptives (OCPs), women do not experience a luteinizing hormone (LH) surge to induce ovulation. Evidence points to the LH surge reducing endogenous opioid tone, and inhibiting this can alter luteal phase sensitivity.[10] Hormonal therapies can therefore impact underlying endogenous pain control systems and alter pain sensitization.

Assessment and Diagnosis of Pain Across the Lifespan

Childhood and Adolescence

Pain assessment depends on developmental stage. In infants and nonverbal children, behavioral cues such as facial expressions, sleep, inactivity, and feeding changes can suggest pain.[12] If the behavior is unclear, pain scales are useful for identification. The most recommended scales in infants include the Neonatal Infant Pain Scale (NIPS) and Face Legs Activity Cry Consolability (FLACC) scale.[12] Alternatively, the Evaluation Enfant Douleur (EVENDOL), COMFORT, and Neonatal Facial Coding System (NFCS) have demonstrated reduced bias.[12] Pain assessment in toddlers and older children can be performed with validated and reliable scales such as the FLACC or Children's Hospital of Eastern Ontario (CHEOPS) scales. However, the EVENDOL, COMFORT, and NFCS scales have lower risk for bias.[12] The COMFORT scale has been validated and adapted for use in PICUs and patients undergoing mechanical ventilation.[12]

Gender differences in pain assessment come into play in childhood when socialization plays a greater role. While girls in childhood have not been shown to have biological differences in pain sensitivity compared to boys, socialization factors are increased for girls. Girls generally have increased verbal skills at a younger age and are encouraged to express emotional vulnerability compared to boys, who may not have the skills or encouragement to express their feelings.[13] This can contribute to girls reporting pain more frequently and at a greater intensity compared to boys in childhood.[13] When possible, self-reporting should be prioritized in assessing pain in children.[12] Self-reported assessment measures can be done in children older than 4 years through the Faces Pain Scale – Revised (FPS-R), the 11-point Numeric Rating Scale (NRS-11), and the Color Analog Scale (CAS) pain scales. If a child presents with intellectual disability, this may prevent self-report, and an observational pain scale is better here alongside caregiver assessments. Scales such as the EVENDOL, CHEOPS, and r-FLACC, are used for children aged 0–7 years old, 1–7 years old, and 4–19 years old, respectively.[12]

When assessing chronic pain in adolescents, it is important to maintain their autonomy and evaluate their relationships with peers. In the 2022 Fit Futures Study, it was found that low levels of social acceptance from peers in early adolescence increase the risk of and is associated with the later development of persistent musculoskeletal pain.[14] The Adolescent

Pediatric Pain Tool (APPT) is a sensitive and reliable tool to gather multiple dimensions of pain in adolescents.[15]

Adulthood and Older Adults

When assessing the female adult, both age and pain severity are important during assessment. Women have been found to include more emotional adjectives such as "disgusting" and "unbearable" as well as vivid sensory language such as "throbbing" when describing pain compared to men.[16]

When assessing older adults, challenges such as cognitive impairment, communication issues, sensory impairments, and underreporting arise. Pain is both underreported and underassessed in older adults due to the assumption that it is a normal part of aging.[7] Therefore, it is important to persistently inquire regarding pain in this population, especially when they present with underlying cognitive impairment since these patients may have difficulty verbally describing their pain.[16] As a person ages, they develop *presbyalgos*, the reduced ability to detect harmful signals due to nervous system losses. The pain threshold is known to increase with age and is more prominent in women. However, there is a reduction in the ability to withstand pain at higher intensities in older individuals as well as longer periods of hyperalgesia after painful stimuli.[7] These are key points when assessing chronic pain to arrive at a diagnosis because they can impact the efficacy of treatment in a population where options are more limited.

Treatment Options with Patient-Centric Approaches

Children and Adolescents

An interdisciplinary approach combining physical, psychosocial, and medical strategies is the most effective gold standard of treatment in children.[2] Pharmaceutical intervention should escalate from first line, and, if opiates are being considered, then co-therapy with over-the-counter analgesics should be implemented to reduce adverse effects.[12]

Adulthood and Older Adults

Age-related changes in pharmacodynamics occur at the receptor and signal transduction levels, and this attenuates the homeostasis mechanisms as well as increases the time to return to a steady state.

Consequently, there is a greater variability in response in the elderly to drugs, and caution needs to be taken with starting doses, titration, and side effects.[7] Concomitantly, functional impairments are frequently present in older adults with chronic pain. Treating the presence of decreased appetite, impaired sleep, depression, and other metrics of quality of life has been found to reduce pain perception and reduce analgesic prescription.[7]

Emerging Trends and Current Research

Current research in gender-specific pain management across the lifespan has laid a foundation for the biological and psychosocial complexity of pain perception changes throughout aging. However, gaps remain in understanding how treatment in women at each stage of life should be tailored. One key area where this is important is hormonal changes and the recommended approaches to treatment of pain in pregnancy, hormone-based therapy, gender-diverse patients, and other instances where hormonal fluctuations directly influence pain. Another area for emerging research is pain assessment tools in pediatric patients and adults that not only better quantify the pain but also can isolate gender-sensitive components. This goes along with research on sex-specific responses to pharmacologic interventions and the best means of approach to managing pain in women. Closing these knowledge gaps expands understanding of the best approaches to improving pain care in women.

Clinical Pearls

- Gender-specific considerations across the lifespan involve adopting strategies that adapt to the biological, psychosocial, and social components of gender in the patient's age group. This can be achieved through a variety of steps, the first of which is to acknowledge differences in pain perception, intensity, and frequency compared to men. The next is to consider hormonal changes in women based on their age and comorbidities and anticipate adjusting medications and plans around hormonal transition periods such as puberty, pregnancy, and menopause.
- Being conscious of holistic approaches, including attention to lifestyle and social components to pain processing, is valuable in the pain assessment.
- Continuing education regarding pain perception variances in gender at different ages can continue to enhance providers' diagnostic accuracy and improved standards of care across the lifespan.

Conclusion

From childhood to old age, gender has a significant influence on the underlying pain experience, reporting, and treatment. Biological, hormonal, psychological, and social factors shape pain processing in women differently at different points of life. These differences are not only clinically significant but also essential to understand to approach diagnosis and treatment. Women continue to face inadequate pain management and delayed care due to the underrepresentation of gender-specific considerations across the lifespan. Incorporating knowledge of gender-informed approaches into pain management and assessment at each age range can bridge this gap and enhance clinical effectiveness. This hopefully creates a personalized, responsive, and compassionate model of care that can improve patient outcomes.

References

1. Chambers C, Taddio A, McMurtry CM, et al. The prevalence of chronic pain in children and adolescents: A systematic review update and meta-analysis. Pain. 2024;165(10):2215–2234.
2. Fisher E, Law E, Darnall BD, et al. Efficacy and safety of pharmacological, physical, and psychological interventions for the management of chronic pain in children: A WHO systematic review and meta-analysis. Pain. 2022;163(1):e1–e19.
3. Li, R., Lopez, D. A., Gupta, M., & Palermo, T. M. (2023). Pubertal development and pain incidence and characteristics in children: A 1-year prospective cohort study of a national sample. *Pain, 164*(12), 2725–2736. https://doi.org/10.1097/j.pain.0000000000002997
4. Nahman-Averbuch et al. (2023) Nahman-Averbuch, H., Harounian, S., Pang, D., et al. (2023). Alterations in pain during adolescence and puberty. *Trends in Neurosciences, 46*(4), 307–317. https://doi.org/10.1016/j.tins.2023.01.004
5. Annastas T, Kawai M, Darnall BD, et al. Characterizing chronic pain in late adolescence and early adulthood: Prescription opioids, marijuana use, obesity, and predictors for greater pain interference. Pain Rep. 2018;3(6):e700.
6. Pandelani FF, Nyalunga SLN, Mogotsi MM, Mkhatshwa VB. Chronic pain: Its impact on the quality of life and gender. Front Pain Res (Lausanne). 2023;4:1253460.
7. Mullins, S., Hosseini, F., Gibson, W., & Thake, M. (2022). Physiological changes from ageing regarding pain perception and its impact on pain management for older adults. *Clinical Medicine, 22*(4), 307–310. https://doi.org/10.7861/clinmed.2022-0221
8. Beach, P. A., Cowan, R. L., Dietrich, M. S., Bruehl, S. P., Atalla, S. W., & Monroe, T. B. (2020). Thermal psychophysics and associated brain activation patterns along a continuum of healthy aging. *Pain Medicine, 21*(9), 1779–1792. https://doi.org/10.1093/pm/pnaa055
9. Failla, M. D., Schmidt, J., Seminowicz, D. A., et al. (2024). Gender differences in pain threshold, unpleasantness, and descending pain modulatory activation across the adult life span: A cross-sectional study. *The Journal of Pain, 25*(4), 1059–1069. https://doi.org/10.1016/j.jpain.2024.01.006
10. Fillingim RB, Edwards RR. The association of hormone replacement therapy with experimental pain responses in postmenopausal women. Pain. 2001;92(1–2):229–234.
11. Athnaiel O, Cantillo S, Paredes S, Knezevic NN. The role of sex hormones in pain-related conditions. Int J Mol Sci. 2023;24(3):1866.
12. Trottier ED, Maharaj S, Ng J, et al. Best practices in pain assessment and management for children. Paediatr Child Health. 2022;27(7):429–448.
13. Chaplin TM. Gender and emotion expression: A developmental contextual perspective. Emot Rev. 2015;7(1):14–21.
14. Jahre H, Grotle M, Smedbråten K, et al. Low social acceptance among peers increases the risk of persistent musculoskeletal pain in adolescents: Prospective data from the Fit Futures Study. BMC Musculoskelet Disord. 2022;23(1):44.
15. Jacob E, Mack AK, Savedra MC, et al. Adolescent pediatric pain tool for multidimensional measurement of pain in children and adolescents. Pain Manag Nurs. 2014;15(3):694–706.
16. Puto G, Repka I, Gniadek A. Gender differences in the quantitative and qualitative assessment of chronic pain among older people. Front Public Health. 2024;12:1344381.

54
Clinical Considerations in Shoulder Osteoarthritis Among Older Women

Carla Demerdjian and Anita Gupta

Introduction

Osteoarthritis (OA) is the most common joint disorder in the aging population and is known to disproportionately affect postmenopausal women. The decreased estrogen levels associated with menopause have been linked to increased levels of inflammation, reduction in cartilage production, and alterations in pain thresholds, which together may contribute to the onset and accelerated progression of OA.[1] Additionally, aging women tend to experience reductions in muscle mass and increased joint laxity, which may worsen existing joint instability and weight-bearing stress, exacerbating the breakdown of articular cartilage.[2]

Although knee and hip OA are more thoroughly discussed in existing literature, shoulder OA of the glenohumeral joint can cause significant functional problems. Basic activities like dressing, cooking, and grooming may frequently be restricted by pain and stiffness, resulting in decreased levels of independence and a lesser quality of life. To optimize patient outcomes, management strategies must focus on targeting both pain and functional restoration, particularly in aging women where muscle loss, comorbidities, and fall risk may cause additional challenges.

Clinical Vignette

A 67-year-old female, presented with progressively worsening left shoulder pain over the past 2 years. The pain was described as an initial waxing and waning ache, which progressed to a constant pain. She complained of sharp exacerbations when reaching above her head or behind her back. She explained struggling with simple daily tasks such as washing her hair, putting on a bra, and comfortably sleeping throughout the night. She reported using topical nonsteroidal anti-inflammatory drugs (NSAIDs) and stretching techniques in attempts to ameliorate the pain, without relief.

On examination, she demonstrated diminished active abduction and external rotation, joint line tenderness, and audible crepitus with movement. Radiographs were consistent with primary shoulder OA, showing moderate glenohumeral joint space narrowing, osteophyte formation, and subchondral sclerosis.

A corticosteroid injection composed of 40 mg triamcinolone acetonide with 1% lidocaine was administered intra-articularly through fluoroscopic guidance. At her follow-up appointment 1 week later, she reported a reduction in pain score from 7/10 to 2/10. She reports that she has been able to return to her normal activities and hobbies. With her pain successfully managed, she began a 6-week physical therapy program aiming to assist in restoring her previous range of motion and strengthening her rotator cuff muscles.

She showed significant functional improvement and reported lasting pain relief at her 6-week follow-up appointment. After being discharged from her program, she continued home exercises and reported increased confidence in managing her symptoms independently.

Treatment Outcomes and Management Strategies

This case highlights how combining interventional and rehabilitative treatments—pain injections and physical therapy, respectively—can effectively manage shoulder OA in aging women by relieving pain and improving functionality. Corticosteroid injections provide rapid pain relief, allowing for more active participation in rehabilitation.

Corticosteroid Injections

Intra-articular corticosteroid injections have persisted as the first-line interventional treatment for moderate to severe OA for several decades. These injections act by reducing synovial inflammation, which is responsible for pain and effusion of joints. Accuracy is significantly improved when injections are performed under ultrasound or fluoroscopic guidance, resulting in enhanced clinical outcomes.[3]

In cases of shoulder OA, corticosteroid injections have been shown to decrease pain levels and enhance functionality of the glenohumeral joint for up to 3 months.[4] However, the relief is generally temporary, and it is advisable to restrict the number of injections (generally ≤3/year) to prevent the potential of cartilage toxicity.[5] Nonetheless, a well-timed injection can significantly enhance the quality of life and facilitate more effective therapy in elderly women demonstrating impaired mobility.

Hyaluronic Acid and Other Injectable Options

Despite being mainly utilized for knee OA, hyaluronic acid (HA) viscosupplementation in the shoulder has yielded varying degrees of success. Although HA injections usually have a delay in therapeutic onset and may not be as effective in more advanced disease, some research indicates that they may provide long-term pain relief that is comparable to corticosteroids.[6]

Novel regenerative therapies such as platelet-rich plasma (PRP) and bone marrow aspirate concentrate are currently under investigation. PRP has been shown in previous studies to mitigate inflammation and aid in healing, but there is conflicting evidence on its role in improving symptoms of shoulder OA, particularly in aging populations.[7]

Table 54.1 Treatment Strategies for Shoulder Osteoarthritis (OA) in Aging Women

Category	Intervention	Mechanism / Approach	Clinical Benefits / Outcomes	Limitations / Considerations
Interventional	Corticosteroid injections	Reduce synovial inflammation; ultrasound/fluoroscopy-guided	Rapid pain relief; improved function up to ~3 months; enables participation in rehabilitation	Temporary effect; ≤3 injections/year; cartilage toxicity risk; recurrence common
Interventional	Hyaluronic acid (viscosupplementation)	Improves joint lubrication and viscoelasticity	Possible longer-term pain relief; may approach steroid efficacy in some cases	Delayed onset; less effective in advanced OA; variable evidence
Regenerative therapies	Platelet-rich plasma (PRP) / bone marrow aspirate concentrate	Anti-inflammatory and regenerative effects	May reduce symptoms and inflammation in some patients	Conflicting evidence; uncertain benefit in elderly OA
Rehabilitative	Physical therapy	ROM exercises, manual therapy, posture correction, strengthening	Improves pain, mobility, and function; enhances outcomes with injections	Requires adherence; gradual improvement; dependent on participation
Rehabilitative	Multimodal rehabilitation programs	Supervised PT followed by home exercise program	Significant improvement in mobility and function when combined with injections	Requires structured guidance and long-term adherence
Pharmacologic	Topical NSAIDs	Local anti-inflammatory action with minimal systemic absorption	Effective for mild–moderate pain; well tolerated in elderly	Limited efficacy in severe OA
Pharmacologic	Oral NSAIDs	Systemic COX inhibition reduces inflammation and pain	Effective analgesia in OA	Risk of GI bleeding, renal impairment, and cardiovascular events; caution in elderly
Lifestyle / Supportive	Weight management, posture correction, fall prevention	Reduces mechanical load and improves biomechanics	Improves overall function and reduces symptom burden	Requires sustained behavioral adherence
Comorbidity optimization	Sarcopenia, osteoporosis, polypharmacy management	Multidisciplinary management of age-related conditions	Improves functional outcomes and reduces complications	Requires coordinated care

Physical Therapy and Exercise

Implementation of physical therapy is vital to maintaining beneficial results from pain injections. Rotator cuff weakness and impaired scapulothoracic rhythm are common in older women, often leading to increased degeneration of the glenohumeral joint. Evidence demonstrates that targeted rehabilitation, including passive range of motion, manual techniques, posture correction, and progressive strengthening, can significantly reduce pain and ameliorate function.[8]

A 2021 review of shoulder OA rehabilitation programs discussed the association of multimodal protocols with significant improvement in mobility and decreases in disability scores, particularly when therapy was introduced after pain levels were decreased via injection.[9] Supervised therapy promotes patient compliance and safety, while the transition to a home-based therapy plan helps the patient sustain long-term benefits.

Pharmacologic and Supportive Strategies

Topical NSAIDs are generally well-tolerated and show efficacy in treatment of mild to moderate symptoms in older adults. Although oral NSAIDs are effective, they carry risks of gastrointestinal bleeding, cardiovascular events, and renal impairment and are advised to be used with caution in the aging population.

Comprehensive care of aging women with OA includes lifestyle modifications, such as promotion of weight management, postural correction, and mitigation of fall risk. Addressing other existing comorbidities often present in this population such as sarcopenia, osteoporosis, and even polypharmacy also contributes to the optimization of functional outcomes.

References

1. Roman-Blas JA, Castañeda S, Largo R, Herrero-Beaumont G. Osteoarthritis associated with estrogen deficiency. Arthritis Res Ther. 2009;11(5):241.
2. Srikanth VK, Fryer JL, Zhai G, Winzenberg TM, Hosmer D, Jones G. A meta-analysis of sex differences in osteoarthritis prevalence. Osteoarthritis Cartilage. 2005;13(9):769–781.
3. Aly AR, Rajasekaran S, Ashworth N. Ultrasound-guided shoulder injections are more accurate and improve clinical outcomes compared to landmark-guided injections: A systematic review and meta-analysis. Br J Sports Med. 2015;49(17):1042–1049. doi:10.1136/bjsports-2014-093573
4. Dogu B, Yucel SD, Sag SY, et al. Efficacy of corticosteroid injection in shoulder osteoarthritis: A randomized, double-blind, placebo-controlled trial. Clin Rheumatol. 2019;38(2):527–534. doi:10.1007/s10067-018-4321-0
5. Kraeutler MJ, Ciccotti MG, Dodson CC, et al. Frequency and impact of corticosteroid injections for shoulder pain: A review. Am J Orthop. 2017;46(3):E138–E143.
6. Papalia R, Franceschi F, Diaz Balzani L, et al. Shoulder viscosupplementation: Evidence for the appropriate indications. Knee Surg Sports Traumatol Arthrosc. 2020;28(10):3255–3265. doi:10.1007/s00167-019-05720-0

7. Chou WY, Ko JY, Wang FS, et al. Clinical outcomes following platelet-rich plasma treatment for rotator cuff tendinopathy and OA. J Shoulder Elbow Surg. 2022;31(1):100–110. doi:10.1016/j.jse.2021.06.032
8. Manske RC, Prohaska D. Physical therapy management of shoulder osteoarthritis: A clinical commentary. Int J Sports Phys Ther. 2017;12(5):806–816.
9. Lin I, Wiles L, Waller R, et al. What does best practice care for musculoskeletal pain look like? Br J Sports Med.2020;54(2):79–86. doi:10.1136/bjsports-2018-099878

PART X
INNOVATIONS AND FUTURE DIRECTIONS

55 Precision Medicine and Personalized Pain Treatment in Women

Rosalynn R. Z. Conic and Lynn Kohan

Introduction

Pain management is typically approached in an algorithmic, "one size fits all" fashion; however this does not account for interindividual variability, including biological, social, and economic characteristics.[1] Thus, therapeutic efficacy is often suboptimal and requires trials of multiple medications, which results in significant disparities in outcomes and reduced quality of life.

As a result, in 2015, a large-scale *precision medicine* (also referred to as *personalized medicine*) research effort was initiated. Precision medicine focuses on tailoring treatment modalities using clinical information, advanced patient data (e.g., genomics, transcriptomics, proteomics, epigenomics, metabolomics), and lifestyle factors (environment) to improve patient care and outcomes. This allows for the identification of unique biomarkers for prognostic and predictive value as well as risk stratification.

While precision medicine is a promising tool, practical application is limited and considered unrealistic in current clinical practice due to the high costs of testing, limited reliable biomarkers, and lack of physician knowledge in interpreting and/or sharing results of testing with the patients. This chapter focuses on the current and emerging applications of personalized and precision medicine approaches to improve the assessment and management of pain in women.

Background

Chronic pain is one of the most prevalent medical conditions worldwide, with women being impacted more frequently secondary to biological and psychosocial differences.[2] Given the magnitude of chronic pain, precision pain medicine becomes particularly important in women due to sex-based differences in pain perception and processing, variations in both pharmacokinetics and pharmacodynamics, traditional underrepresentation of women in clinical pain research trials, and the overall higher prevalence of chronic pain conditions in females.

Biological mechanisms leading to sex differences in pain perception include hormonal influences, genetic and epigenetic factors, and differences in immune function and central sensitization.[3–5] These changes not only lead to the increased prevalence of common chronic pain conditions in women but also how women may respond to treatment, including pharmacologic therapies.

While this significant variability in pain experience and drug response between men and women has been known for some time, it was not until 2009 that a biological pathway difference was identified.[6] Many recent studies suggest a sex-dependent role for many factors within the pain pathway, including neurochemicals, immune factors, receptors, channels, transporters, transcription factors, and signal transduction.[7] The most studied differences in pain processing pathways are T-cell–mediated and microglial-mediated pathways. Specifically, in females, the pain pathway is T-cell–mediated while in males it is microglia-mediated. In females taking exogenous testosterone or those with low T-cell levels, the pain pathway will switch to the microglia pathway.

Furthermore, sex-based differences in genetic polymorphisms of drug-metabolizing enzymes (e.g., cytochrome p450 2D6 [CYP2D6], CYP2C19), opioid receptors (e.g., mu 1 opioid receptor [OPRM1]), and HLA alleles were found, especially relevant for opioids and antidepressants, thus highlighting the need for sex-specific considerations in pain management (Table 55.1).

Table 55.1 Summary of enzymes/biomarkers, their function, and key considerations

Enzyme/Biomarker	Function	Key considerations/ Exceptions
CYP2D6[12]	Breaks medications (including opioids) down into active metabolites	Women may have decreased CYP2D6 activity compared to men—possibly increasing adverse effects
CYP2C19[13]	Impacts metabolism of key medications typically used in pain management (TCAs)	Women may have decreased CYP2C19 activity compared to men—possibly increasing adverse effects
OPRM1 gene (particularly A118G variant)[14]	Opioid sensitivity and emotional response to pain	Women with the G allele may experience a reduced response to opioids and exhibit increased emotional response to pain
ABCB1 (also known as MDR1)[15]	Involved in cellular homeostasis and ATP-dependent translocation of substrates, activates pain inhibition	Women with A-A allele report less pain and disability, lower opioid needs, and increased side effects
Microfibril associated protein 3 (MFAP3)	Component of elastin-associated microfibrils	Decreased expression in those experiencing significant pain, and decreased expression correlates with PTSD
G protein subunit gamma 7 (GNG7)	Plays a role in suppressing pain	Decreased expression in women with depression experiencing significant pain
Guanylate binding protein 1 (GBP1)[11]	Signaling protein related to interferons	Increased expression in women experiencing significant pain, associated with schizophrenia, depression, suicide and PTSD

ATP, adenosine triphosphate; PTSD, posttraumatic stress disorder; TCA, tricyclic antidepressant.

More recently, sex-specific biomarkers such as MFAP3, were identified. There is also increasing recognition of the impact of hormonal fluctuations and transitioning between reproductive periods on women's pain experience.

There is a growing body of evidence for the use of precision tools to improve understanding of these biological differences and optimize treatment, including the study of genetic markers, hormonal profiles, and the use of functional MRI; however, these are yet to become a clinical standard.[8]

Role of Genetic Testing and Biomarkers in Personalized Pain Management

Genetic testing and biomarkers play an emerging role in personalized pain management by identifying individual variability in pain perception, drug metabolism, and response to analgesics. In the case of pharmacogenomics, patients can be identified as poor, intermediate, normal, rapid, and ultrarapid metabolizers; these classifications determine drug efficacy and can assist in medication selection and dosing. Currently, pharmacogenomic testing to identify polymorphisms in CYP2D6, CYP2C19, OPRM1, and ABCB1 can be performed but is far from routine.[1,10] In fact, the Clinical Pharmacogenetics Implementation Consortium (CPIC), which publishes gene–drug dosing guidelines, does not advocate for routine pharmacogenomic testing.[9]

Beyond pharmacogenomics, research into other biomarkers, including those in plasma and cerebrospinal fluid, and sensory testing, shows promise for predicting pain phenotypes and treatment response, but these approaches remain investigational. Next-generation sequencing and multi-omics approaches are expanding the understanding of pain mechanisms and may further refine personalized pain management in the future.[10]

Precision Medicine Strategies Tailored to Women's Pain Conditions

Hormonal fluctuations, specifically in estrogen (increases pain threshold by decreasing inflammation) and progesterone (lower pain sensitivity through increasing gamma aminobutyric acid [GABA] expression in the brain), modulate pain thresholds and analgesic response, making it important to recognize that, depending on the patient's current hormonal state, the pain experience may be different and require different treatment.[4] For example, branched-chain amino acids (BCAAs), phosphatidylinositol (PI(36:2)), and the ratio of PI(36:2) to BCAAs, are associated with increased menstrual pain severity.

Emerging biomarker research, including gene expression profiling, demonstrated some utility of MFAP3, GNG7, GBP1, and other genes in predicting high pain states and treatment responses in women; however, this research remains to be validated.[11] In addition, next-generation sequencing approaches are expanding the identification of pain-related genetic variants, some of which are more prevalent or have different effects in women, further supporting the rationale for sex-specific precision pain management strategies.[10]

Clinical Practice Recommendations

Individualized protocols during hormonal fluctuations may be necessary for some patients, including changes in medication dosing, adding nonopioid analgesics, or considering hormonal therapy. If available, reviewing the patient's pharmacogenomic or biomarker testing can further assist in guiding treatment. For patients who are refractory to treatment, consider initiating pharmacogenomic and biomarker testing if it is available. Finally, some medications modulate enzymes responsible for the breakdown into active metabolites (e.g., duloxetine blocks the CYP2D6 pathway, effectively limiting opioid treatment options to morphine), and it is important to obtain a full medication list, including recently stopped medications.

Conclusion

Personalized and precision medicine is a novel approach to tailoring a diagnostic and therapeutic approach based on biological, genetic, and environmental factors. While scientific advancements in pharmacogenomics and biomarker discovery hold promise, their translation into routine clinical practice is limited by high costs, questionable clinical utility of existing biomarkers, and gaps in provider education. As the field evolves, integrating these precision medicine tools into multidisciplinary, patient-centered care models will be essential to optimizing pain outcomes and reducing disparities in women's health.

References

1. Chadwick A, Frazier A, Khan TW, Young E. Understanding the psychological, physiological, and genetic factors affecting precision pain medicine: A narrative review. J Pain Res. 2021;14:3145–3161. doi:https://doi.org/10.2147/jpr.s3208632
2. Osborne NR, Davis KD. Sex and gender differences in pain. Int Rev Neurobiol. 2022;164:277–307. doi:https://doi.org/10.1016/bs.irn.2022.06.0133
3. Rosen S, Ham B, Mogil JS. Sex differences in neuroimmunity and pain. J Neurosci Res. 2016;95(1–2):500–508. doi:https://doi.org/10.1002/jnr.238314
4. Stieger A, Asadauskas A, Luedi MM, Andereggen L. Women's pain management across the lifespan: A narrative review of hormonal, physiological, and psychosocial perspectives. J Clin Med. 2025;14(10):3427. doi:https://doi.org/10.3390/jcm141034275
5. Liu J, Li Z, Ju J, Chu T, Gao F. Sex differences in the regulation of interleukins in chronic pain: A widely recognized but difficult-to-tackle factor. Int J Mol Sci. 2025;26(8):3835. doi:https://doi.org/10.3390/ijms260838356
6. Sorge RE, LaCroix-Fralish ML, Tuttle AH, et al. Spinal cord toll-like receptor 4 mediates inflammatory and neuropathic hypersensitivity in male but not female mice. J Neurosci. 2011;31(43):15450–15454. doi:https://doi.org/10.1523/jneurosci.3859-11.20117
7. Mogil JS, Parisien M, Esfahani SJ, Luda Diatchenko. Sex differences in mechanisms of pain hypersensitivity. Neurosci Biobehav Rev. 2024;163:105749–105749. doi:https://doi.org/10.1016/j.neubiorev.2024.1057498

8. Godbout-Parent M, Julien N, Nguena Nguefack HL, et al. Changing society, changing research: Integrating gender to better understand physical and psychological treatments used in chronic pain management. Pain. Published online October 9, 2023. doi:https://doi.org/10.1097/j.pain.00000000000030729
9. Bates J, Fudin J, Patel JN. Integrating pharmacogenomics into precision pain management. Support Care Cancer. 2022;30(12):10453–10459. doi:https://doi.org/10.1007/s00520–022-07404–910
10. Kringel D, Lötsch J. Knowledge of the genetics of human pain gained over the last decade from next-generation sequencing. Pharmacol Res. 2025;214:107667. doi:https://doi.org/10.1016/j.phrs.2025.10766711
11. Niculescu AB, Le-Niculescu H, Levey DF, et al. Towards precision medicine for pain: diagnostic biomarkers and repurposed drugs. Mol Psychiatry. 2019;24(4):501–522. doi:https://doi.org/10.1038/s41380–018-0345–512
12. Muriel J, Jordi Barrachina, Guillermo Del Barco, et al. Impact of CYP2D6 genotype on opioid use disorder deprescription: An observational prospective study in chronic pain with sex-differences. Front Pharmacol. 2023;14:1200430. doi:10.3389/fphar.2023.1200430
13. Seeman MV. The pharmacodynamics of antipsychotic drugs in women and men. Front Psychiatry. 2021;12. doi:https://doi.org/10.3389/fpsyt.2021.65090414
14. Trimble E, Kell P, Avella M, France C, Rhudy J. Opioid receptor mu 1 gene (OPRM1) A118G polymorphism and emotional modulation of pain. J Pain Res. 2024;17:489–500. doi:https://doi.org/10.2147/jpr.s44243115
15. Firzana Firfirey, September AV, Shamley D. ABCB1 and OPRM1 single-nucleotide polymorphisms collectively modulate chronic shoulder pain and dysfunction in South African breast cancer survivors. Pharmacogenomics. 2022;23(9):513–530. doi:https://doi.org/10.2217/pgs-2022–0020

Index

For the benefit of digital users, indexed terms that span two pages (e.g., 52–53) may, on occasion, appear on only one of those pages.

D

E

Q

R

S

T

Interventional Pain Medicine for Women's Health